GRAINGER & ALLISON'S

DIAGNOSTIC RADIOLOGY

Multiple Choice Questions

GRAINGER AND ALLISON'S

DIAGNOSTIC RADIOLOGY
Multiple Choice Questions

COMPILED BY

John F. Cockburn
MB, BCh, MRCP, FRCR, FFRRCSI
Consultant Radiologist
General Hospital
St. Helier
Jersey, United Kingdom

Adam W. M. Mitchell
MB, BS, FRCS, FRCR
Lecturer, Interventional Fellow
Department of Interventional Radiology
Hammersmith Hospital
London, United Kingdom

EDITED BY

Ronald G. Grainger
MB, ChB (Hon), MD, FRCP, DMRD,
RFCR, FACR (Hon), FRACR (Hon)
Professor of Diagnostic Radiology
(Emeritus)
University of Sheffield
Honorary Consultant Radiologist
Royal Hallamshire Hospital and
Northern General Hospital
Sheffield, United Kingdom

David J. Allison
BSc, MD, FRCR, FRCP
Professor of Imaging
Imperial College School of Medicine
Hammersmith Hospital
London, United Kingdom

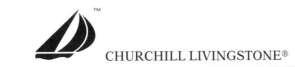
CHURCHILL LIVINGSTONE®

A Division of Harcourt Brace & Company
Edinburgh   London   Philadelphia   Toronto   Montreal   Sydney   Tokyo

CHURCHILL LIVINGSTONE
A Division of Harcourt Brace & Co. Ltd.

© Harcourt Brace & Co. Ltd, 1998

™ ◿ is a registered trademark of Harcourt Brace & Co., Ltd.

First published 1998

ISBN 0–443–05941–1

British Library Cataloguing in Publication Data
A catalogue record for this book is available from the British Library

Library of Congress Cataloging-in-Publication Data
A catalog record for this book is available from the Library of Congress

The Publishers have made every effort to trace the copyright holders for borrowed material. If
they have inadvertently overlooked any they will be pleased to make the necessary
arrangements at the first opportunity.

Printed in the United Kingdom.

Preface

The examination structure in almost all subjects has changed direction dramatically in the last few decades.

Those of us who examined candidates 20 years or more ago realised the very poor return for the many hours and days spent marking essay style answers. Our assessment was arbitrary and subjective, considerably influenced by the lay-out and legibility of the hand writing, resulting in very poor and inadequate discrimination between the candidates, so negating much of the value of the examination.

All this has changed in the last few decades with the introduction, development, refinement and fine tuning of the Multiple Choice Question Assessment (MCQ).

The success of the MCQ structure must *not* indicate that writing well organised, coherent, well-constructed prose, presented in easily read lay-out and hand-writing, is now obsolete. We believe that this facility is most important to any doctor or indeed any educated person.

Diagnostic imaging is an ideal subject for MCQ, for it is composed of several different modalities—conventional X-ray, cross-sectional imaging, CT, MRI, ultrasound, Doppler, radio-isotopes, each with its own technology, imaging anatomy and potential for useful clinically relevant information. No essay style examination can adequately cover these wide-ranging and different modalities, each involving technology, anatomy, physiology and clinical evaluation.

Grainger and Allison's Diagnostic Radiology is a comprehensive text, contributed by over 100 of the world's most eminent radiologists. It is now in its third edition and has been fully accepted internationally as a comprehensive analysis and assessment of current best practice in diagnostic imaging. It has been adopted as the standard text for many trainees preparing for their professional examinations and by their examiners and professional organisations.

In response to repeated requests, we have agreed to design and compose an MCQ book based on Grainger and Allison 3/e, with full answers and cross references to the relevant pages in the main text book.

This MCQ book is specifically designed so that it is not restricted to use with Grainger and Allison 3/e, but can also easily be used by the reader who prefers other parent texts, by utilising both the system-oriented main section of this MCQ book and the randomised test papers in the final section.

Despite an understandably wide spectrum of views among radiology trainees, we are firmly of the opinion that the most difficult part of the MCQ scenario is *composing* questions on clinical imaging to ensure both lack of ambiguity and full agreement on the many potential responses to the questions.

In the 438 MCQs presented here, there will inevitably be several given answers that will raise doubts in the reader. We suggest that these questions be fully discussed with both contemporary and more senior radiologists, for this will be a most valuable learning and teaching experience.

If any reader remains in doubt as to the accuracy of the given answers, we would be pleased to receive appropriate comments and suggestions. Please send these comments to AM with a copy letter to RGG.

We hope that you enjoy the challenge presented by this book, which we have prepared to facilitate your comprehension and retention of the enormous factual content of Clinical Radiology Imaging. The questions are arranged in chapter sequence (as requested by the many people whom we consulted about the format of this book). At the end of the book, there are 120 MCQ randomised questions arranged in blocks of 30 (1 hour), on which you can test your knowledge before sitting the examination.

We wish you every success in your examinations.

JC, AM, RGG and DJA

Editorial Advice on Using This MCQ Book

This MCQ book is carefully based on the third edition of Grainger and Allison's *Diagnostic Radiology*. All of the answers to these MCQs are supplied in the parent book, and every question and answer is cross-referenced from the MCQ book to the chapter and page of the Grainger and Allison third edition. The MCQ book can of course also be used by those persons preferring other parent texts or monographs on specific body systems.

By consensus of many examinees and examiners, this book has been deliberately designed to be used in two different ways—either as a test of the reader's comprehension and retention of information after studying specific chapters in the parent textbook, or as a practice before the actual examination by challenging themselves with either the randomised MCQ papers at the end of the book or those selected from any chosen body system.

Whatever the preferred parent book, the reader should carefully study the appropriate chapter(s) or body systems before attempting the relevant questions in this book.

The last section of this book has 120 randomised questions arranged in blocks of 30 questions (1 hour each), allowing the reader to conduct a simulated examination of 1–4 hours.

Many varied format and marking systems are used by different Examination Boards.

ALWAYS CAREFULLY READ THE INSTRUCTIONS OF YOUR EXAMINATION BOARD AT LEAST TWICE BEFORE ATTEMPTING THE ANSWERS.

This book uses the current format (1997) of the Royal College of Radiologists (UK)—2 papers of 2 hours, each containing 60 randomised questions on imaging and related clinicopathological aspects.

There is a common stem with 5 related questions, each of which should be answered **True** or **False**. Each correct answer gains a point and each incorrect answer loses a point. A **"don't know"** or **no answer** neither gains nor loses a point. **All** of the 5 questions may be True or False, permitting the score for each stem to range from $+5$ to -5.

Our advice to the readers is to develop their own strategy and timing for answering MCQs by extensive practice on many MCQ papers and books. During the actual examination, use the strategy and system which you prefer and with which you are most at ease.

We suggest you practise the following approach:

A Draw three columns for your answers

COLUMN 1	COLUMN 2	COLUMN 3
I know this answer	I think I know this answer, I'm having an educated guess	I don't have a clue

B Whilst practising, always place your answer to each question in one of these columns.

Always mark your confident answers first, but never leave out an answer to any question.

C At the end of the simulated practice examinations, add up your answers in each column and work out your percentage accuracy in each group. Only then can you reach a decision on whether you are a good guesser or not.

Many authorities advise that if you consistently answer about 80% of the questions and about 80% of your answers are correct, it may well be advisable not to attempt the pure guess-work answers in Column 3 as that approach may lose you valuable points.

Most examination boards advise that the examinee enters his/her choice of True or False answers into the question booklet in the first instance, before transferring them to the definitive answer sheet. Ensure that there is very ample time within the examination allocation of time to permit this essential transfer of your data to the answer book. Don't rush this transfer as your examination performance depends on it.

Repeated practice on as many MCQs as you can obtain will much improve your performance.

Don't panic, be methodical, keep to the allotted time and don't cheat in your practice tests.

Enjoy this learning process and Good Luck in the examinations.

JC, AM, RGG, DJA

Acknowledgements

We wish to acknowledge and to thank the many residents and registrars whom we consulted regarding their preferred format of this book, so that it could serve both as an aid to their programmed learning from their preferred textbook and also as a preliminary test before their formal examinations.

We particularly wish to thank Dr Philip Gishen, Clinical Director of Radiology, King's College Hospital, London, and recent Senior Examiner of the Royal College of Radiologists, for his much valued advice and support throughout the development of this book.

JC, AM, RGG, DJA

Contents

1 Imaging Techniques and Modalities   Chapters 1–10 1

2 The Respiratory System   Chapters 11–29 11

3 The Heart and Great Vessels   Chapters 30–44 97

4 The Gastrointestinal Tract   Chapters 45–55 139

5 The Liver, Biliary Tract, Pancreas and Endocrine System   Chapters 56–62 165

6 The Genitourinary Tract   Chapters 63–75 193

7 The Skeletal System   Chapters 76–88 297

8 The Female Reproductive System   Chapters 89–92 403

9 The Central Nervous System   Chapters 93–100 423

10 The Orbit: Ear, Nose & Throat, Face, Teeth   Chapters 101–104 467

11 Angiography, Interventional Radiology & Other Techniques   Chapters 105–108 489

12 The Reticuloendothelial System, Oncology, AIDS   Chapters 109–112 501

Self Assessment Questions 509

1

Imaging Techniques and Modalities

Q 1.1. Concerning the Principles of Magnetic Resonance Imaging

A. The frequency of precession of a nucleus is inversely proportional to the applied magnetic field

B. Spin echo sequences utilize an initial 180° pulse followed at a specific time by a 90° pulse

C. A decrease in mobile proton density is seen in acute demyelination

D. Extracellular methaemoglobin exhibits a high signal on both T1 and T2 images

E. In the STIR sequence, the T1 is reduced to 100–150 ms in order to null the signal from fat

Q 1.2. The Following Statements Apply to Ultrasound

A. Diagnostic ultrasound occupies frequencies between 1 and 20 MHz in the electromagnetic spectrum

B. Ultrasound is propagated through tissue as a transverse wave

C. Time gain compensation allows image brightness for superficial and deep structures to be equalized

D. The prime determinant of the strength of an ultrasound echo is the difference in density between adjacent tissue components

E. A Doppler beam at its highest intensity can cause a significant rise in temperature when directed at a bone surface

A 1.1. *Concerning the Principles of Magnetic Resonance Imaging*

FALSE
A. It is directly proportional as expressed by the Larmor equation: Resonance frequency = Applied field strength × Gyromagnetic ratio.
Ch. 4 Basic Physics, p 64.

FALSE
B. The inversion recovery sequence starts with a 180° pulse followed after a time TI (the inversion time) by a 90° pulse. Spin echo sequences start with a 90° pulse followed at time TE/2 (where TE is the echo time) by a 180° pulse. At a further time TE/2 an echo of the original signal is detected.
Ch. 4 Magnetic Resonance Imaging Basic Physics, p 64.

FALSE
C. Mobile protons are required to yield a detectable signal with most MRI techniques. An increase in mobile protons is seen in many pathological states characterized by an increased signal on T2-weighted images. These include oedema, infection, inflammation, acute demyelination, tumours and cysts.
Ch. 4 Proton Density, p 66.

TRUE
D. Extracellular methaemoglobin has a low T1 value and hence has a high signal on T1 images. It has a relatively high T2 value and hence has a relatively high signal on T2 images.
Ch. 4 T1 and T2, p 67.

TRUE
E. The Inversion Recovery Pulse Sequence
Ch. 4, p 75.

A 1.2. *The Following Statements Apply to Ultrasound*

FALSE
A. Ultrasound is a high-frequency sound wave. It is not part of the electromagnetic spectrum.
Ch. 5 Nature of Ultrasound, p 84.

FALSE
B. Ultrasound is propagated as a longitudinal wave (i.e., tissue moves in the same direction as the wave in a sequence of compression and rarefaction).
Ch. 5 Propagation in Tissue, p 84.

TRUE
C. This technique compensates for reduced signal intensity from deep structures by applying progressively greater amplification to later (deeper) echoes.
Ch. 5 Attenuation, p 84.

FALSE
D. The determinant is **acoustic impedance**. The larger the mismatch in acoustic impedance between adjacent structures, the stronger the echo.
Ch. 5 Echogenicity, p 93.

TRUE
E. Particular care is required during ultrasound examination in pregnancy or in neonatal examination in the vicinity of the skull.
Ch. 5 Safety, p 93.

Q *1.3. Concerning Paediatric Scintigraphy in Bone Conditions*

A. It is possible reliably to differentiate septic arthritis from rheumatoid arthritis using multiphase bone imaging

B. Early osteomyelitis appears as a focus of reduced ^{99m}TcMDP uptake

C. MRI is as sensitive as bone scanning in detecting discitis

D. In Perthe's disease, focal photopenia in an epiphysis means that the loss of the vascular supply to that area must be long-standing

E. Bone scanning is useful for the detection of subtle epiphyseal fractures

Q *1.4. Regarding Scintigraphy in Children*

A. A dilated, unobstructed pelvicaliceal system with preserved renal function will lose half its activity through "wash-out" within 10 minutes of administering a diuretic agent

B. In the presence of reduced renal function, an unobstructed kidney will yield quantitative data which simulates an obstructed system

C. Lack of ^{99m}Tc sulphur colloid uptake by the spleen in an adult is a feature of sickle cell disease

D. Absence of ^{99m}Tc HIDA in the gastrointestinal tract on the images obtained at 24 hours implies the presence of biliary atresia

E. ^{99m}Tc pertechnetate accumulates in Barrett's oesophagus

A 1.3. *Concerning Paediatric Scintigraphy in Bone Conditions*

FALSE   A. Both cause hyperaemic responses early on and a mild non-specific increase in bone uptake may be seen on later images.
Ch. 6B Infection, p 112.

TRUE   B. "Cold" osteomyelitis is caused by the temporary occlusion of small blood vessels owing to the prevention of tracer accumulation by oedema.
Ch. 6B Infection, p 112.

TRUE   C. Both MRI and bone scanning show the changes of infection well before radiographic changes are seen, but scintigraphy offers a wider survey.
Ch. 6B Infection, p 113.

FALSE   D. Transient photopenia can occur in the presence of a joint effusion, and return of uptake is an indication that revascularization is taking place.
Ch. 6B Vascular Disorders, p 113.

FALSE   E. The epiphyses have high physiological uptake of tracer that may mask an underlying fracture.
Ch. 6B Trauma, p 114.

A 1.4. *Regarding Scintigraphy in Children*

TRUE   A. If the washout takes longer than 20 minutes, this indicates obstruction. A value between 10 and 20 minutes is considered non-diagnostic.
Ch. 6B Obstructive Uropathy, p 116.

TRUE   B.
Ch. 6B Obstructive Uropathy, p 116.

TRUE   C. So-called functional asplenia generally occurs between the 2nd and 6th years of life.
Ch. 6B Liver and Spleen, p 117.

FALSE   D. Any cause of severe cholestasis will result in absence of activity in the gastro-intestinal tract.
Ch. 6B Hepatobiliary System, p 118.

TRUE   E. Sites of ectopic gastric mucosa such as Meckel's diverticulum, gastric or enteric duplications and Barrett's oesophagus accumulate this tracer.
Ch. 6B Meckel's Diverticulum and Gastrointestinal Bleeding, p 118.

Q *1.5. The Following Cause Severe Neonatal Cholestasis*

      A. Alpha-1 anti-trypsin deficiency

      B. Cystic fibrosis

      C. Maternal warfarin ingestion

      D. Alagille syndrome

      E. Septo-optic dysplasia

Q *1.6. Concerning the Scintigraphic Investigation of Paediatric Occult Gastrointestinal Bleeding*

      A. Mucoid surfaces of gastric mucosa selectively accumulate the pertechnetate anion after oral administration

      B. Cimetidine and glucagon delay the clearance of pertechnetate from gastric mucosa

      C. Areas of ectopic gastric mucosa parallel the accumulation curve of normal gastric mucosa

      D. A preceding barium follow-through is required for accurate interpretation

      E. Imaging begins at the time of injection of the tracer and continues at 5 minute intervals up to one hour

A *1.5. The Following Cause Severe Neonatal Cholestasis*

TRUE   A. In this condition, there may be a severe neonatal hepatitis that causes intra-hepatic cholestasis.
Ch. 6B Hepatobiliary System, p 118.

TRUE   B. Plugging of the biliary tract by inspissated bile may cause obstruction in the neonate.
Ch. 6B Hepatobiliary System, p 118.

FALSE   C. This is associated with skeletal and neurological anomalies.
Ch. 6B Hepatobiliary System, p 118.

TRUE   D. Affected patients have abnormal faecies, chronic cholestasis, butterfly vertebrae and congenital heart disease. The cholestasis is caused by paucity and hypoplasia of the interlobular bile ducts.
Ch. 6B Hepatobiliary System, p 118.

TRUE   E. This is a form of lobar holoprosencephaly that is associated with neonatal cholestasis.
Ch. 6B Hepatobiliary System, p 118.

A *1.6. Concerning the Scintigraphic Investigation of Paediatric Occult Gastrointestinal Bleeding*

FALSE   A. ^{99m}Tc pertechnetate is administered intravenously.
Ch. 6B Meckel's Diverticulum and Gastrointestinal Bleeding, p 118.

TRUE   B.
Ch. 6B Meckel's Diverticulum and Gastrointestinal Bleeding, p 118.

TRUE   C. This feature assists in the differentiation of such mucosa from other areas that normally accumulate isotope (e.g., the urinary tract).
Ch. 6B Meckel's Diverticulum and Gastrointestinal Bleeding, p 118.

FALSE   D. Barium in the gastrointestinal tract can potentially obscure a suspected area by attenuating its signal.
Ch. 6B Meckel's Diverticulum and Gastrointestinal Bleeding, p 118.

TRUE   E.
Ch. 6B Meckel's Diverticulum and Gastrointestinal Bleeding, p 118.

Q *1.7. False Positive Paediatric Pertechnetate Scans Occur in the Following*

A. Intusussception

B. Crohn's disease

C. Collagenous colitis

D. Hydronephrosis

E. Vesicoureteric reflux

Q *1.8. Regarding Paediatric Thyroid and Cardiopulmonary Scintigraphy*

A. Potassium perchlorate is administered prior to thyroid imaging

B. Hypothyroidism due to enzyme defects in hormone synthesis shows absent or reduced uptake over the thyroid

C. A cold nodule in a child represents a high likelihood of malignancy

D. ^{99m}Tc macroaggregated albumin is used to demonstrate a right to left shunt

E. Krypton 81m is the isotope of choice for the demonstration of air-trapping

A *1.7. False Positive Paediatric Pertechnetate Scans Occur in the Following*

TRUE A. This is a cause of localized hyperaemia and may cause a false positive result.
Ch. 6B Meckel's Diverticulum and Gastrointestinal Bleeding, p 118.

TRUE B. Similarly, this is a cause of localized hyperaemia and may cause a false positive result.
Ch. 6B Meckel's Diverticulum and Gastrointestinal Bleeding, p 118.

FALSE C. This is a disorder characterized by diarrhea affecting elderly patients.

TRUE D. Focal accumulation of tracer in the collecting system of an abnormal kidney may cause a false positive result.
Ch. 6B Meckel's Diverticulum and Gastrointestinal Bleeding, p 118.

TRUE E. Focal accumulation of tracer in the collecting system also occurs in this condition and may cause a false positive result.
Ch. 6B Meckel's Diverticulum and Gastrointestinal Bleeding, p 119.

A *1.8. Regarding Paediatric Thyroid and Cardiopulmonary Scintigraphy*

FALSE A. It is administered following *completion* of the examination to minimize the dose to the gland by reducing iodine uptake.
Ch. 6B Thyroid Imaging, p 121.

FALSE B. Avid trapping in an enlarged gland occurs in such enzyme abnormalities.
Ch. 6B Thyroid Imaging, p 121.

TRUE C.
Ch. 6B Thyroid Imaging, p 121.

TRUE D. Extrapulmonary activity after the administration of a properly prepared intravenous injection implies that such a shunt exists.
Ch. 6B Cardiopulmonary Imaging, p 121.

FALSE E. The half-life of this isotope is too short for this purpose and xenon must be used.
Ch. 6B Pulmonary Ventilation and Perfusion Imaging, p 121.

Q 1.9. Matched Ventilation and Perfusion Defects are Seen in the Following Conditions

    A. Congenital diaphragmatic hernia

    B. Congenital lobar emphysema

    C. Cystic adenomatoid malformation

    D. Pulmonary sequestration

    E. Obliterative bronchiolitis

Q 1.10. Regarding Bone Mineral Density (BMD)

    A. Dual energy X-ray absorptiometry (DXA) uses ^{153}Gd as its X-ray source

    B. Bone mineral density is highly correlated with bone mass

    C. Excessive exercise is associated with preservation of BMD

    D. Aortic calcification can produce erroneous results in the quantification of BMD using DXA

    E. The trabecular bone in Ward's triangle is assessed routinely in femoral neck measurements

A   1.9. Matched Ventilation and Perfusion Defects are Seen in the Following Conditions

TRUE
: A. Owing to the associated pulmonary hypoplasia.
Ch. 6B Pulmonary Ventilation and Perfusion Imaging, p 122.

TRUE
: B. This occurs most commonly in the left upper lobe and right middle and upper lobes, and is a cause of a nonventilated, nonperfused segment of lung.
Ch. 6B Pulmonary Ventilation and Perfusion Imaging, p 122.

TRUE
: C. This appears in several forms as a mass of multiple fluid or air-filled cysts, associated with hypoplasia of the ipsilateral lung.
Ch. 6B Pulmonary Ventilation and Perfusion Imaging, p 122.

TRUE
: D. The lack of ventilation is a consequence of noncommunication with the bronchial tree. Perfusion may be normal (via systemic supply), reduced, or absent, owing to associated hyperaeration of the surrounding lung. A lack of perfusion in the pulmonary phase followed by later evidence of systemic perfusion is characteristic of radionuclide angiography.
Ch. 6B Pulmonary Ventilation and Perfusion Imaging, p 122.

TRUE
: E.
Ch. 6B Pulmonary Ventilation and Perfusion Imaging, p 122.

A   1.10. Regarding Bone Mineral Density (BMD)

FALSE
: A. DXA uses a pencil beam of X-rays from an X-ray tube. Dual photon absorptiometry uses ^{153}Gd as its X-ray source.
Ch. 7 Bone Density Measurement Techniques, p 125.

TRUE
: B. BMD is extremely well correlated with bone mass.
Ch. 7 Bone Density Measurements, p 126.

FALSE
: C. Excessive exercise, osteoporosis, endocrine disorders, smoking and alcohol are some of the factors associated with a low BMD.
Ch. 7 Table 7.2, p 130.

TRUE
: D. Aortic calcification may produce a spurious increase in the calculated BMD.
Ch. 7 Table 7.3, p 133.

TRUE
: E. Femoral neck measurements include the greater trochanter, the femoral neck and Ward's triangle.
Ch. 7 Definition of Terms used in BMD Measurements, p 128.

2

The Respiratory System

Q *2.1. Regarding Chest Radiography*

 A. A lateral decubitus radiograph can detect pleural effusions of less than 20 ml

 B. Expiratory films are mandatory in a patient with a history of foreign body inhalation

 C. Conventional tomography has better spatial resolution than computed tomography (CT)

 D. Reasonable high-resolution CT windows for parenchymal imaging would be: centre +500 and width 1500 HU

 E. CT adrenal imaging is recommended in most patients undergoing CT scanning of a solitary pulmonary nodule

A 2.1. *Regarding Chest Radiography*

FALSE   A. The lateral decubitus projection may be required for the demonstration of pleural fluid and readily distinguishes it from an elevated diaphragm. Generally the smallest amount of fluid that can be detected is not less than 50-100 ml. The patient should be positioned with the side of the putative effusion dependent.
Ch. 11 Standard Techniques, p 201.

TRUE   B. The expiratory film, in a patient with suspected air trapping (e.g., one with a foreign body in a main bronchus) demonstrates poor emptying of the affected side—objective evidence of air trapping. A more sensitive method of demonstrating air trapping is to obtain a radiograph 1 second after a forced expiration (FEV_1).
Ch. 11 Standard Techniques, p 202.

TRUE   C. In centres where CT is not available, linear tomography is useful for the assessment of pulmonary nodules but is unlikely to be helpful in cases in which the plain film is completely normal. The spatial resolution of film/screen radiography far exceeds that of CT, but the latter has superior contrast resolution.
Ch. 11 Tomography, p 202.

FALSE   D. There is a wide range of windows that can be used for lung imaging. (See what you use in your own department and *vary* the settings.) The settings given are better used for bony detail.
Ch. 11 Computed Tomography, p 202.

TRUE   E. The adrenal glands should always be imaged in a case of suspected lung cancer. Adrenal metastases are not uncommon in patients with lung or breast cancer. MRI can be useful in the differentiation of adrenal metastases from non-hyperfunctioning adenomas, though ultimately biopsy may be necessary.
Ch. 11 Computed Tomography, p 203.

Q 2.2. *Regarding the Thymus*

A. Prior to puberty the thymus occupies most of the mediastinum in front of the great vessels as seen on the CXR

B. The CT density (HU) of the thymus tends to decrease with age

C. Thymomas tend to occur in patients less than 20 years of age

D. ACTH is the commonest ectopic hormone to be produced by thymic carcinoid tumours

E. Eighty to ninety percent of patients with thymomas have myasthenia gravis

Q 2.3. *The Following are Normal*

A. A high (relative to muscle) signal intensity of the oesophagus on T2-weighted images of the chest

B. Oesophageal air, as demonstrated on CT, in most patients

C. A 1.5-2.5 cm normal range of excursion of the diaphragm as demonstrated by USS

D. A retrosternal band-like opacity along the lower one third of the anterior chest wall on the lateral radiograph

E. Small nodule(s) in the lower zone(s) with a well-defined lateral border and a less well-defined medial border on a CXR

A 2.2. *Regarding the Thymus*

TRUE A. Prior to puberty, the thymus varies greatly in size giving an extremely wide range of normality. The thymus has two lobes that should be roughly symmetrical in size.
Ch. 12 Normal Chest, p 216.

TRUE B. The size of the gland tends slowly to decrease with age and the gland undergoes fatty replacement which lowers its CT density. By the age of 40 years, the thymus is barely distinguishable from mediastinal fat.
Ch. 12 Normal Chest, p 216.

FALSE C. They are, however, the most common tumour of the anterior mediastinum (remember the 4 "T's": *t*hymoma, *t*eratoma, *t*hyroid enlargement and *t*errible lymphoma). Thymomas are virtually unknown under the age of 20 years.
Ch. 15 Thymic Tumours, p 282.

TRUE D. Carcinoid tumours tend to produce a variety of metabolites, ACTH being the most common in thymic tumours.
Ch. 15 Thymic Tumours, p 282.

FALSE E. Thirty to forty percent of patients with thymoma have myasthenia gravis while only 10% of patients with myasthenia gravis have thymomas.
Ch. 15 Thymic Tumours, p 282.

A 2.3. *The Following are Normal*

TRUE A. On T1 images the oesophagus has a signal intensity similar to that of muscle.
Ch. 15 The Mediastinum, p 284.

TRUE B. Air can be demonstrated along the length of the oesophagus in most patients (80%).
Ch. 15 The Mediastinum, p 284.

FALSE C. The range of movement of the diaphragm, as demonstrated by transabdominal USS, is 2-8.6 cm (mean 5.3 cm).
Ch. 12 The Diaphragm, p 225.

TRUE D. This is the retrosternal fat pad.
Ch. 12 The Retrosternal Line, p 224.

TRUE E. These are the features of the nipple shadow. If there is *any* doubt concerning this diagnosis, a lateral radiograph or a further film with nipple markers should be obtained.

Q 2.4. *The Following Should be Considered as Normal Findings in Chest Imaging*

A. Tracheal cartilage calcification at 20 years of age

B. On the erect CXR the upper-lobe anterior segmental artery and bronchus should have the same diameter

C. Discrete hilar nodes on CT scanning of the chest

D. The right main bronchus and the bronchus intermedius are outlined by air

E. A vascular structure seen between the middle-lobe bronchus and the right lower-lobe bronchus on the lateral CXR

Q 2.5. *Concerning Pulmonary Consolidation*

A. The consolidation associated with pulmonary sarcoidosis is due to granulomata within the alveoli

B. A segmental distribution is characteristic

C. Desquamative insterstitial pneumonitis (DIP) is a predominantly interstitial process producing alveolar compression

D. There is usually associated loss of volume

E. Early changes include acinar nodules/shadows 1-4 mm in diameter

A 2.4. *The Following Should be Considered as Normal Findings in Chest Imaging*

FALSE A. Normal calcification does not occur before the age of 40. Calcification in younger patients is generally related to metabolic disorders (e.g., hyperparathroidism and renal failure).
Ch. 12 The Central Airways, p 209.

TRUE B. The anterior upper-lobe bronchus and artery have the same diameter (4-5 mm). If a vessel is greater than 1.5 times its accompanying bronchus, it should be considered abnormal.
Ch. 12 The Central Airways, p 209.

FALSE C. Normal lymph nodes cannot be recognised as discrete structures on a plain film or a CT scan.
Ch. 12 The Central Airways, p 209.

TRUE D.
Ch. 12 The Hila, p 209.

FALSE E. There is no vascular structure between these entities.
Ch. 12 The Hila, p 212.

A 2.5. *Concerning Pulmonary Consolidation*

FALSE A. The granulomata are in the interstitium and they enlarge and compress the alveoli (in a manner similar to lymphoma). Radiologically, this process cannot readily be distinguished from alveolar/airspace consolidation.
Ch. 13 Consolidation, p 233.

FALSE B. Consolidation doesn't respect segments.
Ch. 13 Consolidation, p 233.

FALSE C. DIP occurs in both compartments of the secondary pulmonary lobule.
Ch. 13 Consolidation, p 233.

FALSE D. There is an isovolumetric replacement of alveolar gas by fluid (exudate or transudate) within the secondary pulmonary lobule. Significant abnormal *loss* of pulmonary volume is termed collapse.
Ch. 13 Consolidation, p 233.

FALSE E. An acinar nodule is consolidation within the acinus which measures 5-10 mm. If small nodules are demonstrated infection may well be the cause, (e.g., miliary TB).
Ch. 13 Consolidation, p 233.

Q *2.6. The Following are Causes of an Air Bronchogram on the CXR*

A. Nonobstructive collapse

B. Passive atelectasis

C. Lymphoma

D. Progressive massive fibrosis

E. Alveolar cell carcinoma

Q *2.7. The Following are Associated with "Expansive" Consolidation*

A. Consolidation secondary to a neoplasm

B. Mycobacterium avium-intracellulare infection

C. Drowning

D. Klebsiella pneumonia

E. Pneumococcal pneumonia

A 2.6. *The Following are Causes of an Air Bronchogram on the CXR*

TRUE   *A.*
                  Ch. 13 Table 13.3, p 231.

TRUE   *B.* This is a form of non-obstructive collapse.
                  Ch. 13 Table 13.3, p 231.

TRUE   *C.* The alveoli are collapsed owing to expansion of the interstitium; this produces radiological changes that are identical to those seen in other forms of consolidation.
                  Ch. 13 Table 13.3, p 231.

TRUE   *D.* An uncommon cause of an air bronchogram.

TRUE   *E.*
                  Ch. 13 Table 13.3, p 231.

A 2.7. *The Following are Associated with "Expansive" Consolidation*

TRUE   *A.* The neoplasm is an endobronchial tumour (commonly a central squamous cell tumour) which obstructs the flow of lobar bronchial fluid; secretions accumulate and expand the pulmonary lobe.
                  Ch. 13 Consolidation, p 233.

FALSE   *B.* This bacterium is commonly found in association with Pneumocystis carinii infection in patients with **AIDS**.
                  Ch. 13 Consolidation, p 233.

FALSE   *C.* Expansive consolidation is occasionally referred to as the "drowned lung," but it has no association with drowning.

TRUE   *D.*
                  Ch. 13 Consolidation, p 233.

TRUE   *E.*
                  Ch. 13 Consolidation, p 233.

Q *2.8. A Morgagni Hernia*

    A. Commonly presents in childhood after streptococcal infections

    B. Occurs through a defect in the posterior pleuroperitoneal fold

    C. Contains large bowel in over 90% of cases

    D. May extend into the pericardium

    E. Is optimally diagnosed with an oral water-soluble contrast medium study

A 2.8. *A Morgagni Hernia*

FALSE   A. *Bochdalek* hernias present in childhood, often after a streptococcal infec- ·
tion.
Ch. 14 Diaphragmatic Hernias, p 273.

FALSE   B. Morgagni hernias occur through a defect in the right *anterior* hemidiaphragm.
Ch. 14 Diaphragmatic Hernias, p 273.

FALSE   C. Fat and mesentery tend to pass through the defect; large bowel only does
so occasionally.
Ch. 14 Diaphragmatic Hernias, p 273.

TRUE   D.
Ch. 14 Diaphragmatic Hernias, p 273.

FALSE   E. As the large bowel is the hollow organ most commonly found within the
hernia, study *per rectum* is the most appropriate method of investigation.
Ch. 14 Diaphragmatic Hernias, p 273.

Q *2.9. Regarding Pleural Effusions*

A. Lamellar effusions are a feature of ARDS

B. Rupture of the upper third of the oesophagus commonly gives rise to a left-sided effusion

C. Unilateral right-sided effusions are associated with ascites

D. The lateral radiograph is the most sensitive method for detecting a pleural effusion

E. Chylothorax is characterised by its low density when imaged by CT

A 2.9. Regarding Pleural Effusions

FALSE   A. In patients with ARDS the primary pathology is capillary leakage that permits leakage of fluid into the alveoli. The fact that the pulmonary venous pressure and the capillary wedge pressure are not elevated accounts for the relative absence of septal lines and lamellar effusions.
Ch. 14 Lamellar Effusion, p 260.

FALSE   B. The upper third of the oesophagus is adjacent to the mediastinal surface on the right, whereas the lower third tends to lie to the left and is adjacent to the left infero-medial pleural surface. These anatomical relationships determine the probable location of any fluid collection resulting from an oesophageal perforation.
Ch. 14.

TRUE   C. Most bilateral effusions are transudates, though SLE, metastases, pulmonary embolism and lymphoma are all exceptions to the rule. Right-sided effusions, with ascites, are seen in Meig's syndrome. Disease adjacent to the diaphragm can produce an effusion on the corresponding side (e.g., pancreatitis and left-sided effusion and hepatic abscess and right-sided effusion).
Ch. 14 Pleural Effusion, p 258.

FALSE   D. There are many methods for demonstrating pleural effusions (not forgetting the lateral decubitus film, which is especially helpful in patients with suspected subpulmonary effusion); USS is a very sensitive method that can detect extremely small volumes of fluid.
Ch. 14 Pleural Effusion, p 258.

FALSE   E. Although chylothorax contains a large amount of lipid it also contains other proteins and macromolecules. The fat content is certainly not sufficient significantly to lower the HU of an effusion. (A little bit of knowledge does not always go a long way.)
Ch. 14 Chylothorax, p 265.

Q 2.10. *Diaphragmatic Paralysis*

A. Should be imaged using USS rather than fluoroscopy

B. Occurs with brachial plexus trauma

C. Can be assumed when screening demonstrates paradoxical movement of the hemidiaphragm

D. In the presence of a normal CXR (AP and lateral), a CT scan of the chest is superfluous

E. Lateral screening is preferential to AP screening when diaphragmatic paralysis is suspected

A *2.10. Diaphragmatic Paralysis*

FALSE   A. USS may well demonstrate paralysis, but it is user dependent and can only assess one side at a time, making it less sensitive than fluoroscopy.
Ch. 14 Diaphragmatic Movement and Paralysis of the Diaphragm, p 271.

TRUE   B. The diaphragm is supplied by the cervical nerves from C3, 4 and 5. Any process that interrupts the neuromuscular pathway to the diaphragm can produce diaphragmatic paralysis (e.g., phrenic nerve interruption or painful inhibition caused by inflammatory irritation). Severe trauma, such as brachial plexus avulsion (C5-T1), can be associated with damage to the phrenic nerve.
Ch. 14 Diaphragmatic Movement and Paralysis of the Diaphragm, p 271.

FALSE   C. An important mimic of phrenic paresis is eventration of the diaphragm, usually on the left. In a small but significant number of "normal" individuals, no cause for phrenic paresis can be found. This usually occurs on the right and is thought by some to be the legacy of a previous neuritis.
Ch. 14 Diaphragmatic Movement and Paralysis of the Diaphragm, p 273.

TRUE   D. A CT scan is unlikely to demonstrate the cause of the paralysis.
Ch. 14 Diaphragmatic Movement and Paralysis of the Diaphragm, p 273.

TRUE   E. Lateral screening enables both the left and right hemidiaphragms to be assessed at the same time, enabling real-time paradox to be visualised. By asking the patient to sniff, the maximum amount of paradox can be demonstrated.
Ch. 14 Diaphragmatic Movement and Paralysis of the Diaphragm, p 273.

Q *2.11. Concerning Bronchopleural Fistulae*

A. There is a frequent association with recurrent pneumothoraces

B. When post surgical they tend to occur in the first 24-48 hours

C. They should be suspected in patients in whom an air-fluid level is demonstrable on the erect CXR one month following a pneumonectomy

D. Air leak occurs more frequently following lobectomy than pneumonectomy

E. They are associated with necrotizing pulmonary infection

A 2.11. *Concerning Bronchopleural Fistulae*

FALSE   A. Bronchopleural fistulae differ from pneumothorax in that the communication with the pleural space is via the airways rather than the distal air spaces. They occur in two settings: the breakdown of an anastomosis, and in necrotizing pulmonary infections.
Ch. 14 Bronchopleural Fistula, p 266.

FALSE   B. The radiological changes that occur after removal of a lung are:

Day 1—vacant hemithorax, trachea in the midline.
Day 2 to several weeks—fluid fills the hemithorax and the trachea shifts to the surgical side.
Months—a small amount of air may reside in the apex of the thorax without any significance.
Bronchopleural fistulae, in this situation, occur at 10–14 days.
Ch. 14 Bronchopleural Fistula, p 266.

FALSE   C. Any drop in the fluid level by more than 20 mm, the reappearance of air or shift of the mediastinum away from the surgical side, suggests a bronchopleural fistula. (Early fistulae are usually due to poor surgical technique and late fistulae to infection or tumour at the stump.)
Ch. 25 Pneumonectomy, p 474.

TRUE   D. Following a lobectomy, the vacant space is occupied by air and fluid. If an increase in the air-fluid level occurs, it is usually due to a parenchymal air leak through the lung sutures.
Ch. 25 Lobectomy, p 474.

TRUE   E. Any necrotizing pulmonary infection, particularly in the mechanically ventilated and immunocompromised patient, can produce peripheral lung infarction and bronchopleural fistula(e).
Ch. 14 Bronchopleural Fistula, p 266.

Q *2.12. Concerning Neurogenic Tumours of the Thorax*

    A. Neuroblastoma does not occur in the anterior mediastinum

    B. A thoracic neuroblastoma is likely to be of higher stage (i.e., INSS 3 or 4) than an abdominal tumour

    C. Nerve-sheath tumours are generally spherical

    D. Calcification in a tumour suggests that it is more likely to be benign than malignant

    E. Lateral thoracic meningoceles almost always communicate with the subarachnoid space

Q *2.13. Concerning the Erect Chest Radiograph*

    A. Mediastinal emphysema is associated with pneumoperitoneum in 5-10% of patients

    B. Mediastinal emphysema forms discrete pockets and locules of air

    C. Pneumomediastinum per se is of little clinical significance

    D. Acute severe asthma produces pneumomediastinum in about 50% of patients

    E. Pharyangeal perforation is commonly associated with pneumomediastinum

A   2.12. *Concerning Neurogenic Tumours of the Thorax*

FALSE   A. Neuroblastomas can occur anywhere; generally from or around the sympathetic chain. They commonly arise in the adrenal gland or pararenal tissue or in the posterior hemithorax.
Ch. 15 Mediastinal Masses, p 280.

FALSE   B. Thoracic neuroblastomas are generally of lower stage (i.e., INSS 1 and 2).

TRUE   C. Nerve-sheath tumours are normally spherical whereas *ganglioneuromas* tend to be sausage-shaped and lie parallel to the vertebral column.
Ch. 15 Neurogenic Tumours, p 292.

FALSE   D. Tumour calcification has no bearing on the nature of the tumour.
Ch. 15 Neurogenic Tumours, p 292.

TRUE   E. A meningocele is an extension of the theca containing CSF within the subarachnoid space and will therefore fill with contrast medium during myelography though MRI is now the investigation of choice. A lateral thoracic meningocele is a rare lesion that can present as an asymptomatic mass that may cause pressure deformity of bone. It is commonly associated with neurofibromatosis.
Ch. 15 Lateral Thoracic Meningocele, p 294.

A   2.13. *Concerning the Erect Chest Radiograph*

FALSE   A. Pneumomediastinum is classically associated with *retroperitoneal* gas rather than *intraperitoneal* gas.
Ch. 15 Mediastinal Emphysema, p 299.

FALSE   B. Mediastinal emphysema tends to present as a poorly defined, streaky, low-density pattern on the frontal CXR that should be differentiated from pneumopericardium and pneumothorax.
Ch. 15 Mediastinal Emphysema, p 299.

TRUE   C. Pneumomediastinum per se is of little clinical significance, but a cause should be sought in all cases, as this may influence treatment and further investigations.
Ch. 15 Mediastinal Emphysema, p 299.

FALSE   D. This is a well-recognized but uncommon finding (< 5%).
Ch. 15 Mediastinal Emphysema, p 299.

FALSE   E. Pneumomediastinum is a well-recognized but uncommon occurrence in pharyngeal perforation.
Ch. 15 Mediastinal Emphysema, p 299.

Q *2.14. Regarding the Radiology of Pneumonia*

    A. A pleural effusion commonly occurs with Legionella pneumonia.

    B. Chest radiographic changes occur in 25% of cases of brucellosis

    C. Moderately sized pleural effusions are a common radiographic feature of Mycoplasma pneumonia

    D. Leptospira interrogans infection causes a haemorrhagic pneumonia with small pleural effusions

    E. The pattern of consolidation suggests the microbe in most cases

Q *2.15. Concerning the Complications of Pneumonia*

    A. In patients who have not undergone drainage or biopsy procedures hydropneumothorax is caused by *Clostridium perfringens*

    B. Pulmonary gangrene is suspected when a large irregular cavity containing an irregular intracavitary body develops within a pneumonia

    C. Cavitation is not a feature of amoebic pneumonia

    D. Empyema is a complication of thoracic actinomycosis

    E. Lobar expansion is often a feature of Klebsiella pneumoniae infection

A 2.14. *Regarding the Radiology of Pneumonia*

TRUE A. This occurs in as many as 50% of cases, but is not a dominant feature.
Ch. 16 Pulmonary Infections in Adults, p 307.

FALSE B. Despite the common occurrence of respiratory symptoms, *radiological* changes are rare in brucellosis.
Ch. 16 Brucellosis, p 308.

FALSE C. On PA radiography, effusions are rarely a feature as they are small and transient.
Ch. 16 Mycoplasma Pneumonia, p 309.

TRUE D. Pulmonary involvement is variably reported as occuring in 11-67% of cases. It is manifest as bilateral ground-glass opacities, which resolve after about two weeks.
Ch. 16 Leptospirosis, p 311.

FALSE E.

A 2.15. *Concerning the Complications of Pneumonia*

TRUE A. Gas-forming organisms (e.g., *Bacteroides fragilis* and *Clostridium perfringens*) may rarely cause a hydropneumothorax. The most common causative agents are *Staphylococcus aureus*, Gram negative and anaerobic organisms.
Ch. 16 Hydropneumothorax, p 311.

TRUE B. Gangrene occurs when pneumonia causes thrombosis within intrapulmonary vessels. Most cases have been associated with Klebsiella and Streptococcal pneumonia.
Ch. 16 Pulmonary Gangrene, p 311.

FALSE C. Cavitation most commonly occurs in Staphylococcal, Gram negative (Klebsiella, Proteus, Pseudomonas), anaerobic and mycobacterial infections. Less common causes are fungal, amoebic and helminth-associated pneumonias.
Ch. 16 Abscess Formation, p 311.

TRUE D. This infection spreads across fascial planes and from a primary lung focus may penetrate into the pleural cavity, chest wall or pericardium.
Ch. 16 Actinomycosis, p 319.

TRUE E. Enlargement of an affected lobe by Klebsiella pneumoniae is said to be characteristic of that organism.
Ch. 16 Volume Changes, p 312.

Q *2.16. Concerning Pulmonary Tuberculosis*

    A. An isolated pleural effusion is a manifestation of primary tuberculosis

    B. Cavitation is a common manifestation of primary tuberculosis

    C. In 95% of cases, the initial lesion arises in the apicoposterior segment of an upper lobe or the apical segment of a lower lobe

    D. Miliary spread is more commonly a result of primary than post-primary tuberculosis

    E. A pleural effusion in post-primary infection carries a worse prognosis than one occurring in primary tuberculosis

Q *2.17. Regarding Hydatid Disease in the Lung*

    A. Cysts are more often than not ruptured at the time of presentation

    B. Intrapulmonary hydatid masses almost never calcify

    C. Rupture of an intrapulmonary cyst always leads to an air-fluid level

    D. Cyst rupture may be followed by the complete expectoration of its contents.

    E. Unruptured cysts usually occur in the upper zones

A 2.16. *Concerning Pulmonary Tuberculosis*

TRUE   A. Subpleural foci can give rise to a pleural effusion, which may be the only manifestation of the disease.
Ch. 16 Primary Tuberculosis, p 313.

FALSE   B. The occurrence of cavitation in primary tuberculosis is uncommon and indicates progressive primary disease.
Ch. 16 Consolidation, p 314.

TRUE   C. Isolated involvement of the anterior segment of an upper lobe virtually excludes the diagnosis.
Ch. 16 Major Radiological Findings, p 315.

FALSE   D.
Ch. 16 Miliary Tuberculosis, p 317.

TRUE   E. In post-primary infection, the effusion is usually an empyema, which leads to pleural scarring, calcification and, occasionally, chest wall involvement.
Ch. 16 Pleural Effusion, p 317.

A 2.17. *Regarding Hydatid Disease in the Lung*

TRUE   A. Two-thirds are ruptured at presentation.
Ch. 16 Hydatid Disease, p 324.

TRUE   B. Unlike in the mediastinum or abdomen where calcification is common.
Ch. 16 Hydatid Disease, p 324.

FALSE   C. If the endocyst and ectocyst membranes remain intact and only the pericyst ruptures, the net effect is a ring opacity with a rounded central homogeneous density and a crescent of air superiorly. The appearance then resembles a mycetoma.
Ch. 16 Hydatid Disease, p 324.

TRUE   D. The "empty cyst" sign.
Ch. 16 Hydatid Disease, p 324.

FALSE   E. Most are situated in the mid and lower zones.
Ch. 16 Hydatid Disease, p 324.

Q 2.18. *Regarding Pulmonary Involvement in AIDS*

    A. Pneumatoceles associated with *Pneumocystis carinii* infection gradually resolve after the pneumonia has been successfully treated

    B. Pneumothoraces associated with Pneumocystis infection are usually rapidly reabsorbed

    C. Aspergillus fungus is isolated in at least 75% of AIDS patients undergoing bronchial lavage

    D. Bacterial pneumonia is more common than Pneumocystis pneumonia

    E. Cavitation does not occur in pulmonary Kaposi's sarcoma

Q 2.19. *The Following are Common Features of Large Airway Obstruction*

    A. Hyperinflation

    B. Hypoinflation

    C. A normal inspiratory chest radiograph

    D. Bronchogenic cyst formation

    E. A bronchocele

A *2.18. Regarding Pulmonary Involvement in AIDS*

TRUE

    A. They sometimes persist as chronic, thin-walled, air-filled cavities.
       Ch. 16 Pneumocystis Carinii, p 326.

FALSE

    B. Pneumothoraces are serious complications of this infection and are very difficult to treat. Bronchopleural fistula is common and re-expansion of the lung may not occur.
       Ch. 16 Pneumocystis Carinii, p 326.

FALSE

    C. Despite it being increasingly recognized as a pathogen in AIDS patients, Aspergillus is still relatively infrequently isolated.
       Ch. 16 Aspergillosis, p 331.

TRUE

    D. *Streptococcus pneumoniae* and Haemophilus influenzae are the most common pulmonary pathogens in AIDS.
       Ch. 16 Pyogenic Organisms, p 333.

TRUE

    E.
       Ch. 16 Kaposi's Sarcoma, p 334.

A *2.19. The Following are Common Features of Large Airway Obstruction*

TRUE

    A.
       Ch. 17 Table 17.1, p 343.

TRUE

    B.
       Ch. 17 Table 17.1, p 343.

TRUE

    C.
       Ch. 17 Table 17.1, p 343.

FALSE

    D.
       Ch. 17 Table 17.1, p 343.

TRUE

    E.
       Ch. 17 Table 17.1, p 343.

Q 2.20. *Concerning Middle-Lobe Collapse*

    A. Increasing collapse may be accompanied by radiological signs of apparent improvement

    B. Minor depression of the horizontal fissure (five to ten degrees) is a reliable sign

    C. Contact (of the collapsed lobe) with the lower sternum is a useful sign

    D. On CT the collapsed lobe is seen to have a triangular shape with a laterally pointed apex that is retracted from the chest wall

    E. It cannot be differentiated from lingular collapse on the lateral radiograph

Q 2.21. *Regarding Lobar Collapse*

    A. The more collapsed a lobe is, the more opaque it appears on the chest radiograph

    B. Apparent reduction in the size of the hilum occurs in lower-lobe collapse

    C. In compensatory hyperinflation, the affected hyperinflated lung fails to deflate normally on expiration

    D. Rounded atelectasis is most common in the lower lobes

    E. In left upper-lobe collapse the lower lobe may expand to reach the level of the apex of the hemithorax

A 2.20. *Concerning Middle-Lobe Collapse*

TRUE   A. The signs of middle-lobe collapse tend to become less obvious, on the frontal radiograph, with progressive collapse.
Ch. 17 Collapse, p 344.

FALSE   B. Depression of the horizontal fissure of up to 10 degrees below the horizontal should be regarded as normal.
Ch. 17 Collapse, p 344.

TRUE   C. This feature aids in the differentiation of fluid within the major fissure from collapse.
Ch. 17 Collapse, p 344.

TRUE   D.
Ch. 17 Collapse, p 344.

FALSE   E. Lingular collapse has no minor fissure to give a clear upper border to the increased density, and the shift of the oblique fissure is often relatively small.
Ch. 17 Collapse, p 344.

A 2.21. *Regarding Lobar Collapse*

FALSE   A. The opacity of a collapsed lobe depends on the amount of retained fluid/secretions in that lobe and not on the volume of the lobe.
Ch. 18 Opacity of the Collapsed Lobe, p 359.

TRUE   B. The lower-lobe artery is obscured by the collapsed lower lobe and the interlobar artery (which contributes to the hilar shadow) is rotated out of profile. This causes a reduction in the apparent size of the hilum.
Ch. 18 Hilar Vascular Alterations, p 359.

FALSE   C. By definition there is no air trapping
Ch. 18 Compensatory Overinflation, p 362.

TRUE   D. Other lobes may also be affected, and the condition is not uncommonly bilateral.
Ch. 18 Rounded Atelectasis, p 363.

TRUE   E. When this happens, the superior border of the collapsed upper lobe may be outlined by air. The expanded lower lobe may also appear as a superomedial lucency that separates the collapsed upper lobe from the aorta. The combination of these findings is referred to as a "Luftsichel."
Ch. 18 Rounded Atelectasis, p 363.

Q *2.22. Concerning Chronic Bronchitis and Emphysema*

    A. A normal CXR is found in 40-60% of patients

    B. Over-inflation and pulmonary plethora are radiological features present in the affected areas of the lung

    C. The "dirty chest" is a typical finding

    D. Upper-zone blood diversion is found in some cases of emphysema

    E. Well-defined cysts on HRCT are a feature

Q *2.23. Pulmonary Parenchymal Involvement by Lymphoma*

    A. Occurs in approximately 30% of cases at presentation

    B. Occurs more frequently in non-Hodgkin's disease than in Hodgkin's disease

    C. Tends to be high grade when the lung is the primary site

    D. When associated with a pleural effusion, generally signifies extension into the pleura

    E. Is common in patients with normal hilar and mediastinal nodes and extra-thoracic disease

A 2.22. *Concerning Chronic Bronchitis and Emphysema*

TRUE A.
Ch. 19 *Chronic Bronchitis and Emphysema, p 369.*

FALSE B. The lungs tend to be *oligaemic* owing to destruction of blood vessels and alveolar walls.
Ch. 19 *Chronic Bronchitis and Emphysema, p 369.*

TRUE C. This describes the constellation of radiographic findings, which includes irregular pulmonary nodules and bronchial-wall thickening found in chronic bronchitis.
Ch. 19 *Chronic Bronchitis and Emphysema, p 369.*

TRUE D. When the emphysema is predominantly basal, there is increased blood flow to the upper zones (e.g., in alpha-1 antitrypsin deficiency). This should not be mistaken for the changes of left sided cardiac failure. Signs of air trapping and low diaphragms are usually present with basal emphysema that is severe enough to cause redistribution of blood flow.
Ch. 19 *Chronic Bronchitis and Emphysema, p 369.*

FALSE E. Emphysema does not produce cysts. It is defined as areas of low attenuation that originate at the centre of the pulmonary lobule (centriacinar emphysema) or large areas of low attenuation with a paucity of vessels (panacinar emphysema). These lesions do not have walls lined by endothelium.
Ch. 19 *Chronic Bronchitis and Emphysema, p 369.*

A 2.23. *Pulmonary Parenchymal Involvement by Lymphoma*

FALSE A. Only 10-15% present with extra-nodal pulmonary parenchymal involvement.
Ch. 20 *Malignant Lymphoma, p 390.*

FALSE B. Hodgkin's disease occurs three times more frequently in the pulmonary parenchyma than non-Hodgkin's disease.
Ch. 20 *Malignant Lymphoma, p 390.*

FALSE C. Primary lymphoma of the lung is very uncommon. When it occurs, it is generally low grade (small lymphocytic).
Ch. 20 *Malignant Lymphoma, p 390.*

FALSE D. Pleural effusions tend to be caused by hilar obstruction rather than by trans-pulmonary spread and usually resolve when the hilar adenopathy resolves.
Ch. 20 *Malignant Lymphoma, p 390.*

FALSE E. Extra-thoracic disease and normal hilar nodes in association with a solitary pulmonary nodule suggest that the nodule is not lymphomatous in nature.
Ch. 20 *Malignant Lymphoma, p 390.*

Q *2.24. Concerning Lymphoid Diseases of the Lungs*

A. Pseudolymphoma has the same histological features as lymphocytic interstitial pneumonitis (LIP)

B. Solitary mass pseudolymphoma is associated with HIV infection and AIDS

C. Lymphodenopathy is a well recognized feature of uncomplicated lymphocytic interstitial pneumonitis

D. Lymphoid granulomatosis is frequently a premalignant condition

E. Leukaemic infiltrates are demonstrated on the plain CXR in approximately 30-60% of patients with leukaemia

Q *2.25. Regarding Pulmonary Neoplasms*

A. Bronchial carcinoid tumours do not metastasize

B. Bronchial carcinoids are more likely to produce Cushing's syndrome than the carcinoid syndrome

C. Calcification in bronchial carcinoid can be demonstrated in only 5-10% of patients on CT

D. Pulmonary hamartomas commonly present in the fourth decade

E. There is an association of pulmonary chondromata and intraadrenal tumours in Carney's triad

A 2.24. *Concerning Lymphoid Diseases of the Lungs*

TRUE   A. Pseudolymphoma and LIP share the same histological features. Pseudolymphoma, however, is a solitary mass whereas LIP tends to be a diffuse disease.
Ch. 20 Lymphocytic Interstitial Pneumonitis (LIP), p 392.

FALSE   B. *Lymphocytic interstitial pneumonitis* is often associated with AIDS and Sjogren's Syndrome.
Ch. 20 Pseudolymphoma and LIP, p 392.

FALSE   C. If lymphadenopathy is demonstrated in patients with LIP, lymphomatous change should be suspected.
Ch. 20 Lymphocytic Interstitial Pneumonitis, p 392.

TRUE   D. Malignant transformation occurs in 50% of patients with lymphoid granulomatosis.
Ch. 20 Lymphoid Granulomatosis, p 392.

FALSE   E. Notwithstanding the fact that leukaemic pulmonary infiltrates are frequently found at autopsy, the chest radiograph is normal in most patients with leukaemia.
Ch. 20 Leukaemia, p 393.

A 2.25. *Regarding Pulmonary Neoplasms*

FALSE   A. Although bronchial carcinoid tumours are classified as "benign" tumours they do metastasize.
Ch. 20 Bronchial Carcinoid, p 388.

TRUE   B. The carcinoid syndrome is extremely rare in patients with bronchial carcinoid whereas Cushing's syndrome, though uncommon, is more frequently encountered.
Ch. 20 Bronchial Carcinoid, p 388.

FALSE   C. Calcification, as demonstrated on CT, occurs in up to 35% of patients.
Ch. 20 Bronchial Carcinoid, p 388.

TRUE   D.
Ch. 20 Bronchial Carcinoid, p 388.

FALSE   E. Carney's triad consists of pulmonary chondroma (ta), extra-adrenal paragangliomata and gastric epitheloid leiomyosarcoma.
Ch. 20 Pulmonary Hamartoma, p 389.

Q *2.26. Concerning the Radiology of Bronchogenic Carcinoma*

A. Tumours that have more than 90 degrees of circumferential contact with the aorta should be regarded as irresectable

B. Mediastinal fat plane obliteration suggests irresectability of the tumour

C. MRI has proved to be of little help in distinguishing T3 from T4 tumours

D. Contact with the visceral pleura is often associated with pain

E. All Pancoast's tumours should be imaged with MRI if there is no obvious bone destruction

Q *2.27. Concerning the Diagnosis and Staging of Lung Cancer*

A. A negative CXR with positive cytology suggests a better prognosis than a positive CXR with positive cytology

B. Approximately 30-40% of potentially visible primary peripheral pulmonary cancers had been missed on at least one previous CXR in the NCI (National Cancer Institute) screening programme

C. The TNM classification does not apply to small-cell cancer of the lung

D. The sensitivity and specificity of nodal enlargement, as demonstrated by CT, tend to be better in Europe and Japan than in the USA

E. Pre-operative nodal sampling (biopsy) should be undertaken in nodes < 10 mm in transaxial diameter if they receive lymph from the region of the tumour

A 2.26. *Concerning the Radiology of Bronchogenic Carcinoma*

FALSE   A. Glazier in 1989 suggested that tumours having less than 90 degrees contact with the aorta are resectable. Read this section very carefully.
Ch. 20 Spread of Tumour, p 382.

TRUE   B. Fat plane invasion suggests irresectability, although in isolation, it should not preclude the patient from undergoing a potentially curative operation.
Ch. 20 Spread of Tumour, p 382.

FALSE   C. MRI is the method of choice for examining the subcarinal region (see TNM staging system in Grainger and Allison) as the scans are obtained coronally. This is superior to CT scanning in the axial plane with image reconstruction.
Ch. 20 Spread of Tumour, p 382.

FALSE   D. There is no sensory innervation of the visceral pleura. Contact with the parietal pleura produces pain.
Ch. 20 Spread of Tumour, p 382.

TRUE   E. Coronal MRI views are mandatory in Pancoast's tumours.
Ch. 20 Spread of Tumour, p 382.

A 2.27. *Concerning the Diagnosis and Staging of Lung Cancer*

TRUE   A. This is probably a reflection of the small size of the tumour, though the true reason for this phenomenon is unknown.
Ch. 20 Early Diagnosis of Bronchial Carcinoma, p 382.

FALSE   B. The NCI found 45 out of 50 lesions were missed on the previous radiographs (i.e., 90%).
Ch. 20 Early Diagnosis of Bronchial Carcinoma, p 382.

TRUE   C. TNM is used for all non–small cell pulmonary cancers.
Ch. 20 Table 20.1, p 383.

TRUE   D. This finding is probably due to the higher prevalence of coincidental histoplamosis in the USA, which gives erroneous false positive nodes.
Ch. 20 Spread of Tumour, p 382.

FALSE   E. Pre-operative nodal sampling should only be undertaken in patients in whom the transaxial node diameter is greater than 10 mm.
Ch. 20 Spread of Tumour, p 382.

Q 2.28. Concerning Bronchogenic Carcinoma

A. Massive hilar or mediastinal adenopathy is a well recognized feature of large cell carcinoma

B. Large cell carcinomas are manifest as a solitary peripheral nodule in 60-70% of cases

C. Cavitation is seen in up to 5% of adenocarcinomas

D. Consolidation/collapse of the lung is most frequently seen with squamous carcinoma of the lung

E. Bronchiolo-alveolar cell carcinoma is usually indistinguishable from other types of carcinoma in the frontal radiograph

Q 2.29. Concerning Peripheral Primary Bronchogenic Tumours

A. Peripheral tumours are much less common than central lesions

B. Lobulation is a common finding

C. Demonstration of a peripheral shadow or "tail" is pathognomonic of malignancy

D. In the United Kingdom, calcification of the pulmonary mass is present in about 20% of tumours investigated with CT

E. Serial radiographs may demonstrate a doubling of the tumour *diameter* within 30-490 days (median 120 days)

A 2.28. *Concerning Bronchogenic Carcinoma*

TRUE   A. Massive hilar adenopathy is frequently seen with both small and large cell carcinomas.
Ch. 20 Radiographic Patterns Based on Cell Type, p 379.

TRUE   B. Adenocarcinoma occurs as a small peripheral nodule in 72% cases and a large cell carcinoma in 63%.
Ch. 20 Radiographic Patterns Based on Cell Type, p 379.

TRUE   C. Cavitation is seen in 12% of squamous cell tumours and in 6% of adenocarcinomas and large cell carcinomas.
Ch. 20 The Peripheral Tumour, p 376.

TRUE   D. Squamous cell carcinomas are frequently central lesions and therefore tend to produce collapse/consolidation more often than other lesions.
Ch. 20 The Central Tumour, p 377.

TRUE   E. Beware. Bronchiolo-alveolar cell carcinomas may well grow very slowly with doubling times > 18 months.
Ch. 20 Radiographic Patterns Based on Cell Type, p 379.

A 2.29. *Concerning Peripheral Primary Bronchogenic Tumours*

FALSE   A. Approximately 60% of bronchogenic tumours are central in location; 40% are peripheral.
Ch. 20 Peripheral Tumours, p 376.

TRUE   B. Lobulation is commonly found in peripheral tumours and represents localized peripheral growth of the tumour.
Ch. 20 Peripheral Tumours, p 376.

FALSE   C. The streak or tail shadow is a non-specific finding.
Ch. 20 Peripheral Tumours, p 376.

FALSE   D. Calcification is demonstrated in about 6-10% of tumours on CT (U.K < 5% and the USA 13%).
Ch. 20 The Solitary Pulmonary Mass, p 397.

FALSE   E. The tumour doubles in *volumes* during this period. If the tumour doubles in volume, the diameter increases by 26%.
Ch. 20 The Solitary Pulmonary Mass, p 397.

Q 2.30. *Bronchogenic Carcinoma*

    A. May present with multiple primary tumours in 10-15% of patients

    B. Is very rare under the age of 25 years

    C. Typically presents clinically with pneumonia or, radiologically, as a solitary pulmonary nodule

    D. Is typically asymptomatic in about 40-60% of patients

    E. In the superior sulcus may present with brachial plexus neuropathy

Q 2.31. *Pulmonary Metastasis (Metastases)*

    A. Are solitary in about 50% of asymptomatic patients

    B. Are more easily demonstrated on a low kV radiograph than a high kV radiograph

    C. Are the most likely cause of multiple lesions less than 1 cm in diameter in an asymptomatic patient

    D. When demonstrated on the CXR always require further imaging with CT

    E. Can be imaged with 99 mTc FDG

A 2.30. *Bronchogenic Carcinoma*

FALSE
A. Multiple primary tumours occur in much less than 1% of patients.
Ch. 20 Bronchial Carcinoma, p 375.

TRUE
B. Bronchogenic carcinoma is extremely rare below 35 years and virtually unknown below 25 years.
Ch. 20 Bronchial Carcinoma, p 375.

TRUE
C. These are the two most common findings at presentation.
Ch. 20 Bronchial Carcinoma, p 375.

FALSE
D. About 25% of patients with bronchogenic carcinoma are asymptomatic.
Ch. 20 Bronchial Carcinoma, p 375.

TRUE
E. The superior sulcus is the groove in the apex of the lung formed by the subclavian vessels (cf. Pancoast's tumour).
Ch. 20 Bronchial Carcinoma, p 375.

A 2.31. *Pulmonary Metastasis (Metastases)*

FALSE
A. A solitary metastasis is only demonstrated in about 2-6% of such patients.
Ch. 20 Metastases, p 393.

FALSE
B. Small metastases are often "whited out" on the low kV films.
Ch. 20 Metastases, p 393.

FALSE
C. Another diagnosis should be sought as noncalcified metastases are infrequently seen when < 1 cm.
Ch. 20 Metastases, p 393.

FALSE
D. CT may be helpful as a few patients may be suitable for resection.
Ch. 20 Metastases, p 393.

FALSE
E. FDG (Fluorodeoxyglucose) emits gamma rays from fluorine and is imaged using PET scanners.
Ch. 20 Metastases, p 393.

Q 2.32. *Concerning Pulmonary Haemorrhage*

    A. Haemoptysis is a common presentation

    B. Air-space shadowing tends to clear within 5-10 days

    C. There is an increase in the KCO_2

    D. Systemic lupus erythematosis nephritis with pulmonary haemorrhage is associated with antiglomerular basement membrane antibodies

    E. Cardiac enlargement is an important sign when deciding the aetiology of pulmonary haemorrhage

Q 2.33. *The Following Features Suggest That Pulmonary Oedema is Non-Cardiogenic in Nature*

    A. Septal lines

    B. Increased pulmonary blood volume

    C. Central and peripheral distribution of lung opacities

    D. Enlarged cardiac silhouette

    E. The presence of basal pulmonary crackles prior to any changes on the CXR

A 2.32. *Concerning Pulmonary Haemorrhage*

FALSE　　　A. Haemoptysis is an uncommon presentation in patients with pulmonary haemorrhage as bleeding occurs below the mucociliary escalator of the bronchial tree. The blood in the alveoli clears via macrophage breakdown.
Ch. 21 Diffuse Pulmonary Haemorrhage, p 410.

TRUE　　　B. Pulmonary oedema clears within 24-48 hours; pulmonary infection tends to clear within 5-30 days.
Ch. 21 Diffuse Pulmonary Haemorrhage, p 410.

FALSE　　　C. There is increased uptake in the KCO. Haemoglobin avidly takes up carbon monoxide, providing a sensitive means of detecting fresh intra-alveolar haemorrhage.
Ch. 21 Diffuse Pulmonary Haemorrhage, p 410.

FALSE　　　D. *Goodpasture's disease* is classically associated with antiglomerular basement antibodies.
Ch. 21 Diffuse Pulmonary Haemorrhage, p 410.

FALSE　　　E.
Ch. 21 Pulmonary Haemorrhage, p 410.

A 2.33. *The Following Features Suggest That Pulmonary Oedema is Non-Cardiogenic in Nature*

FALSE　　　A.
Ch. 21 Table 21.4, p 407.

TRUE　　　B.
Ch. 21 Table 21.4, p 407.

FALSE　　　C.
Ch. 21 Table 21.4, p 407.

FALSE　　　D.
Ch. 21 Table 21.4, p 407.

FALSE　　　E.
Ch. 21 Pulmonary Oedema, p 403.

Q 2.34. *The Following are Commonly Associated with Unilateral or Bilateral Hilar Adenopathy*

     A. Sarcoidosis

     B. Post-primary TB

     C. Thermophilic actinomycetes spore inhalation

     D. Castleman's disease (giant lymph node hyperplasia)

     E. Primary pulmonary lymphangiectasia

Q 2.35. *Concerning the Pulmonary Eosinophilias*

     A. A peripheral eosinophil count of less than 500 mm^{-3} does not exclude the diagnosis

     B. The pulmonary infiltrates with eosinophilia (PIE) syndrome is associated with *Schistosoma japonicum*

     C. There is an association with bronchoceles

     D. Chlorpromazine is associated with pulmonary eosinophilia

     E. Chronic pulmonary eosinophilia associated with allergic bronchopulmonary aspergillosis produces upper-zone fibrosis

A 2.34. *The Following are Commonly Associated with Unilateral or Bilateral Hilar Adenopathy*

TRUE   A. Forty percent of patients with intra-thoracic sarcoidosis have adenopathy on the CXR at the time of diagnosis. Garland's triad (i.e., bilateral hilar and right paratracheal adenopathy) is present in 75-90% of patients with intra-thoracic sarcoid adenopathy.
Ch. 21 Table 21.8, p 417.

FALSE   B. Adenopathy is a feature of primary TB.
Ch. 21 Table 21.8, p 417.

FALSE   C. Thermophilic actinomycetes from forced air equipment causes a hypersensitivity pneumonitis. Nodal enlargement is only rarely demonstrated on the CXR in patients with mushroom worker's lung.

FALSE   D. Castleman's disease tends to produce mediastinal adenopathy (middle and posterior) rather than hilar enlargement. Some cases may be indistinguishable from lymphoma.
Ch. 21 Lymphoid Disorders of the Lungs, p 424.

FALSE   E. Primary pulmonary lymphangiectasia produces subpleural cysts, thickening of the interlobular septa and ectatic lymph channels; there is no obstruction to the flow of lymph. Nodal enlargement is not a feature of this disease.
Ch. 27 Lymphangiectasis, p 501.

A 2.35. *Concerning the Pulmonary Eosinophilias*

TRUE   A. The definition of pulmonary eosinophila is "an eosinophilic pulmonary infiltrate usually, but not always, associated with excess eosinophils in the peripheral blood."
Ch. 21 Pulmonary Eosinophilia, p 424.

FALSE   B. It is normally found with *S. haematobium* and *S. mansoni,* not *S. japonicum*.
Ch. 21 Table 21.14, p 424.

TRUE   C. Bronchoceles are a characteristic finding in patients with advanced allergic bronchopulmonary aspergillosis (ABPA).
Ch. 21 Allergic Bronchopulmonary Aspergillosis, p 424.

FALSE   D.
Ch. 21 Table 21.14, p 424.

TRUE   E.
Ch. 21 Pulmonary Eosinophilia, p 424.

Q *2.36. The Following Are Associated Upper-Zone Pulmonary Fibrosis*

      A. Extrinsic allergic alveolitis

      B. *Mycobacterium kansasi*

      C. Wegener's granulomatosis

      D. Mycoplasma infections

      E. Berylliosis

Q *2.37. Concerning Pulmonary Oedema*

      A. Mendelson's syndrome produces changes on the CXR within 24 hours

      B. Fresh-water drowning can usually be differentiated from salt-water drowning on the CXR

      C. Air-space shadowing in drug abusers tends to clear within a few hours following treatment

      D. Withdrawal of 200 ml of a pleural effusion can produce pulmonary oedema

      E. After head injury the distribution of pulmonary oedema is commonly symmetrical

A 2.36. *The Following Are Associated Upper-Zone Pulmonary Fibrosis*

TRUE A.

Ch. 21 Table 21.12, p 414.

TRUE B.

Ch. 21 Table 21.12, p 414.

FALSE C.

Ch. 21 Table 21.12, p 414.

FALSE D.

Ch. 21 Table 21.12, p 32.

TRUE E. The findings are extremely similar to those seen in sarcoidosis.
Ch. 21 Table 21.12, p 414.

A 2.37. *Concerning Pulmonary Oedema*

TRUE A. Mendelson's syndrome results from the inhalation of acidic gastric contents. The mortality is high.
Ch. 21 Pulmonary Oedema Due to Microvascular Injury, p 408.

FALSE B. There is no significant difference between the two. The increase in capillary permeability produces a proteinaceous exudate in addition to the oedematous transudate; there is subsequent hyaline membrane formation and fibrosis.
Ch. 21 Pulmonary Oedema Due to Microvascular Injury, p 408.

TRUE C. However, if the air-space shadowing is complicated by aspiration, the clearing may take longer.
Ch. 21 Pulmonary Oedema Due to Microvascular Injury, p 408.

TRUE D. The withdrawal of any amount of fluid from the pleural cavity can produce pulmonary oedema, though this is very unusual when small volumes are withdrawn.
Ch. 21 Pulmonary Oedema Due to Microvascular Injury, p 408.

FALSE E.

Ch. 21 Pulmonary Oedema Due to Microvascular Injury, p 408.

Q 2.38. *Regarding Diffuse Pulmonary Disease*

    A. In patients with fibrosing alveolitis the presence of subpleural and ground-glass shadowing (as demonstrated by HRCT) suggests the likelihood of a good response to steroid treatment

    B. Langerhan's cell histiocytosis has an equal sex incidence

    C. The cysts demonstrated on HRCT in patients with Langerhan's cell histiocytosis have no visible walls

    D. Adenopathy on the plain CXR is a common feature of Langerhan's cell histiocytosis

    E. Lymphangiomyomatosis (LAM) is almost exclusively confined to females

Q 2.39. *Concerning Pulmonary Parenchymal Disease Caused by Organic Material—Extrinsic Allergic Alveolitis (EAA)*

    A. It is commonly associated with eosinophilia

    B. It produces lower-zone changes in the acute phase

    C. It can produce a honeycomb lung

    D. It produces a distribution of fibrosis similar to that seen with interstitial pneumonitis (fibrosing alveolitis)

    E. It is invariably associated with finger clubbing

A *2.38. Regarding Diffuse Pulmonary Disease*

TRUE   A. This is equivalent to DIP (Desquamative Interstitial Pneumonitis).
Ch. 21 Fibrosing Alveolitis or Diffuse Interstitial Pneumonia, p 413.

FALSE   B. Males are more frequently affected than females in the proportions of 4:1.
Ch. 21 Histiocytosis X, p 413.

FALSE   C. Wall visibility defines a cyst.
Ch. 21 Fig. 21.15, p 414.

FALSE   D. This is a rare feature of LCH on the plain CXR and should suggest an alternative diagnosis.
Ch. 21 Histiocytosis X, p 413.

TRUE   E. LAM and tuberose sclerosis may produce similar changes in the lungs, which include large volume lungs, multiple cysts and small pleural effusions. They are both exclusive to females.
Ch. 21 Tuberose Sclerosis and Lymphangiomyomatosis, p 415.

A *2.39. Concerning Pulmonary Parenchymal Disease Caused by Organic Material—Extrinsic Allergic Alveolitis (EAA)*

FALSE   A. There is no such association.
Ch. 21 Damage to Lung Parenchyma by Organic Material, p 411.

TRUE   B. This is the description of the classical changes, though many patients do not show any changes on the initial radiograph. The changes, in the acute phase, range from loss of clarity of the pulmonary vessels, to a hazy ground-glass appearance which can progress to look like frank pulmonary oedema.
Ch. 21 Damage to Lung Parenchyma by Organic Material, p 411.

TRUE   C. Any pulmonary disease that produces fibrosis can produce a honeycomb pattern.
Ch. 21 Damage to Lung Parenchyma by Organic Material, p 411.

FALSE   D. Interstitial pneumonitis (fibrosing alveolitis) classically produces fibrosis in the lower zones whereas the fibrosis produced by EAA is typically in the upper zones.
Ch. 21 Damage to Lung Parenchyma by Organic Material, p 411.

FALSE   E. Fibrosis secondary to fibrosing alveolitis can produce finger clubbing but not invariably so.
Ch. 21 Fibrosing Alveolitis or Diffuse Interstitial Pneumonia, p 413.

Q 2.40. *Regarding Sarcoidosis*

A. Radiological parenchymal changes occur in 50-70% of patients

B. The most common parenchymal pattern consists of areas of patchy consolidation

C. By characterizing the type of pulmonary parenchymal pattern, it is possible to predict if and where any fibrosis will occur

D. Bronchovascular beading is a very sensitive sign of sarcoidosis

E. If a large effusion is demonstrated in a patient with sarcoidosis, another diagnosis should be sought

Q 2.41. *The Following Are Features of Collagen Vascular Disease in the Chest*

A. Basal pulmonary fibrosis occurs in more than 30% of patients with systemic lupus erythematosis

B. Pleural effusion is the most common radiographic manifestation of rheumatoid disease

C. Caplan's nodules occur in patients who have been exposed to silicone

D. The fibrosis demonstrated in patients with systemic sclerosis can be readily differentiated from other causes of basal fibrosis

E. The apparent reduction in lung volume in patients with dermatomyositis and polymyositis is commonly due to basal fibrosis

A 2.40. *Regarding Sarcoidosis*

TRUE
    A. There are three types of parenchymal change: reversible, nonreversible (equivalent to mixed) and fibrotic.
        Ch. 21 Sarcoidosis, p 416.

FALSE
    B. The three types of parenchymal shadowing are multiple rounded or irregular small 2-4 mm nodules (75-90%), patchy consolidation (10-20%) and 10-40 mm nodules (2%).
        Ch. 21 Sarcoidosis, p 416.

FALSE
    C. No such prediction can be made.
        Ch. 21 Sarcoidosis, p 416.

TRUE
    D. The finding of bronchovascular beading is very sensitive and specific for sarcoidosis. The phenomenon is characterized by 1-5 mm nodules in the perilymphatic region (along the bronchovascular bundles, interlobular septa and subpleural space).
        Ch. 21 Sarcoidosis, p 416.

TRUE
    E. Pleural effusions occur in only 2% of patients with sarcoidosis and are generally small when present.
        Ch. 21 Sarcoidosis, p 416.

A 2.41. *The Following Are Features of Collagen Vascular Disease in the Chest*

FALSE
    A. In most series, the incidence of such fibrosis is less than 3% in SLE. Apparent loss of lung volume may occur owing to diaphragmatic myopathy.
        Ch. 21 Systemic Lupus Erythematosis, p 419.

TRUE
    B. In a significant minority of patients, the pleural disease antedates the arthritis, though most patients have a positive latex test.
        Ch. 21 Rheumatoid Disease, p 420.

FALSE
    C. Caplan's syndrome, originally described in Welsh miners, is a disease entity in which nodules rapidly appear in crops when patients with rheumatoid arthritis have been exposed to silica. *Silicone* is an unrelated prosthetic material.
        Ch. 21 Rheumatoid Disease, p 420.

FALSE
    D. One must look for other features of systemic sclerosis on the radiograph such as an air oesophagogram, calcinosis, basal pneumonia (secondary to aspiration) and a possible lipoid pneumonia (low-density fat globules may well be demonstrated on CT).
        Ch. 21 Systemic Sclerosis, p 421.

FALSE
    E. Basal fibrosis does occur in these conditions, however, as well as diaphragmatic myopathy.
        Ch. 21 Dermatomyositis, p 422.

Q 2.42. *Regarding Sarcoidosis*

A. The most common presentation in the UK is one of bilateral hilar adenopathy

B. A stage III presentation is when the CXR demonstrates a pulmonary opacity in the absence of any hilar adenopathy

C. Asymmetrical mediastinal adenopathy occurs in less than 10% of patients

D. Nodal enlargement disappears within 6-12 months in over 80% of cases

E. 10-20% of patients develop intrapulmonary opacities on CXR prior to nodal enlargement

Q 2.43. *The Following Is Associated with Eggshell Hilar Nodal Calcification*

A. Coalworker's pneumoconiosis

B. Amyloidosis

C. Histiocytosis

D. Tuberculosis

E. Scleroderma

A 2.42. *Regarding Sarcoidosis*

FALSE   A. *Erythema nodosum* is the most common presenting feature in the UK.
            Ch. 21 Sarcoidosis, p 416.

TRUE   B. Stage I = Lymphadenopathy.
            Stage II = Lymphadenopathy + parenchymal opacity.
            Stage III = Parenchymal opacity alone.
            The lower the stage at presentation, the better the prognosis.
            Ch. 21 Sarcoidosis, p 416.

TRUE   C. As confirmed by CT, marked asymmetry is sufficiently unusual as to bring
            the diagnosis into question.
            Ch. 21 Sarcoidosis, p 416.

TRUE   D. Ninety-five percent of patients (who have had nodal enlargement) have no
            nodal adenopathy 12 months after their initial CXR.
            Ch. 21 Sarcoidosis, p 417.

FALSE   E. This is not true for pulmonary sarcoidosis.
            Ch. 21 Sarcoidosis, p 416.

A 2.43. *The Following Is Associated with Eggshell Hilar Nodal Calcification*

TRUE   A.
            Ch. 22 Silicosis, p 438.

TRUE   B.
            Ch. 22 Silicosis, p 438.

FALSE   C. No. *Histoplasmosis* may cause glandular calcification.
            Ch. 22 Silicosis, p 438.

FALSE   D. TB often produces hilar nodal calcification but this is not usually eggshell
            in type
            Ch. 22 Silicosis, p 438.

TRUE   E.
            Ch. 22 Silicosis, p 438.

Q 2.44. Industrial/Occupational Lung Disease

    A. Is a group of disorders that results solely from inorganic dust exposure

    B. When due to coal worker's pneumoconiosis (CWP), is characterized by discrete nodules (1-4 mm) often most profuse in the upper zones

    C. May be associated with large spiculated intra-pulmonary masses (1-10 cm) in the late phase of the disease

    D. Induces extensive fibrosis when produced by silica (SiO_2)

    E. Is treated with antibiotics in some instances

Q 2.45. Regarding Asbestos-Related Thoracic Disease

    A. The short fibres of crocidolite are more likely to induce chest disease than the longer fibres of chrysotile

    B. Classical signs of asbestosis are the "holly leaf" pleural plaque and the diaphagmatic calcification

    C. Malignancy should be suspected in all patients who develop a pleural effusion

    D. Malignant mesotheliomas usually arise independently from pleural plaques

    E. Severe pulmonary asbestosis tends to affect the whole lung

A 2.44. Industrial/Occupational Lung Disease

FALSE   A. The disorders may also result from exposure to *organic* dusts. There are five main categories of industrial lung disease, namely: Occupational Asthma, Byssinosis, Extrinsic Allergic Alveolitis, Pneumoconioses and Toxic Fume Exposure.
Ch. 22 The Pneumoconioses Due to Mineral Dust, p 437.

TRUE   B. In patients with pure CWP, there is little associated fibrosis.
Ch. 22 Coal Worker's Pneumoconiosis, p 437.

TRUE   C. This is the description of Progressive Massive Fibrosis. The differential diagnosis for these masses includes TB and bronchial carcinoma
Ch. 22 Progressive Massive Fibrosis, p 437.

TRUE   D. The pneumoconioses produced by *silicates* tend not to exhibit marked fibrosis. The inhalation of *silica* (SiO_2), however, tends to a marked fibrotic reaction. The radiological picture of *silica* pneumoconiosis is one of macules that are similar to those seen with CWP but larger and more densely fibrotic.
Ch. 22 Silicosis, p 438.

TRUE   E. The zoonoses, although not part of the five main categories of industrial lung disease, may be acquired by workers; some of these can be treated with antibiotics (e.g., *Chlamydia psittaci*).
Ch. 22 Zoonoses, p 442.

A 2.45. Regarding Asbestos-Related Thoracic Disease

TRUE   A. The shorter fibres are the more "penetrating" and are therefore associated with a higher risk of thoracic disease.
Ch. 22 Asbestosis, p 439.

FALSE   B. *Asbestosis* is specific for the lungs and refers to pulmonary and not pleural fibrosis induced by asbestos exposure.
Ch. 22 Table 22.2, p 437.

TRUE   C. Any asbestos worker that develops a pleural effusion should be investigated for a pleural or pulmonary malignancy before diagnosing a benign effusion.
Ch. 22 Asbestosis, p 439.

TRUE   D. Malignant mesotheliomas generally presents with pain and dyspnoea. Two-thirds of the patients also present with pleural effusions. Rib destruction is demonstrated in 15% of patients.
Ch. 22 Asbestosis, p 439.

FALSE   E. Unlike coal worker's pneumoconiosis (CWP), the upper zones tend to be spared in asbestosis, even in the most severe cases.
Ch. 22 Asbestosis, p 439.

Q *2.46. The Diagnosis of Pulmonary Thromboembolism*

A. Can be made by ventilation/perfusion scanning using ^{99m}Tc as the sole radionuclide

B. Should never be made when there is a matched ventilation/perfusion defect

C. Is extremely unlikely (less than 5% false negative rate) in patients with a "low probability" ventilation/perfusion scan using the PIOPED criteria

D. Can be excluded or made in the majority of patients by means of ventilation/perfusion scanning

E. Can be made by pulmonary angiography when other tests are inconclusive

A 2.46. *The Diagnosis of Pulmonary Thromboembolism*

TRUE

A. In most centres, ^{99m}Tc-labelled microspheres are used as the perfusion agent and ^{81m}Krypton as the ventilation agent. If Krypton is not available, technegas (^{99m}Tc labelled carbon particles) can be used instead.
Ch. 23 Radionuclide Studies in Pulmonary Embolus, p 450.

FALSE

B. A ventilation/perfusion mismatch is the most likely finding in thromboembolism. However, if pulmonary infarction has occurred, both the ventilation and the perfusion will be reduced in that area of the lung. It is important to note that the underventilation may not be as marked as the under-perfusion because of the effect of surrounding ventilation.
Ch. 23 Radionuclide Studies in Pulmonary Embolus, p 450.

FALSE

C. The false negative rate was 15% in the PIOPED study.
Ch. 23 Radionuclide Studies in Pulmonary Embolus, p 450.

FALSE

D. In a major study, only 13% of patients were in the high probability group and 14% in the normal group; therefore the majority of patients were in the "indeterminate" or "low" probability groups.
Ch. 23 Radionuclide Studies in Pulmonary Embolus, p 450.

TRUE

E. This is one of the indications for pulmonary angiography in young and otherwise healthy patients in whom the risks of pulmonary angiography are extremely low.
Ch. 23 Radionuclide Studies in Pulmonary Embolus, p 450.

Q 2.47. The Radiological Signs of Pulmonary Thromboembolism Include

A. A normal chest radiograph

B. Westermark's sign—alteration of the pulmonary vasculature distal to an embolus

C. Fleischner's sign—dilation of a main pulmonary vessel by back pressure or clot

D. Hampton's hump—a shallow hump-shaped lesion on the pleural surface due to a pulmonary infarct

E. Demonstrable effusions in most cases of pulmonary infarction

Q 2.48. Concerning Pulmonary Thromboembolism

A. Of the patients surviving for one hour following acute pulmonary embolism and in whom the correct diagnosis has not been made, 30% will die

B. Haemoptysis occurs in more than 60% of patients with an acute pulmonary embolus

C. Right-sided cardiac failure occurs when more than 50% of the pulmonary vasculature has been occluded by embolus

D. Five to 10% of patients with acute pulmonary embolism may develop chronic pulmonary hypertension

E. The classical ECG findings of pulmonary embolism include sinus tachycardia, right axis deviation, $S_1Q_3T_3$ and ST changes

A 2.47. *The Radiological Signs of Pulmonary Thromboembolism Include*

FALSE

A. In the PIOPED study (Prospective Investigation of Pulmonary Embolus Diagnosis), the CXR was abnormal in most patients (88%) with known pulmonary embolism. However, this was also true of those who did not have pulmonary embolism.
Ch. 23 The Imaging of Pulmonary Thromboembolism, p 449.

TRUE

B.
Ch. 23 The Imaging of Pulmonary Thromboembolism, p 449.

TRUE

C.
Ch. 23 The Imaging of Pulmonary Thromboembolism, p 449.

TRUE

D. Remember that most pulmonary infarctions are not humped, triangular or wedge-shaped. They have a variety of shapes depending on their orientation and the degree of surrounding haemorrhage.
Ch. 23 The Imaging of Pulmonary Thromboembolism, p 449.

TRUE

E. The size of an effusion is generally related to the size of the infarct, though in some patients inconspicuous or surprisingly small infarcts may be associated with extremely large effusions.
Ch. 23 The Imaging of Pulmonary Thromboembolism, p 449.

A 2.48. *Concerning Pulmonary Thromboembolism*

TRUE

A. Eighty-nine percent of patients survive the first hour and 29% of these are correctly diagnosed and treated with anticoagulants. Of these 29%, only 8% will die (2.3% of the original 89%). Of the 71% of patients in whom the diagnosis is not made, 30% would be 21% of the original 89%).
Ch. 23 Pulmonary Thromboembolism, p 446.

FALSE

B. Haemoptysis occurs in only 17% of patients with pulmonary embolism.
Ch. 23 Pulmonary Thromboembolism. Clinical Features and Physiological Facts, p 447.

TRUE

C. Right-sided heart failure occurs when approximately 50% of the pulmonary vasculature is occluded by acute pulmonary embolism. The maximum pressure that the right ventricle can develop is 45 mm Hg; values above this will produce rapid-onset, right-sided cardiac failure.
Ch. 23 Pulmonary Embolism, p 448.

TRUE

D. Pulmonary hypertension is uncommon and usually follows recurrent small pulmonary emboli.
Ch. 23 Pulmonary Embolism, p 448.

TRUE

E. A radiologist should still remember some medical basics.

Q 2.49. *Concerning Patients with Traumatic Injury to the Chest*

    A. It is important to demonstrate all rib fractures employing additional views if necessary

    B. The finding of a 1st rib fracture may signify severe trauma

    C. Pulmonary contusion is usually seen without rib fractures

    D. A localized pulmonary haematoma usually resolves within 2-4 days

    E. Fat embolism is usually indistinguishable from ARDS

A 2.49. *Concerning Patients with Traumatic Injury to the Chest*

FALSE   A. Ten to 15% of rib fractures are missed on the frontal CXR; these missing fractures should only be sought if their detection would alter the management of the patient.
Ch. 24 The Thoracic Cage, p 459.

TRUE   B. Such a fracture is an important marker of major trauma that can include upper-limb vascular injuries, brachial plexus injuries, bronchial rupture and myocardial trauma.
Ch. 24 The Thoracic Cage, p 459.

TRUE   C. Pulmonary *contusion* results in extravasation of blood into the alveoli which is followed by oedema. It seldom causes any respiratory embarrasment, even when severe.
Ch. 24 The Lung, p 460.

FALSE   D. Pulmonary contusion resolves within 5-10 days. A localized pulmonary *haematoma* may take months, or even years, to resolve.
Ch. 24 The Lung, p 460.

TRUE   E. Patients with fat embolism generally tend to develop arterial hypoxaemia prior to any changes on the frontal CXR. The radiological change is one of diffuse air-space shadowing; if this feature is seen in isolation, there is a wide differential diagnosis, which includes ARDS.
Ch. 24, The Lung, p 460.

Q *2.50.* *Concerning Traumatic Aortic Rupture*

    A. It is rare in patients over 65 years of age

    B. It occurs just proximal to the innominate artery in about 30% of cases

    C. It kills most patients before they reach hospital

    D. It can produce a pseudoaneurysm that is very likely to rupture within 5 years of diagnosis

    E. It requires an aortogram when there is a high index of suspicion, regardless of the CXR findings

A *2.50. Concerning Traumatic Aortic Rupture*

TRUE

A. It is also uncommon in children.
Ch. 24 The Mediastinum, p 462.

TRUE

B. In the remainder, it occurs distal to the left subclavian artery.
Ch. 24 The Mediastinum, p 462.

TRUE

C.

Ch. 24 The Mediastinum, p 462.

TRUE

D. Of those patients surviving the initial injury, 30% die within the first 24 hours and 90% within 12 months. 10% of patients who survive longer than 12 months will develop a pseudoaneurysm.
Ch. 24 The Mediastinum, p 462.

TRUE

E. There are many well-described radiological signs of aortic rupture that include a left apical pleural cap, displacement of the trachea to the right, widening of the mediastinum and loss of clarity of the mediastinal structures (e.g., the aortic knuckle). If sufficient doubt remains, aortography should be performed.
Ch. 24 The Mediastinum, p 462.

Q (2.51.) *Regarding the CXR in the Post-Operative Patient*

A. About 10% of patients develop visible atelectases after major abdominal surgery

B. Post-operative atelectasis is not usually an infective process

C. Miliary atelectasis can be detected as multiple fine nodules (2-3 mm) throughout the lungs

D. Aspiration pneumonitis tends to clear spontaneously and entirely within 3 days

E. In the presence of a pulmonary capillary wedge pressure below 15 mm Hg, air-space shadowing is unlikely to be due to cardiac failure

A 2.51. Regarding the CXR in the Post-Operative Patient

FALSE
A. Post-operative atelectasis occurs in nearly 50% of patients undergoing major abdominal surgery. The most common finding is linear *plate atelectasis* (Fleischner's plate atelectasis).
Ch. 25 Atelectasis, p 467.

TRUE
B. However, if affected areas are not treated promptly, with appropriate measures such as suction, mobilization, analgesia, physiotherapy and deep breathing, they may rapidly become secondarily infected.
Ch. 25 Atelectasis, p 467.

FALSE
C. Miliary or micro-atelectasis tends not to produce any parenchymal abnormality. The lungs appear to be reduced in volume and the patients tend to be hypoxaemic.
Ch. 25 Atelectasis, p 467.

FALSE
D. 1-2 days—progression of air-space shadowing.
5-7 days—stabilization and regression.
7-14 days—complete clearance.
Ch. 25 Aspiration Penumonitis, p 468.

TRUE
E. The first signs of interstitial pulmonary oedema are perihilar haze, peribronchial cuffing and fluid in the interlobular septa (Kerley A + B lines). These tend to occur at *pulmonary capillary wedge pressures* of 20-25 mm Hg.
Ch. 25 Pulmonary Oedema, p 469.

Q 2.52. *Concerning Adult Respiratory Distress Syndrome*

    A. The CXR remains normal for the first 12 hours after the insult

    B. By 48 hours, the lungs are haemorrhagic and oedematous

    C. After several days, hyaline membranes form within the distal air spaces

    D. The patient is usually symptomatic prior to any gross changes on the CXR

    E. A pulmonary arterial pressure (PAP) measurement is more useful than a wedge-pressure measurement in differentiating ARDS from pulmonary oedema

Q 2.53. *Concerning External Therapeutic Chest Radiation*

    A. Symptomatic reactions are uncommon when less than 25% of the lung is irradiated

    B. Prednisolone potentiates the pulmonary reaction to chest radiation

    C. The changes of radiation pneumonitis tend to be demonstrated on the CXR at 2-3 months

    D. Radiation fibrosis is always preceded by radiation pneumonitis on the frontal CXR

    E. The fibrotic stage tends to stabilize at 12-24 months

A 2.52. *Concerning Adult Respiratory Distress Syndrome*

TRUE
A. Although the CXR remains normal, fibrin deposition, platelet microemboli and areas of haemorrhage all occur, and these can be demonstrated microscopically.
Ch. 25 ARDS, p 472.

TRUE
B. The radiographic changes (alveolar shadowing) now reflect the microscopic changes.
Ch. 25 ARDS, p 472.

TRUE
C. Hence the name adult hyaline membrane disease.
Ch. 25 ARDS, p 472.

FALSE
D. Symptoms tend to occur on the 2nd day after the insult. At this time, there are usually moderate/gross changes on the CXR.
Ch. 25 ARDS, p 472.

FALSE
E. Although the PAP may be helpful, it is more useful to know the pulmonary capilliary wedge pressure, which is a reflection of the left atrial and pulmonary venous pressure.
Ch. 25 ARDS, p 472.

A 2.53. *Concerning External Therapeutic Chest Radiation*

TRUE
A. Hence, the field size and dose are kept to a minimum.
Ch. 25 Radiation Therapy, p 479.

FALSE
B. Chemotherapeutic agents such as actinomycin D, bleomycin, adriamycin and cyclophosphamide can potentiate the effects of irradiation when given simultaneously or sequentially. *Steroids* suppress symptoms.
Ch. 25 Radiation Therapy, p 479.

TRUE
C. The initial changes are those of air-space consolidation confined to the region of the radiotherapy port and there may be associated volume loss within the region. Changes can occur within one week of irradiation and range from consolidation to permanent fibrosis.
Ch. 25 Radiation Pneumonitis, p 479.

FALSE
D. There are many patients who have demonstrable radiation pneumonitis. A significant number, however, will have no changes on the CXR. Pneumonitis following DXT is always present, but it is not always demonstrable on the frontal radiograph.
Ch. 25 Radiation Fibrosis, p 479.

TRUE
E. From time to time, the fibrotic stage can be difficult to differentiate from tumour recurrence or lymphangitis: CT may be helpful in difficult cases.
Ch. 25 Radiation Fibrosis, p 479.

Q *2.54. Concerning the CXR in the Critically Ill Person*

A. On the supine view, air in the medial aspect of the pleural space may have the same appearance as a pneumomediastium or pneumopericardium

B. In a patient with a suspected pneumothorax, a negative supine film does not effectively exclude the diagnosis

C. Small pleural effusions are frequently demonstrated in patients who have undergone upper abdominal surgery

D. In patients who have undergone CAB (Coronary Artery Bypass) surgery, a rapidly enlarging cardiac silhouette in the absence of cardiac failure suggests serious pericardial haemorrhage

E. In patients who have undergone CAB surgery, subdiaphragmatic air in the immediate post-operative period suggests perforation of an intra-abdominal viscus

A 2.54. Concerning the CXR in the Critically Ill Person

TRUE

    A. On the supine view, air may collect in a number of places including the lateral and medial margins of the lungs, the subpulmonary space and in the pulmonary fissures.
Ch. 25 Extrapulmonary Air, p 472.

TRUE

    B. If a pneumothorax is suspected, an upright or decubitus film must be obtained.
Ch. 25 Extrapulmonary Air, p 472.

TRUE

    C. Such small post-operative effusions are of little significance and tend to disappear over 3-4 days.
Ch. 25 Pleural Effusion, p 473.

TRUE

    D. Most patients develop mediastinal widening following CAB surgery (usually less than a 50% increase over the pre-operative diameter). Re-operation is rapidly required when the increase in mediastinal diameter is greater than 70%.
Ch. 25 Cardiac Surgery, p 475.

FALSE

    E. This finding is usually caused by inadvertent disruption of the xiphisternal attachment of the diaphragm. It is benign and self-limiting.
Ch. 25 Cardiac Surgery, p 475.

Q 2.55. Regarding Lung Transplantation

A. Acute rejection is the first demonstrable complication following a lung transplant on the CXR

B. In patients who have undergone transbronchial biopsy, focal nodule(s) in the central portions of lung may be demonstrated

C. The primary reason for lung transplant failure is bronchial dehiscence

D. Bronchial dehiscence is rarely visible on the frontal CXR

E. Chronic lung rejection is defined as obliterative bronchiolitis or accelerated arteriosclerosis or both

Q 2.56. Concerning Ectopic or Hamartomatous Development of the Lung

A. Cystic adenomatoid malformation of the lung (CAM) is a lesion containing all the components of normal lung

B. The mass of CAM is always predominantly cystic

C. Occasionally CAM may present with a large single cyst

D. The cysts of CAM may communicate with the bronchial tree

E. Pulmonary hypoplasia is an associated finding in some patients

A *2.55. Regarding Lung Transplantation*

FALSE

    A. During the first 10 days following a lung transplant, *oedema* tends to be the most common complication. *Acute rejection* is the predominant event over the next 3 months. *Airways dehiscence* occurs from the second week to the second month. *Infection* can occur at any time.
Ch. 26 Fig. 26.1, p 484.

FALSE

    B. Post biopsy nodules are seen in the *outer* ⅓ of the lungs on the PA radiograph. They generally resolve within 2 weeks.
Ch. 26 Manifestations Related to Specific Surgical and Management Techniques, p 485.

TRUE

    C. Steroids and cyclosporin have reduced this complication. When this complication occurs, however, fatal infection is not infrequent.
Ch. 26 Airway Dehiscence, p 486.

TRUE

    D. Plain films can sometimes identify parabronchial air collections or lobar collapse. The primary use of the CXR is to exclude other causes of pulmonary embarassment.
Ch. 26 Airway Dehiscence, p 486.

TRUE

    E. These findings must be taken in context with the changes in respiratory function.
Ch. 26 Acute and Chronic Rejection, p 487.

A *2.56. Concerning Ectopic or Hamartomatous Development of the Lung*

FALSE

    A. CAM does not contain cartilage.
Ch. 27 CAM, p 502.

FALSE

    B. CAM contains both solid and cystic components that vary in their relative proportions and may present with differing radiological pictures.
Ch. 27 CAM, p 502.

TRUE

    C. Multiple cysts are usually seen in CAM, though a large single cyst (termed a unicameral cyst) may predominate or may exist in isolation.
Ch. 27 CAM, p 502.

TRUE

    D. The cysts may or may not communicate with the bronchial tree—eventually most do.
Ch. 27 CAM, p 502.

TRUE

    E. This is due to compression of the underlying lung *viz.* unilateral pulmonary hypoplasia.
Ch. 27 CAM, p 502.

Q 2.57. Cystic Adenomatoid Malformation (CAM)

A. Can have radiological appearances similar to those of a Bochdelek hernia on the CXR

B. Can usually be distinguished from bowel by chest USS

C. Can be readily diagnosed antenatally at 37 weeks

D. Usually presents with oligohydramnios in late pregnancy

E. Appears similar to congenital lobar emphysema (CLE) on CXR

Q 2.58. The Following May Appear on the CXR as Multiple Lung Cysts in Children

A. Pulmonary sequestration

B. Lymphocytic interstitial pneumonitis

C. Congenital lobar emphysema

D. Pulmonary interstitial emphysema

E. A bronchogenic cyst

A 2.57. Cystic Adenomatoid Malformation (CAM)

TRUE A. The differential diagnosis of a multiloculated cystic mass in the lung should include a Bochdalek hernia. A Bochdalek hernia (*B* for Bochdaleck, B for back (posterior), B for babies) must be distinguished from CAM. In the case of a hernia, the plain AXR will demonstrate a paucity of gas filled bowel loops in the abdomen which clinically and radiologically appears scaphoid; in CAM the abdominal gas pattern is usually normal.
Ch. 27 CAM, p 502.

TRUE B. Bowel loops undergoing peristalsis are readily seen in most cases.
Ch. 27 CAM, p 502.

TRUE C. The hemithorax containing the CAM may show:

Antenatal USS	Type of CAM
Multiple cysts up to 10 cm	I
Multiple small cysts < 1.5 mm	II
Solid lung	III

Ch. 27 CAM, p 502.

FALSE D. The mass tends to compress the mediastium and thus the oesophagus. In over 50% of pregnancies with affected fetuses, polyhydramnios is present.

TRUE E. In CLE, the lung is emphysematous. The lung in CAM contains no pulmonary vessels, though a few internal cyst strands may be seen. The findings may appear similar on plain radiography; CT scanning may differentiate between the two.
Ch. 27 CAM, p 502.

A 2.58. The Following May Appear on the CXR as Multiple Lung Cysts in Children

TRUE A.
Ch. 27 Table 27.5, p 497.

FALSE B. This tends to produce poorly defined nodules and is frequently encountered in children with HIV infection.
Ch. 27 Table 27.5, p 497.

TRUE C.
Ch. 27 Table 27.5, p 11.

TRUE D.
Ch. 27 Table 27.5, p 11.

FALSE E. This is generally single.
Ch. 27 Table 27.5, p 497.

Q *2.59. The Following Pulmonary Abnormalities are Associated with Other Congenital Anomalies in More Than 50% of Patients*

    A. Intralobar pulmonary sequestration

    B. Secondary pulmonary lymphangiectasis

    C. Cystic adenomatoid malformation (CAM)

    D. Tracheobronchomegaly

    E. Swyer-James-McLeod Syndrome

Q *2.60. Concerning Congenital Pulmonary Anomalies*

    A. Swyer-James' Syndrome is the commonest congenital pulmonary anomaly

    B. Tracheal agenesis is incompatible with life

    C. Bronchial stenosis may be produced by an aberrant left main pulmonary artery

    D. Bronchial atresia tends to present in the older child or the adult

    E. The normal trachea expands 50% in diameter during expiration whereas in children with tracheomalacia there is an expansion of 70% or greater

A *2.59. The Following Pulmonary Abnormalities are Associated with Other Congenital Anomalies in More Than 50% of Patients*

FALSE

A. *Extra-lobar* pulmonary sequestration is associated with other anomalies in >60% of cases that present under the age of one year.
Ch. 27 Table 27.4, p 495.

TRUE

B. This disorder is usually associated with severe congenital heart disease.
Ch. 27 Congenital Lymphangiectasia, p 501.

FALSE

C. In 25% of cases with CAM there are associated chromosomal or visceral abnormalities.

FALSE

D. Mounier-Kuhn Syndrome presents in the fourth decade and may rarely be associated with Ehlers-Danlos Syndrome.

FALSE

E. This is an acquired disorder of the lungs, usually secondary to a viral infection causing bronchiolitis obliterans.
Ch. 27 Pulmonary Artery Aplasia, p 501.

A *2.60. Concerning Congenital Pulmonary Anomalies*

FALSE

A. The Swyer-James' syndrome is an acquired disease resulting from an infection in infancy causing bronchiolitis obliterans.
Ch. 27 Congenital Pulmonary Anomalies, p 493.

TRUE

B.
Ch. 27 Tracheobronchial Agenesis and Stenosis, p 494.

TRUE

C. The aberrant left main pulmonary artery arises from the right main pulmonary artery and passes behind the trachea, in front of the oesophagus, indenting the oesophagus anteriorly on its right side. This forms a pulmonary artery sling.
Ch. 27 Tracheobronchial Agenesis and Stenosis, p 494.

TRUE

D. This condition most frequently involves the segmental upper-lobe bronchus but may be demonstrated in the lower lobes.
Ch. 27 Bronchial Atresia, p 494.

FALSE

E. Replace the words "expands" and "expansion" by "narrows" and "narrowing" and you have the correct definition.
Ch. 27 Tracheobronchomalacia, p 494.

Q 2.61. Concerning Pulmonary Hypoplasia and Pulmonary Agenesis

A. On clinical and radiological examination, unilateral agenesis presents with a symmetrically developed thorax

B. It is commonly an isolated abnormality

C. All of the following can contribute to pulmonary hypoplasia: oligohydrammios, hypoperfusion, thoracic cage restriction and decreased respiratory movements

D. The Potter syndrome comprises the following: renal agenesis, abnormal facies, pulmonary hypoplasia and truncus arteriosus

E. A left-sided primary pulmonary hypoplasia may be indistinguishable from left upper-lobe collapse

Q 2.62. Concerning the Pulmonary Vasculature

A. Secondary lymphangiectasis is a reversible condition

B. Pulmonary arteriovenous malformations are a feature of Noonan's syndrome

C. The pulmonary arteriovenous malformations in patients with hereditary haemorrhagic telangiectasia are usually not amenable to coil embolization therapy

D. Patients with pulmonary artery aplasia can be distinguished from those with the Swyer-James-McLeod syndrome by the absence of air trapping

E. Pulmonary artery atresia is incompatible with life

A 2.61. *Concerning Pulmonary Hypoplasia and Pulmonary Agenesis*

TRUE   A. The radiographic appearance is indistinguishable from that of total lung collapse. The chest wall is normal.
Ch. 27 Pulmonary Agenesis, p 495.

FALSE   B. No. It's more commonly associated with other fetal developmental abnormalities.
Ch. 27 Pulmonary Agenesis, p 495.

TRUE   C. Primary pulmonary hypoplasia is idiopathic. *Secondary* pulmonary hypoplasia can be produced by any one or combination of the above.
Ch. 27 Pulmonary Agenesis, p 495.

FALSE   D. Truncus arteriosus is not a feature of the Potter syndrome.
Ch. 27 Pulmonary Hypoplasia, p 496.

TRUE   E. A helpful feature in the differentiation of the two conditions is the presence of a wedge of tissue orientated towards the hilum.
Ch. 27 Primary Pulmonary Hypoplasia, p 496.

A 2.62. *Concerning the Pulmonary Vasculature*

TRUE   A. Patients with this disorder have severe pulmonary venous hypertension that is usually caused by obstructed total anomalous pulmonary venous return or by the hypoplastic left heart syndrome.
Ch. 27 Congenital Lymphangiectasis, p 501.

FALSE   B. *Noonan's syndrome* can produce lymphangiectasis as part of a diffuse lymphangiectasia. There are associated cardiac defects. *Pulmonary arteriovenous malformations* can present in isolation or as part of the Hereditary Haemorrhagic Telangiectasia syndrome.
Ch. 27 Congenital Lymphangiectasis, p 501.

FALSE   C. The lesions in HHT are generally multiple and are large enough to embolize.
Ch. 27 Pulmonary Arteriovenous Malformations of the Lung, Fig. 27.12, p 501.

TRUE   D.
Ch. 27 Pulmonary Artery Aplasia, p 501.

FALSE   E. Pulmonary atresia is compatible with life. It can be regarded as an extreme form of Fallot's disease.
Ch. 35 Pulmonary Artery Atresia with Intact Ventricular Septum, p 697.

Q *2.63. In Patients with the Scimitar Syndrome*

    A. Only the right lung is involved

    B. The anomalous vein drains into the inferior vena cava

    C. The diagnosis should be confirmed by arteriography

    D. Most cases present in the young

    E. The hallmark of this condition is a hypoplastic lung

Q *2.64. Congenital Lobar Emphysema (CLE)*

    A. Is characterized by small cysts in the affected lung

    B. May present with complete opacification of the affected lobe

    C. Affects the lower lobes in more than 25% of cases

    D. Can resemble a tension pneumothorax

    E. Requires surgical treatment in most cases

A 2.63. In Patients with the Scimitar Syndrome

TRUE

A. If the left lung is involved the patient is likely to have abnormal visceral situs.
Ch. 27 Scimitar Syndrome, p 496.

TRUE

B. This anomalous vein can be demonstrated by USS, CXR, angiography, CT and MRI.
Ch. 27 Scimitar Syndrome, p 496.

FALSE

C. If necessary, a CXR and CT are usually all that is necessary to confirm the diagnosis.
Ch. 27 Scimitar Syndrome, p 496.

FALSE

D. Most cases present as adults; when demonstrated in the young, the Scimitar syndrome is usually incidental to other problems (e.g., congenital heart disease).
Ch. 27 Scimitar Syndrome, p 496.

TRUE

E. Occasionally, the abnormal draining vein cannot be demonstrated but the diagnosis of the Scimitar syndrome should always be entertained in patients with a hypoplastic right lung.
Ch. 27 Scimitar Syndrome, p 496.

A 2.64. Congenital Lobar Emphysema (CLE)

FALSE

A. CLE refers to an over-inflated lobe that compresses normal adjacent lung. Cysts are not a feature.
Ch. 27 CLE, p 496.

TRUE

B. Although the precise cause of CLE has not been fully established, it is believed that there is some defect in the bronchial supporting structures. This theory is supported by the occasional case in which fetal lung fluid is trapped within the lobe resulting in an opaque, expanded lobe that converts to the classical form when the fluid is drained or absorbed.
Ch. 27 CLE, p 496.

FALSE

C. The lower lobes are affected in fewer than 2% of cases.
Ch. 27 CLE, p 496.

TRUE

D. The only distinguishing feature may be the faint vascular markings that are not present in a tension pneumothorax.
Ch. 27 CLE, p 496.

FALSE

E. In most cases, treatment is expectant in the hope of improvement with time and growth.
Ch. 27 CLE, p 496.

Q 2.65. *The Following Features Occur with Approximately Equal Frequency in Patients with Intra-Lobar and Extra-Lobar Pulmonary Sequestration*

    A. No connection to the tracheobronchial tree

    B. Recurrent pneumonia

    C. A similar blood supply

    D. A lower lobe predominance

    E. Other associated congenital abnormalities

Q 2.66. *Concerning Intra-Lobar Sequestration*

    A. The sequestration is contained within the normal lung

    B. Males and females are equally affected

    C. The majority of patients present before the age of 20 years

    D. The sequestration may drain into the portal vein

    E. 20–30% of patients present with clubbing

A 2.65. *The Following Features Occur with Approximately Equal Frequency in Patients with Intra-Lobar and Extra-Lobar Pulmonary Sequestration*

TRUE   *A.*
                  Ch. 27 Pulmonary Sequestration, p 498.

FALSE   *B.* This occurs more frequently in *intra*-lobar pulmonary sequestration.
                  Ch. 27 Pulmonary Sequestration, p 498.

TRUE   *C.* Both intra and extra-lobar pulmonary sequestrations are supplied by a systemic artery, usually from the aorta or a bronchial artery.
                  Ch. 27 Pulmonary Sequestration, p 498.

TRUE   *D.* Sequestrations are very rare in the middle (lingula) and upper lobes.
                  Ch. 27 Pulmonary Sequestration, p 498.

FALSE   *E.* It is very rare for *intra*-lobar sequestration to be associated with other congenital abnormalities.
                  Ch. 27 Pulmonary Sequestration, p 498.

A 2.66. *Concerning Intra-Lobar Sequestration*

TRUE   *A.* It is also contained within the normal pleural envelope.
                  Ch. 27 Pulmonary Sequestration, p 498.

TRUE   *B.* Males are more frequently affected with *extra*-lobar sequestration (4 M : 1 F).
                  Ch. 27 Pulmonary Sequestration, p 498.

FALSE   *C.* Eighty percent present after the age of 20 years, whereas 60% of patients with *extra*-lobar sequestration present below the age of one year.
                  Ch. 27 Pulmonary Sequestration, p 498.

FALSE   *D.* An *extra*-lobar sequestration drains to systemic veins and portal venous drainage has also been documented. An *intra*-lobar sequestration always drains into the pulmonary veins.
                  Ch. 27 Pulmonary Sequestration, p 498.

FALSE   *E.* Clubbing is not a recognised feature, though patients could potentially become clubbed if the sequestration undergoes chronic sepsis.
                  Ch. 27 Pulmonary Sequestration, p 498.

Q *2.67. Regarding the Radiology of the Thymus*

A. An abrupt angulation of the trachea away from the aortic arch at the level of the thoracic inlet is a sign of thymic enlargement

B. Absence of a thymic shadow on the frontal CXR in the first 24 hours of life suggests immunodeficiency

C. Thymic enlargement is a normal finding following recovery from a period of stress.

D. The thymic silhouette enlarges in the upright position on deep inspiration

E. After the age of 5 years, visualization of the thymus on CXR is abnormal

A 2.67. *Regarding the Radiology of the Thymus*

FALSE

A. This is a sign of an expiratory film and occurs owing to the pliability of the infant trachea. Thymic enlargement does not cause this appearance.
Ch. 28 The Normal Chest, p 506.

TRUE

B. Thymic aplasia is associated with T-cell immunodeficiency in DiGeorge's syndrome. In the first 24 hours, the normal thymus may rapidly involute and be invisible on standard radiographs.
Ch. 28 The Normal Chest, p 506.

TRUE

C. So-called thymic rebound.
Ch. 28 The Normal Chest, p 506.

FALSE

D. It becomes smaller in the upright position and with inspiration.
Ch. 28 The Normal Chest, p 506.

FALSE

E. It is an expected finding up to the age of two and becomes progressively less often visible up to the age of eight. After eight years of age, the thymus is rarely seen on frontal CXR but its presence is not necessarily abnormal.
Ch. 28 The Normal Chest, p 506.

Q *2.68. Concerning Paediatric Diaphragmatic Disorders*

    A. Bochdalek hernias are the most common intrathoracic fetal anomaly

    B. Morgagni hernias are most commonly seen anteromedially on the left

    C. After repair of a Bochdalek hernia, the mediastinum remains shifted to the contralateral side

    D. Diaphragmatic eventration is not associated with pulmonary hypoplasia

    E. The scaphoid abdomen usually differentiates diaphragmatic hernia from cystic adenomatoid malformation of the lungs

A 2.68. *Concerning Paediatric Diaphragmatic Disorders*

TRUE
    A. Patients symptomatic at birth may have Bochdalek hernias which are usually left-sided and account for over 80% of congenital diaphragmatic hernias.
    Ch. 28 Diaphragmatic Hernias, p 508.

FALSE
    B. They are anteromedially sited more commonly on the *right* and often contain liver, fat or transverse colon. The presentation is usually in older children.
    Ch. 28 Diaphragmatic Hernias, p 508.

TRUE
    C. When the abdominal contents have been returned to the abdomen, and the diaphragmatic hiatus repaired, the mediastinum remains shifted to the contralateral side because of associated ipsilateral pulmonary hypoplasia. This may be a permanent feature.
    Ch. 28 Diaphragmatic Hernias, p 508.

FALSE
    D. Respiration may be severely compromised as a result of pulmonary hypoplasia in both eventration and diaphragmatic paralysis.
    Ch. 28 Eventration and Diaphragmatic Paralysis, p 508.

TRUE
    E. When the bowel contents are in the chest a scaphoid abdomen (seen on lateral abdominal and CXR) results. Other helpful signs are continuity between intraluminal bowel gas in the abdomen and the chest, an abnormally positioned nasogastric tube, and the characteristic changes produced by the injection of a small amount of air into the gastrointestinal tract.
    Ch. 28 Diaphragmatic Hernias, p 508.

Q 2.69. *Concerning the Radiology of Paediatric Chest Disorders*

    A. Pneumonia with pleural effusion in a child less than 1 year of age usually indicates a staphylococcal infection

    B. Pneumatoceles are most commonly caused by *Klebsiella* pneumonia

    C. The presence of pneumatoceles usually implies ongoing destruction of lung parenchyma

    D. Air trapping in severe viral bronchiolitis commonly results in pneumothorax

    E. Hilar adenopathy is commonly associated with Mycoplasma pneumonia

A 2.69. *Concerning the Radiology of Paediatric Chest Disorders*

TRUE   A. Pleural fluid is usually due to a bacterial or mycoplasma infection. In the very young, staphylococcus is the most common cause.
Ch. 28 Pulmonary Infection, p 510.

FALSE   B. Staphyloccal pneumonia is the most common cause in childhood. *Pneumococcus*, *E. coli* and *Klebsiella* are common causes in the older patient, along with trauma.
Ch. 28 Pulmonary Infection, p 510.

FALSE   C. Pneumatoceles occur during the healing phase following pulmonary infection and usually represent regional obstructive hyperinflation.
Ch. 28 Pulmonary Infection, p 510.

FALSE   D. Viral lower respiratory infections rarely result in pneumothorax despite the severity of air trapping.
Ch. 28 Infections Due to Viruses, p 512.

FALSE   E. Hilar adenopathy is a rare association which, if prominent, should make one consider tuberculosis as a cause. Small pleural effusions occur in 20% of cases of Mycoplasma pneumonia.
Ch. 28 Mycoplasma, p 514.

Q *2.70. Regarding Thoracic Manifestations of HIV Infection in Children*

A. A sudden increase in the size of hilar nodes is likely to be due to involvement by Kaposi's sarcoma

B. Pneumatoceles are a manifestation of Pneumocystis carinii infection (PCP)

C. Lymphocytic interstitial pneumonitis (LIP) indicates the diagnosis of AIDS in a young child

D. LIP is mimicked by tuberculous infection

E. T-cell lymphoma is the commonest thoracic malignancy in paediatric patients with AIDS

Q *2.71. Regarding Airway Obstruction in Children*

A. A smooth, concentric narrowing of the sub-glottic trachea is a normal expiratory finding

B. In acute epiglottitis, the sub-glottic trachea usually appears normal on radiography

C. About 75% of inhaled foreign bodies lodge in the right main bronchus

D. In the presence of air trapping, contralateral mediastinal shift is best seen with an inspiratory film

E. Pneumomediastinum is commonly caused by inhaled foreign bodies

A 2.70. Regarding Thoracic Manifestations of HIV Infection in Children

FALSE   A. This is a sign which occurs most commonly with *B-cell lymphoma*. Kaposi's sarcoma is overwhelmingly associated with homosexual intercourse and is very rarely seen in the paediatric population.
Ch. 28 Paediatric Pulmonary Infection with Human Immunodeficiency Virus, p 514.

TRUE   B. Cavitation, pneumatoceles and pneumothorax all occur in paediatric PCP.
Ch. 28 Paediatric Pulmonary Infection with Human Immunodeficiency Virus, p 514.

TRUE   C. Under the age of 13 years this condition, which is part of the spectrum of pulmonary lymphoid hyperplasia, defines the onset of AIDS in HIV positive children.
Ch. 28 Paediatric Pulmonary Infection with Human Immunodeficiency Virus, p 514.

TRUE   D. A diffuse interstitial infiltrate and hilar lymphadenopathy may occur in untreated pulmonary tuberculosis.
Ch. 28 Paediatric Pulmonary Infection with Human Immunodeficiency Virus, p 514.

FALSE   E. *B-cell lymphoma* is the most common thoracic malignancy in these patients. Pulmonary leiomyosarcoma has been reported to be a manifestation of paediatric AIDS.
Ch. 28 Paediatric Pulmonary Infection with Human Immunodeficiency Virus, p 514.

A 2.71. Regarding Airway Obstruction in Children

FALSE   A. This is a sign of laryngotracheobronchitis (croup) and is demonstrated on AP and lateral films of the trachea.
Ch. 28 Inflammatory lesions producing upper airway obstruction, p 517.

TRUE   B. Oedema and swelling of the epiglottis and aryepiglottic folds are the radiological hallmarks of this condition. The diagnosis is usually a clinical one, with radiology reserved for atypical or doubtful cases.
Ch. 28 Epiglottitis, p 518.

FALSE   C. There is no predilection for either side.
Ch. 28 Inhaled Foreign Body, p 518.

FALSE   D. An *expiratory* film best demonstrates air trapping caused by obstruction.
Ch. 28 Inhaled Foreign Body, p 518.

FALSE   E. Pneumothorax and pneumomediastinum are rarely caused by inhaled foreign bodies.
Ch. 28 Inhaled Foreign Body, p 518.

Q *2.72. Bilateral Airspace Shadowing in a 1-Week-Old Neonate Occurs Commonly in the Following Conditions*

    A. Retained fetal lung fluid

    B. Aspiration of clear amniotic fluid

    C. Respiratory distress syndrome (RDS)

    D. Cystic adenomatoid malformation

    E. Congenital pulmonary venolobar syndrome (Scimitar syndrome)

A   2.72. *Bilateral Airspace Shadowing in a 1-Week-Old Neonate Occurs Commonly in the Following Conditions*

FALSE

A. This simulates interstitial pulmonary oedema. It resolves within 48 hours after birth.
Ch. 28 Retained Fetal Lung Fluid, p 523.

FALSE

B. This usually clears within 48 hours and is often indistinguishable from retained fetal lung fluid. The management of these two conditions is identical.
Ch. 28 Aspiration of Clear Amniotic Fluid, p 522.

TRUE

C. Alveolar collapse is the mechanism behind the bilateral "consolidation" seen in this condition.
Ch. 28 Respiratory Distress Syndrome, p 520.

FALSE

D. There is almost always a well-defined unilateral mass.
Ch. 28 Respiratory Distress in the Newborn Baby, p 520.

FALSE

E. Unilateral hypogenetic lung and partial anomalous venous return are the main components of this syndrome. The right lung is always involved in Scimitar syndrome. The contralateral lung is affected only if there is an associated cardiac anomaly.

3

The Heart and Great Vessels

Q *3.1. Regarding Uncorrected Transposition of the Great Arteries (UTGA)*

A. UTGA is the commonest type of congenital heart disease causing central cyanosis at or shortly after birth

B. Isolated UTGA has a better prognosis than one complicated by a VSD

C. The heart size is usually normal at birth

D. Is associated with pulmonary plethora and prominent main pulmonary artery

E. Indomethacin is given at birth to maintain ductal patency

A 3.1. *Regarding Uncorrected Transposition of the Great Arteries (UTGA)*

TRUE   *A.* In UTGA, the aorta arises from the right ventricle. The pulmonary artery arises from the left ventricle. The infant becomes cyanosed at or shortly after birth. In Fallot's tetralogy, which is more frequent than UTGA, cyanosis usually occurs at 2-6 years of age.
Ch. 35 Transposition of the Great Arteries, p 706.

FALSE   *B.* UTGA requires an additional anomaly in order for the systemic and pulmonary circulations to communicate. This is most commonly a VSD.
Ch. 35 Transposition of the Great Arteries, p 707.

TRUE   *C.* This is because UTGA does not impose a major fetal haemodynamic problem.
Ch. 35 Transposition of the Great Arteries, p 708.

FALSE   *D.* The pulmonary trunk is almost always unidentifiable on frontal CXR as it lies in the midline posteriorly in uncorrected TGA, and posteriorly to the right in corrected TGA. The combination of unobtrusive pulmonary arteries and plethoric lungs in a cyanotic child is very suggestive of uncorrected TGA.
Ch. 35 Transposition of the Great Arteries, p 708.

FALSE   *E.* Indomethacin is used to effect ductal closure. In order to prevent this in UTGA and other conditions, Prostaglandin E infusion is used.
Ch. 35 Transposition of the Great Arteries, p 709.

Q 3.2. Regarding Transposition of the Great Arteries

A. UTGA is usually associated with right-sided aortic arch

B. Angiocardiography is mandatory to decide UTGA treatment

C. Corrected TGA is less common than UTGA

D. The cardiac contour of CTGA is suggestive of an "egg on its side"

E. MRI is useful for post-operative follow-up

A 3.2. *Regarding Transposition of the Great Arteries*

FALSE
    A. Important causes of a right-sided aortic arch are as follows:
Truncus arteriosus 40%
Tetratology of Fallot 30%
Tricuspid atresia 10%
Probably less than 5% UTGA have a right aortic arch.
Ch. 35 Transposition of the Great Arteries, p 707.

FALSE
    B. Continuity of LV and pulmonary artery as well as continuity of RV and aorta is easily seen on cardiac ultrasound. Doppler can demonstrate the shunt of an associated VSD and pulmonary stenosis can also be assessed by doppler ultrasound.
Ch. 35 Transposition of the Great Arteries, p 708.

TRUE
    C. CTGA accounts for only 15% of TGA. CTGA is often associated with conduction defects and atrio-ventricular valve incompetences. In CTGA, the patient is not usually cyanosed because oxygenated blood returning from the lungs via the pulmonary veins travels to the left atrium *and thence to the inverted right ventricle and thence to the transposed aorta,* This is made possible by the position of the right ventricle to the left of the left ventricle. In other words, the transposed aorta and pulmonary artery are "corrected" by the inversion of the ventricles which now connect both to the wrong atrium and to the wrong arterial outflow.
Ch. 35 Corrected Transposition of the Great Arteries, p 710.

TRUE
    D. The cardiac contour of CTGA is characterized by a long prominent ascending aortic convexity forming the left border of the superior mediastinum. In this position, the aortic arch is curving anti-clockwise. In contrast, the "egg on its side" appearance is caused by UTGA, in which right atrial enlargement is largely responsible for the cardiac shape, and the ascending aorta is small, midline and often not border-forming, causing a narrow vascular pedicle in the frontal view.
Ch. 35 Corrected Transposition of the Great Arteries, p 710.

TRUE
    E. Serial MRI after the Mustard procedure allows repeated noninvasive assessment of right ventricular and tricuspid valve function and complements cardiac ultrasound information.
Ch. 35 Corrected Transposition of the Great Arteries, p 710.

Q 3.3. *Concerning Tricuspid Atresia*

A. The right ventricle is small and hypoplastic

B. There is usually a concave pulmonary bay

C. The left atrium is enlarged

D. A VSD is often present

E. Pulmonary plethora cannot co-exist

A 3.3. *Concerning Tricuspid Atresia*

TRUE   A. There is no communication between right atrium and right ventricle. There is a large interatrial right to left shunt through an ASD. Blood gets to the lungs from right atrium to left atrium to left ventricle, thence through a VSD into the hypoplastic right ventricle or via a PDA.
Ch. 35C Tricuspid Atresia, p 691.

TRUE   B. As the amount of blood flow from the hypoplastic right ventricle is small, the pulmonary artery is usually correspondingly reduced in size. Cyanosis often occurs soon after birth.
Ch. 35C Tricuspid Atresia, p 692.

TRUE   C. This is due to the large right to left interatrial shunt via the obligatory ASD or associated patent foramen ovale.
Ch. 35C Tricuspid Atresia, p 692.

TRUE   D. If no VSD is present, the right ventricle is rudimentary, and blood gets to the lungs via a PDA or via large bronchial arterial branches arising from the descending aorta. If a VSD is present, a shunt from left ventricle to right ventricle enables the right ventricle to supply the pulmonary artery.
Ch. 35C Tricuspid Atresia, p 692.

FALSE   E. There is an associated transposition of the great arteries in 20-30%. When this is present, proximal pulmonary arterial enlargement and pulmonary plethora may occur as the pulmonary artery then arises from the large left ventricle, receiving more than 50% of cardiac output.
Ch. 35C Tricuspid Atresia, p 693.

Q 3.4. Regarding Tetralogy of Fallot (TF)

    A. It usually presents as cyanosis at birth

    B. Right ventricular hypertrophy is present in utero

    C. Pulmonary arterial stenosis may be associated

    D. It is uniformly fatal unless operated on in early childhood

    E. Oesophageal notching indicates severe pulmonary stenosis or atresia

A 3.4. *Regarding Tetralogy of Fallot (TF)*

FALSE   A. TGA and tricuspid atresia (TA) are the main congenital cardiac causes of cyanosis at or very soon after birth. TF is usually acyanotic at birth, because the pulmonary/infundibular stenosis is often not very severe at this stage. Progressive RVOT obstruction occurs, however, due to increasing fibroelastosis. Cyanosis usually occurs by 4 years of age.
Ch. 35C Tetralogy of Fallot, p 693.

FALSE   B. Right ventricular outflow tract obstruction does not cause RV hypertrophy in the fetal circulation because blood flow to the lungs is very small.
Ch. 35C Tetralogy of Fallot, p 693.

TRUE   C. Stenosis most commonly occurs proximally in the infundibulum of the right ventricle. Valvular and post-valvular stenoses are also common.
Ch. 35C Tetralogy of Fallot, p 693.

FALSE   D. Survival without surgical correction is not uncommon, even to early adulthood.
Ch. 35C Tetralogy of Fallot, p 693.

TRUE   E. If pulmonary stenosis is very severe, bronchial arterial hypertrophy may occur. This is a cause of posterio-lateral indentations on the oesophagus, visible on barium swallow.
Ch. 35C Tetralogy of Fallot, p 696.

Q 3.5. *Concerning the Eisenmenger Reaction*

A. It is almost always preceded by a large left to right shunt

B. In Eisenmenger ASD, the heart size may reduce when the left-to-right shunt reverses

C. The pulmonary veins are enlarged in VSD Eisenmenger

D. Is associated with the Eisenmenger complex

E. Central pulmonary arterial calcification is a characteristic feature of severe pulmonary artery hypertension in Eisenmenger reaction

A 3.5. *Concerning the Eisenmenger Reaction*

FALSE   A. In the case of a large *VSD*, a torrential left to right shunt does not develop because in the early postnatal period, the pulmonary arterioles retain fetal high resistance to flow. This maintains a high RV pressure which often equals that of the LV leading to a balanced (bidirectional) shunt. An early Eisenmenger reaction develops when a further increase in pulmonary arterial pressure due to arteriolar intimal hyperplasia occurs. In *ASD*, Eisenmenger reaction is always preceded by a large left to right shunt.
Ch. 35C Pulmonary Arteriolar Obstruction—Eisenmenger Reaction (ASD), p 698.

TRUE   B.
Ch. 35C Pulmonary Arteriolar Obstruction—Eisenmenger Reaction (ASD), p 698.

FALSE   C. This does not occur as there is no increase in pulmonary blood flow.
Ch. 35C Pulmonary Arteriolar Obstruction—Eisenmenger Reaction (ASD), p 698.

TRUE   D. The Eisenmenger complex consists of a high ventricular septal defect, overriding aorta and right ventricular hypertrophy without right ventricular outflow tract obstruction. The original left to right shunt causes reactive pulmonary arteriolar muscular and intimal thickening. Shunt reversal usually occurs in early adulthood.
Ch. 35C Pulmonary Arteriolar Obstruction—Eisenmenger Reaction (ASD), p 698.

TRUE   E. This may be associated with pathognomonic curvi-linear ductal calcification in the case of Eisenmenger PDA. The central pulmonary arteries may be affected by curvi-linear calcification in severe pulmonary hypertension of Eisenmenger reaction.
Ch. 35C Patent Ductus Arteriosus, p 699.

Q 3.6. *In Total Anomalous Pulmonary Venous Drainage*

A. All cardiac chambers contain blood with about the same oxygen content

B. An ASD is essential for survival

C. Total anomalous pulmonary veins most commonly drain directly into the right atrium

D. Pulmonary venous hypertension is greatest with supracardiac drainage

E. In some varieties of anomalous pulmonary venous drainage, pulmonary oedema may occur with a normal sized heart

A 3.6. *In Total Anomalous Pulmonary Venous Drainage*

TRUE
    A. This is because there is admixture of systemic venous and pulmonary venous blood in the right atrium which receives all of the venous drainage (both systemic and pulmonary) to the heart. This is usually about 90% saturated and hence the patient is often slightly cyanosed.
Ch. 35C Total Anomalous Pulmonary Venous Drainage, p 700.

TRUE
    B. In order for oxygenated blood returning from the lungs to reach the systemic circulation, an ASD (often associated with a patent foramen ovale) must be present (*viz* tricuspid atresia).
Ch. 35C Total Anomalous Pulmonary Venous Drainage, p 700.

FALSE
    C. The most common pattern of drainage is supradiaphragmatic, and supracardiac (i.e., the right and left pulmonary veins) meet behind the left atrium to form a large vein that ascends vertically in front of the left hilum to drain into the left brachiocephalic vein that joins the superior vena cava.
Ch. 35C Total Anomalous Pulmonary Venous Drainage, p 700.

FALSE
    D. Obstruction of veins by septae or kinking occurs in less than 10% of supracardiac TAPVD. By contrast, the vast majority of infracardiac TAPVD has obstructed pulmonary venous return, often via the portal vein.
Ch. 35C Total Anomalous Pulmonary Venous Drainage, p 701.

TRUE
    E. Infracardiac drainage is usually obstructed and causes intense pulmonary venous congestion and oedema. The heart size may be normal, because pressure (not volume) overload of the right ventricle is the dominant haemodynamic feature.
Ch. 35C Total Anomalous Pulmonary Venous Drainage, p 702.

Q 3.7. *Regarding Congenital Cardiac Anomalies*

  A. Partial anomalous pulmonary venous drainage may be associated with a vertical density on the left of the upper mediastinum on CXR

  B. Partial anomalous pulmonary venous drainage affects the right lung more frequently than the left

  C. Situs inversus is more likely to have an associated cardiac anomaly if there is also dextrocardia

  D. There is a left to right shunt in hypoplastic left heart syndrome

  E. The VSDs producing loud cardiac murmurs usually transmit a large shunt

A 3.7. *Regarding Congenital Cardiac Anomalies*

TRUE

A. An anomalous left upper lobe vein may be seen as a soft tissue density parallel to the left upper mediastinum entering the left brachiocephalic vein. This variant of PAPVD is often associated with a secundum ASD.
Ch. 35D Anomalous Pulmonary Venous Drainage, p 721.

TRUE

B. The scimitar (anomalous lobar vein) is seen almost always on the right side. Anomalous pulmonary venous drainage occurs about twice as commonly on the right than on the left.
Ch. 35D Anomalous Pulmonary Venous Drainage, p 721.

FALSE

C. Situs inversus + dextrocardia is much less likely to have a morphological anomaly than the much rarer situs inversus + laevocardia.
Ch. 35D Primary Dextrocardia, p 728.

TRUE

D. There is a left to right shunt through an ASD which diverts pulmonary venous blood usually from the small left atrium into the right atrium and thence to the right ventricle. There is also a more distal right to left shunt: e.g., a patent ductus arteriosus conducts blood from left pulmonary artery to the descending aorta.
Ch. 35D Hypoplastic Left Heart Syndrome, p 723.

FALSE

E. Muscular ventricular septal defects often produce a loud murmur, but they are usually small and transmit a small left to right shunt.
Ch. 35B Muscular VSD (Maladie de Roger), p 682.

Q 3.8. Concerning Truncus Arteriosus

A. It is caused by failure of the interventricular septum to develop

B. Causes a boot-shaped heart

C. A single semilunar valve is usually present

D. Either pulmonary plethora or oligaemia may be seen

E. Is a cause of unequal pulmonary blood flow

Q 3.9. Concerning VSD

A. Most occur in the muscular septum

B. VSD with pulmonary hypertension reliably produces an abnormal mediastinal silhouette

C. VSD may be demonstrated angiocardiographically in the LAO position after direct injection into the main pulmonary artery

D. Eisenmenger reaction occurs more commonly with ASD than VSD

E. Right ventricular hypertrophy may cause functional infundibular stenosis

A 3.8. Concerning Truncus Arteriosus

FALSE   A. This anomaly is caused by failure of the fetal truncus arteriosus to be divided into aorta and pulmonary artery by the spiral septum. The truncus receives the output of both ventricles because of the presence of a high VSD below its origin.
Ch. 35C Persistent Common Truncus Arteriosus, p 704.

TRUE   B. There is a concave pulmonary bay (not in Type 1), biventricular hypertrophy with elevation of the cardiac apex and very often a high right-sided aortic arch.
Ch. 35C Persistent Common Truncus Arteriosus, p 704.

TRUE   C. At the base of the truncus is a dysplastic valve that usually has three leaflets but sometimes more. It is generally incompetent and massive regurgitation into the ventricles can cause heart failure.
Ch. 35C Persistent Common Truncus Arteriosus, p 705.

TRUE   D. In Type 1, the pulmonary arteries are usually large and pulmonary plethora is present. In Types 2 and 3, pulmonary oligaemia is usually present.
Ch. 35C Persistent Common Truncus Arteriosus, p 704.

TRUE   E. This is especially true if there is hemitruncus, where one lung is supplied by a pulmonary artery arising normally from the right ventricle, and the other abnormally from the aorta.
Ch. 35C Persistent Common Truncus Arteriosus, p 706.

A 3.9. Concerning VSD

FALSE   A. The membranous septum is the most common site of VSD (80%).
Ch. 35B Membranous VSD, p 682.

FALSE   B. The CXR may show no significant chamber enlargement due to the balanced ventricular pressures, relatively small shunt and absence of volume overload.
Ch. 35B Muscular VSD (Maladie de Roger), p 683.

TRUE   C. If the catheter tip is left in the main pulmonary artery, a prolonged angiographic run will demonstrate the left to right shunt after return of blood from the lungs.
Ch. 35B Angiocardiography, p 683.

FALSE   D. VSD is the most common cause of shunt reversal secondary to increase in pulmonary vascular resistance.
Ch. 35B Obstructive Pulmonary Arterial Hypertension, p 686.

TRUE   E. This results in the development of Fallot's tetralogy disordered haemodynamics with cyanosis, usually occurring about 3-5 years of age.
Ch. 35B Essential Component of More Complex Anomalies, p 685.

Q *3.10. Regarding Patient Ductus Arteriosus (PDA)*

    A. The CXR appearance mimics that of VSD

    B. Ductus closure in a premature infant is promoted by both oxygen therapy and prostaglandin infusion

    C. Ductus closure precipitates the onset of cyanosis in Fallot's tetralogy

    D. Calcification of the PDA usually indicates severe pulmonary arterial hypertension

    E. PDA is the most common cause of an extracardiac left to right shunt

A *3.10. Regarding Patient Ductus Arteriosus (PDA)*

TRUE   A. Enlargement of both ventricles and the left atrium occurs accompanied by proximal pulmonary arterial enlargement and prominence of pulmonary vasculature. These findings are nonspecific signs of a left to right shunt. ASD will also simulate this picture apart from left atrial enlargement, which occurs late if at all.

Ch. 35B Patent Ductus Arteriosus, p 686.

FALSE   B. Oxygen therapy promotes closure by reducing the hypoxia of respiratory distress syndrome in the premature infant that delays PDA closure. Indomethacin promotes ductus closure by acting as a prostaglandin antagonist—prostaglandins are ductus dilators not ductus closers.

Ch. 35B Patent Ductus Arteriosus, p 686.

TRUE   C. A patent ductus in Fallot's physiology allows pulmonary arterial filling from the aorta, thus reducing pulmonary oligaemia. Ductus closure thus reduces pulmonary blood flow precipitating or exacerbating cyanosis.

Ch. 35B Patent Ductus Arteriosus, p 686.

TRUE   D.

Ch. 35B Patent Ductus Arteriosus, p 687.

TRUE   E.

Ch. 35B Patent Ductus Arteriosus, p 686.

Q 3.11. Regarding MRI of the Cardiovascular System

A. Blood moving at 5 cm/sec yields no signal on spin-echo sequences

B. Nonturbulent blood flow on gradient echo sequences has a uniformly high signal

C. Pericardium is readily distinguished from pericardial effusion

D. Spin echo is the method of choice for imaging an aortic dissection flap

E. Implantable pacemakers are generally not a contraindication to MRI

A 3.11. Regarding MRI of the Cardiovascular System

TRUE   A. Blood moving at a rate of more than 3 cm per second gives no signal, whereas slower-moving blood can be isointense with surrounding tissue. A signal void is used as a determinant of patency in coronary bypass grafts, though small volumes of blood moving backwards and forwards can cause the same appearance.
Ch. 34 Coronary Arteries and Coronary Artery bypass Grafts, p 641.

TRUE   B. When turbulence is present (e.g., stenotic valves), signal loss is evident in the region of the valve cusps and beyond.
Ch. 34 Detection of Turbulence, p 639.

FALSE   C. Normal fibrous pericardium has a low signal on T1 and T2-weighted images. Pericardial fluid exhibits a high signal on T2-weighted images; however, because cardiac motion causes turbulent motion within it, areas of signal loss are seen, which makes it difficult to distinguish between fluid and pericardium.
Ch. 34 The Pericardium, p 643.

FALSE   D. A thin flap will not be imaged in this sequence unless there is a column of static blood in the false lumen which contrasts with the lack of signal in the true lumen due to the flow of blood. A gradient echo sequence demonstrates the flap best as a thin sliver of low signal. Velocity mapping will demonstrate differential flow velocities in each lumen, confirming the diagnosis.
Ch. 34 Aortic Dissection, p 644.

FALSE   E. They represent an absolute contraindication.
Ch. 34 Limitations of MR Imaging, p 651.

Q *3.12. Regarding Noninvasive Cardiac Imaging*

    A. Sternal wires cause less artefact in gradient echo than in spin-echo MRI sequences

    B. Protons resonate at the same frequency regardless of tissue type

    C. A left ventricular ejection fraction of 65% indicates hypokinesia

    D. Increased ejection fraction in the presence of a low cardiac output suggests the presence of a ventricular septal defect (VSD) or mitral incompetence

    E. A left ventricular aneurysm may be seen to contract in systole on Echocardiography

A 3.12. *Regarding Noninvasive Cardiac Imaging*

FALSE   A. Metals cause areas of signal drop-out owing to distortion of the local magnetic field. This defect is small for spin-echo images but is more significant in gradient echo images.

Ch. 34 Coronary Arteries and Coronary Artery Bypass Grafts, p 641.

FALSE   B. Differences between the resonance frequencies of protons in different chemical milieux form the basis of chemical shift imaging. Protons in fatty tissue resonate at a lower frequency than protons in water. On this basis, STIR image sequences can suppress fat by effectively filtering out these lower frequency protons.

Ch. 34 Proton Chemical Shift Imaging, p 635.

FALSE   C. The normal left ventricle ejects about two thirds of its volume. Severe impairment is indicated by an ejection fraction of less than 30%

Ch. 37A Ejection Fraction, p 759.

TRUE   D. This combination of findings indicates that although the left ventricle is emptying adequately, not all of the blood is contributing to the cardiac output. Shunting into the right ventricle through a VSD may be responsible. Regurgitation into the left atrium through an incompetent mitral valve is another cause of this phenomenon.

Ch. 37A Ejection Fraction, p 759.

FALSE   E. True ventricular aneurysms do not contract as they are fibrous. Ventricular pseudoaneurysms do not contract either.

Ch. 37A Echocardiography, p 768.

Q 3.13. *Distinct Enlargement of the Heart Silhouette on CXR Within 5 Days of*
    M. Infarction is Expected in

   A. Dressler's syndrome

   B. Acquired VSD

   C. Papillary muscle rupture

   D. Pulmonary embolism

   E. Myocardial rupture

A 3.13. *Distinct Enlargement of the Heart Silhouette on CXR Within 5 Days of Infarction is Expected in*

FALSE A. Post-myocardial infarction syndrome is characterized by fever, pericarditis, pneumonitis and pleural effusion. Enlargement of the cardiac silhouette usually begins 2-3 weeks post infarction and often responds to steroids.
Ch. 37A Dressler's Syndrome, p 763.

TRUE B. This may occur several days to three weeks after a myocardial infarction. There is usually no pulmonary oedema (*viz.* papillary muscle rupture) unless gross volume overload occurs.
Ch. 37A Post-infarction Mitral Regurgitation, p 769.

FALSE C. There is sudden gross mitral valve regurgitation with a clinical picture similar to that of ruptured septum. Rapid onset pulmonary oedema unresponsive to medical management is seen on CXR. There is little or no increase in the heart size.
Ch. 37A Post-infarction Mitral Regurgitation, p 769.

FALSE D.

TRUE E. Usually occurs within a few days of infarction and has an almost 100% mortality.
Ch. 37A Rupture of the Heart, p 766.

Q 3.14. *Regarding Implanted Cardiac Devices and Valves*

A. On a frontal CXR, a pacing wire projected over the apex of the right ventricle may be located within left hepatic vein, middle cardiac vein, coronary sinus or right ventricle

B. A pacing wire tip within 3 mm of the epicardial fat pad indicates myocardial perforation

C. A mitral valve prosthesis is usually more vertically oriented than an aortic valve prosthesis

D. Transthoracic Doppler Echocardiography is more useful for identifying regurgitation in the mitral than in the aortic valve

E. Patients whose prosthetic valves have metallic struts should not undergo MRI

A 3.14. *Regarding Implanted Cardiac Devices and Valves*

TRUE   A.

Ch. 40 Pacemaker Not Functioning, p 815.

FALSE   B. Myocardial perforation can be confidently diagnosed only when the tip of the wire lies within the fat pad. A tip lying within 3 mm of the fat pad indicates penetration of myocardium, and echocardiography is then useful to identify the exact location of the tip of the wire and to assess any accompanying pericardial effusion.

Ch. 40 Myocardial Perforation, p 817.

TRUE   C. In addition, the mitral prosthesis lies more inferiorly and posteriorly and is also more likely to be viewed en face on the frontal view.

Ch. 41 Diagnostic Imaging Studies Following Valve Implantation, p 826.

FALSE   D. Ultrasound is more useful for aortic valve analysis as the identification and quantification of mitral valve dysfunction is hampered by the interposition of the prosthesis between transducer and left atrium regardless of which praecordial window is used.

Ch. 41 Doppler Echocardiography, p 831.

FALSE   E. The only valves thought to represent a contraindication to MRI are the older Starr-Edwards valves. All other valves are considered safe for exposure to diagnostic strength magnetic fields.

Ch. 41 Effect of Magnetic Resonance on the Prosthetic Valve, p 835.

Q 3.15. *The Causes of an Enlarged Left Atrium Include*

        A. Obstruction to left ventricular emptying

        B. PDA

        C. Tricuspid atresia

        D. Aortopulmonary window

        E. Nonrheumatic mitral incompetence

Q 3.16. *Reduced Prominence of the Main Pulmonary Artery on the PA Chest Radiograph Is Caused by the Following*

        A. Tetralogy of Fallot

        B. Tricuspid atresia

        C. Uncorrected transposition of the great arteries

        D. Truncus arteriosus

        E. Pulmonary valvular stenosis

A 3.15. *The Causes of an Enlarged Left Atrium Include*

TRUE   A. Aortic stenosis, aortic coarctation and HOCM may all raise the LV filling pressure with secondary enlargement (mild) of the left atrium. Left atrial myxoma may cause left atrial enlargement secondary to mitral valve obstruction.
Ch. 30 Causes of Selective Left Atrial Enlargement, p 566.

TRUE   B. A left to right shunt through PDA increases blood flow through left atrium and left ventricle and may therefore cause a moderately enlarged left atrium.
Ch. 35B Patent Ductus Arteriosus, p 686.

TRUE   C. There is an obligatory right atrial to left atrial shunt.
Ch. 35C Tricuspid Atresia, p 691.

TRUE   D. Because of the increased output of LA and LV as in PDA.
Ch. 35B Aortopulmonary Window, p 688.

TRUE   E. The most common cause of left atrial enlargement is rheumatic mitral valve disease, either regurgitant or stenotic. Marked enlargement of the left atrial appendage is nearly always due to rheumatic mitral disease. Nonrheumatic mitral incompetence causes enlargement of the main left atrial chamber but rarely of the appendage.
Ch. 36 Plain Film Radiography, p 736.

A 3.16. *Reduced Prominence of the Main Pulmonary Artery on the PA Chest Radiograph Is Caused by the Following*

TRUE   A. Right ventricular outflow obstruction in this condition causes the main pulmonary artery to be underdeveloped.
Ch. 35C Radiology, p 694.

TRUE   B. The pulmonary bay is markedly concave, and there is pulmonary oligaemia with narrow sparse vessels.
Ch. 35C Radiology, p 692.

TRUE   C. The superior mediastinum is classically narrow on the PA chest radiograph and wide on the lateral view because both the ascending aorta and pulmonary artery tend to lie in the midline. The pulmonary trunk is not border forming on the PA film.
Ch. 35C Radiology, p 708.

TRUE   D. There is a deeply concave pulmonary bay with small hila and an upturned apex, which when a right-sided aortic arch is present produces the classic "sitting duck" appearance on the PA chest radiograph.
Ch. 35C Persistent Common Truncus Arteriosus, p 704.

FALSE   E. Post-stenotic dilation is almost invariable in this condition, leading to *increased* prominence of the main pulmonary artery and left pulmonary artery.
Ch. 35D Pulmonary Valve Stenosis, p 718.

Q 3.17. Concerning Coarctation of the Aorta

A. Notching of the superior border of the ribs is often prominent in the level of D4-D12 segments.

B. Coarctation is frequently accompanied by a dysplastic aortic valve.

C. When coarctation is accompanied by an aberrant right subclavian artery, there is characteristically unilateral notching on the right side.

D. The kink at the coarctation site points backwards towards the ligamentum arteriosum insertion into the pulmonary artery.

E. Coarctation is more frequent in males, and is also a feature of Turner's syndrome in the female.

Q 3.18. Concerning Atrial Septal Defect (ASD)

A. With a large ASD, the right to left shunt is usually big

B. ASD is associated with both Down's syndrome and Holt-Oram syndrome

C. In ASD, there is often aberrant pulmonary venous drainage to the left lung

D. In ostium primum ASD, all of these features may be present—ASD, VSD, mitral incompetence, tricuspid incompetence, left ventricle to right atrium shunt

E. ASD with high flow commonly causes Eisenmenger reaction before the age of 10 years

A 3.17. *Concerning Coarctation of the Aorta*

FALSE
    A. *Inferior* border of the ribs are notched due to the tortuosity and dilatation of the intercostal arteries carrying blood retrogradely into the dorsal aorta.
Ch. 43 Coarctation, p 859.

TRUE
    B. The dysplastic, usually bicuspid, aortic valve may become severely thickened and calcified, resulting in valvar stenosis in later life.
Ch. 43 Coarctation, p 860.

FALSE
    C. As the aberrant right subclavian artery arises below the coarctation, it delivers low pressure blood to the right axilla and arm. Therefore, it cannot support a collateral circulation with reversed flow through the right intercostal arteries.
Ch. 43 Fig. 43.11, p 860.

FALSE
    D. The kink in the aorta is forwards toward the pulmonary artery.
Ch. 43 Coarctation, p 859.

TRUE
    E.
Ch. 43 Coarctation, p 860.

A 3.18. *Concerning Atrial Septal Defect (ASD)*

FALSE
    A. The left to right shunt is usually big.
Ch. 35B Ostium Secundum or Fossa Ovalis Defect, p 677.

TRUE
    B. Holt-Oram syndrome involves congenital heart disease (often ASD) and abnormalities of the upper limbs.
Ch. 35B Skeletal Features, p 667.

FALSE
    C. The more frequent aberrant drainage is to the right lung.
Ch. 35B Associations of Atrial Septal Defect, p 680.

TRUE
    D. Ostium primum ASD involves a major defect of development of the atrial and ventricular septa and the cushions which form the atrio-ventricular valves.
Ch. 35B Endocardial Cushion Defects, p 677.

FALSE
    E. Rarely before 20 or even 30 years of age.
Ch. 35B Radiology, p 678.

Q 3.19. *Concerning Cardiomyopathy*

    A. Dilated cardiomyopathy is mimicked by end-stage aortic stenosis

    B. Endocardial biopsy should be performed in a young patient with acute onset heart failure, pyrexia and respiratory symptoms

    C. Endocardial fibroelastosis causes mitral stenosis

    D. Hypertrophic cardiomyopathy often presents with atypical angina

    E. Endomyocardial fibrosis causes subendocardial hyperreflectivity on ultrasound

Q 3.20. *Concerning Atrial Myxoma*

    A. The diagnosis can be established by histological examination of a peripheral embolectomy specimen

    B. Enlargement of the atrial appendage is common

    C. The tumour arises from the upper part of the interatrial septum

    D. The tumour is more reflective than intracavitary thrombus

    E. Whorls of calcium, when present, are pathognomonic

A 3.19. Concerning Cardiomyopathy

TRUE   A. The aortic valve must be examined in detail in any patient with a large heart and low-output failure, as the response to aortic valve replacement is excellent.
Ch. 39 Echocardiography, p 799.

TRUE   B. This is a description of viral myocarditis that is accompanied by rising titres of Coxsackie, Influenza or other viruses.
Ch. 39 Viral Myocarditis, p 799.

FALSE   C. In this potentially lethal childhood condition, deposition of collagen and elastic tissue occurs on the inside of the left ventricle. This encroaches on the mitral valve causing regurgitation.
Ch. 39 Miscellaneous Conditions, p 801.

TRUE   D. This condition, characterized by asymmetrical septal hypertrophy and systolic anterior motion of the mitral valve, is associated with left ventricular hypertrophy which may be such that its blood supply is outstripped, resulting in chest pain.
Ch. 39 Hypertrophic Cardiomyopathy, p 802.

TRUE   E.
Ch. 39 Restrictive Cardiomyopathy, p 805.

A 3.20. Concerning Atrial Myxoma

TRUE   A.
Ch. 39 Left Atrial Myxoma, p 806.

FALSE   B. Unlike rheumatic mitral valve disease, the atrial appendage rarely enlarges in the presence of a left atrium enlarged by myxoma obstruction.
Ch. 39 Plain Film Radiography, p 806.

FALSE   C. The site of attachment of the tumour is the *lower* part of the interatrial septum. This accounts for its propensity to protrude into either the right or left ventricle during atrial systole.
Ch. 39 Cardiac Catheterization and Angiocardiography, p 807.

TRUE   D. Although thrombus is occasionally pedunculated, it usually occurs in an enlarged fibrillating atrium when it appears as an immobile, sessile, echopoor mass. It is more echogenic if calcification is present.
Ch. 39 Cross-sectional Echocardiography, p 807.

FALSE   E. Whorls of calcium are characteristic of *ventricular* fibromas that are usually left-sided. Myxomas rarely calcify; when they do, this pattern is not a feature.
Ch. 39 Fibroma, p 808.

128

Q 3.21. *Imaging in Cardiac Trauma*

A. In traumatic haemopericardium, the amount of fluid in the pericardial space required to cause tamponade is larger than in chronic effusion

B. Blunt trauma causes myocardial infarction

C. Traumatic myocardial pseudoaneurysms calcify in 70-80% of cases

D. Traumatic pericarditis calcifies and rarely causes cardiac restriction

E. The aortic valve is the valve most commonly affected in cardiac trauma

Q 3.22. *Regarding the Radiology of the Pericardium*

A. A cystic structure arising within the pericardium containing layered calcific deposits is suggestive of a bronchogenic cyst

B. Bilateral hilar overlay occurs in pericardial effusion

C. Chylous pericarditis usually has a negative Hounsfield number on CT

D. Pericardial calcification and thickening are pathognomonic of constrictive pericarditis

E. Malignant mesothelioma is the commonest primary pericardial malignancy

A 3.21. *Imaging in Cardiac Trauma*

FALSE   A. Rapid collection of blood occurs in trauma, allowing no time for the pericardial space to enlarge to accommodate it.
Ch. 39 Echocardiography, p 809.

TRUE   B. This may go on to cause ventricular aneurysm or rupture, valvular regurgitation or acquired septal defect.
Ch. 39 Echocardiography, p 809.

FALSE   C. They may calcify if present for several years, but calcification is considerably less common than with LV aneurysms associated with ischaemic heart disease.
Ch. 39 False Aneurysms, p 809.

TRUE   D. Restriction is rare after post-traumatic calcification of the pericardium.
Ch. 39 Pericardium, p 810.

TRUE   E. Leading to aortic incompetence.
Ch. 39 Valve Disruptions, p 810.

A 3.22. *Regarding the Radiology of the Pericardium*

TRUE   A. This appearance differs from that of simple pericardial cysts that do not contain layered calcific debris.
Ch. 42 Intrapericardial Bronchogenic Cyst, p 840.

TRUE   B. The pulmonary arteries can be seen through the globular mediastinal enlargement. If the enlargement is due to the heart, the hila are displaced laterally and are not overlayed.
Ch. 42 Pericarditis, p 842.

FALSE   C. The Hounsfield number of chylous pericarditis fluid is similar to that of transudate.
Ch. 42 CT and MRI, p 842.

FALSE   D. These features also occur in pericarditis that is not necessarily constrictive. In about 10% of cases of constrictive pericarditis, they are absent. The hallmark of constrictive disease is limited diastolic ventricular filling, often associated with a tubular morphology of the right ventricle.
Ch. 42 Radiology of Constrictive Pericarditis, p 845.

TRUE   E. It presents with haemorrhagic effusion and tamponade. The relationship to asbestos exposure is not clear.
Ch. 42 Pericardial Neoplasms, p 847.

Q *3.23. Concerning Congenital Anomalies of the Thoracic Aorta*

    A. An aberrant right subclavian artery causes an anterolateral indentation of the oesophagus as seen on a barium swallow

    B. In right-sided aortic arch mirror-image branching is associated with cyanotic congenital heart disease in nearly all cases

    C. In right-sided aortic arch not associated with congenital heart disease, the descending aorta passes to the left of the spine behind the oesophagus

    D. In a double aortic arch, the right arch is usually the larger of the two

    E. The most common cause of a tight vascular ring is a right-sided aortic arch with an aberrant left subclavian artery

A *3.23. Concerning Congenital Anomalies of the Thoracic Aorta*

FALSE   A. The indentation is *posterior* as the aberrant vessel runs behind the oesophagus, running upwards and to the right.
Ch. 43 Aberrant Right Subclavian Artery, p 855.

TRUE   B. Most commonly Tetralogy of Fallot (30-40%), Truncus arteriosus (30-40%) and Tricuspid atresia (15-25%). It is rare in transposition.
Ch. 43 Right Aortic Arch, p 855.

TRUE   C. In this circumstance ("right circumflex retro-oesophageal arch"), the left subclavian artery passes anteriorly to the oesophagus forming a vascular ring. The descending aorta in other cases may descend to the right of the spine without forming a vascular ring.
Ch. 43 Aberrant Left Subclavian Artery, p 855.

TRUE   D. The ascending aorta bifurcates anterior to the trachea to form a larger, more cephalad right arch and a smaller left arch. These two unite behind the oesophagus to form the descending aorta, which usually descends to the left of the spine.
Ch. 43 Double Aortic Arch, p 857.

FALSE   E. While this *is* the most common cause of a vascular ring, it does not usually require surgical intervention. The most common *tight* ring is a Type 1 double aortic arch in which both arches are patent.
Ch. 43 Double Aortic Arch, p 857.

Q 3.24. *Regarding Obstructive Disease of the Thoracic Aorta*

A. A bicuspid aortic valve is the most common cause of congenital valvular stenosis

B. Supravalvular aortic stenosis is associated with peripheral pulmonary artery stenosis

C. Preductal coarctation usually presents early in life

D. The aortic arch region in pseudocoarctation is usually more prominent on the frontal radiograph than it is in true coarctation

E. Rib notching occurs as a result of pseudocoarctation

Q 3.25. *Causes of Rib Notching Include*

A. Takayasu's arteritis

B. Tetralogy of Fallot

C. Vena caval obstruction

D. Osteogenesis imperfecta

E. Achondroplasia

A 3.24. *Regarding Obstructive Disease of the Thoracic Aorta*

TRUE   A. Most cases of bicuspid aortic valve do not cause problems until the valve thickens and calcifies in early adulthood.
Ch. 43 Aortic Valve Stenosis, p 858.

TRUE   B. In *Williams' syndrome* elfin facies, hypercalcaemia, mental retardation, dwarfism, supravalvular aortic stenosis and peripheral pulmonary artery stenosis occur.
Ch. 43 Aortic Valve Stenosis, p 859.

TRUE   C. This is the so-called *infantile form* which is associated with hypoplasia of the aortic portion between the left subclavian artery and the ductus. Pre-ductal coarctation is usually associated with a PDA transmitting a right to left shunt.
Ch. 43 Coarctation, p 859.

TRUE   D. Marked elongation and kinking of the aorta results in a prominent aortic knuckle superiorly and a kinked descending aorta inferiorly.
Ch. 43 Coarctation, p 860.

FALSE   E. There is no obstruction to arterial flow, therefore, no rib notching or delay in radio-femoral pulsation or upper limb hypertension.
Ch. 43 Coarctation, p 860.

A 3.25. *Causes of Rib Notching Include*

TRUE   A. This may causes aortic obstruction at any level and intercostal arterial vascular collateral vascular arterial enlargement.
Ch. 43 Table 43.2, p 861.

TRUE   B. Cyanotic congenital heart disease with pulmonary oligaemia predisposes to rib notching because of enlarged collateral aortic intercostal arteries.
Ch. 43 Table 43.2, p 861.

TRUE   C. Both superior and inferior vena caval obstruction may rely on the enlargement of intercostal venous collaterals for the maintenance of adequate venous drainage.
Ch. 43 Table 43.2, p 861.

FALSE   D. This causes "ribbon ribs" but not rib notching.
Ch. 43 Table 43.2, p 861.

FALSE   E. This is a cause of wide ribs with prominent costo-chondral junctions. Rib notching is not a feature.
Ch. 43 Table 43.2, p 861.

Q 3.26. Regarding Aortic Dissection

A. Most aortic dissections have a discernible entry and exit site

B. The detection of an intimal flap is pathognomonic of the condition

C. Pericardial and pleural fluid collections are associated with a worse prognosis

D. MRI is particularly useful as, in addition to showing the aortic flap, it allows the function of the aortic valve to be assessed

E. Although CT, MRI and echocardiography are very useful diagnostic techniques, aortography still remains the "gold standard" with accuracy approaching 100%

Q 3.27. The Following Chest Radiographic Signs are Commonly Associated with Aortic Transection

A. Normal chest film

B. Left apical cap

C. Deviation of trachea to the left

D. Widening of the right paratracheal stripe

E. Deviation of a naso-gastric tube to the right

A *3.26. Regarding Aortic Dissection*

TRUE

    A. These are referred to as complete, as opposed to incomplete dissections in which the exit site is not demonstrable.
    Ch. 43 Aortic Dissection, p 861.

TRUE

    B. A double lumen is also pathognomonic.
    Ch. 43 Aortic Dissection, p 862.

TRUE

    C. These imply that rupture of the aorta has occurred.
    Ch. 43 Aortic Dissection, p 862.

TRUE

    D. In addition, it allows the accurate measurement of the aortic valve which is important in planning valve replacement.
    Ch. 43 Aortic Dissection, p 865.

TRUE

    E.
    Ch. 43 Aortic Dissection, p 862.

A *3.27. The Following Chest Radiographic Signs are Commonly Associated with Aortic Transection*

TRUE

    A. As many as 30% of cases have a normal CXR on admission.
    Ch. 43 Traumatic Tear, p 867.

TRUE

    B. An extrapleural haematoma at the apex can be left or right-sided.
    Ch. 43 Traumatic Tear, p 867.

FALSE

    C. The mediastinal haematoma causes displacement of the trachea to the right.
    Ch. 43 Traumatic Tear, p 867.

TRUE

    D. Due to the superior tracking of extravasated mediastinal blood.
    Ch. 43 Traumatic Tear, p 867.

TRUE

    E. This is particularly useful as it is not influenced by the often anteroposterior supine positioning of the patient.
    Ch. 43 Traumatic Tear, p 867.

Q 3.28. *Concerning Cardiac Intervention*

    A. Percutaneous pulmonary balloon valvoplasty is the treatment of choice for pulmonary stenosis

    B. The choice of balloon size is more critical for pulmonary stenosis than for aortic stenosis

    C. There is a high mortality from balloon dilation of critical aortic stenosis in neonates

    D. Coil embolization of patent ductus arteriosus is used to close small ducts

    E. Balloon valvoplasty of acquired mitral stenosis is performed after dilating a track made through the interatrial septum

A 3.28. *Concerning Cardiac Intervention*

TRUE

A. This is now the treatment of choice for all patients with pulmonary valve stenosis.
Ch. 44 Pulmonary Valvoplasty, p 871.

FALSE

B. The balloon size for aortic dilation is chosen to be no bigger than the aortic annulus because aortic regurgitation is not well tolerated. In contrast, the balloon size for pulmonary valvoplasty can be 30% greater than the pulmonary valve annulus as regurgitation is much less of a problem.
Ch. 44 Aortic Valvoplasty, p 873.

TRUE

C. The mortality from balloon dilatation of this condition is similar to that of surgery.
Ch. 44 Critical Aortic Stenosis, p 873.

TRUE

D. Various types of coil have been used for this purpose, the best of which is probably the Jackson detachable coil which allows controlled coil deployment and removal if necessary.
Ch. 44 Occlusion of the Patent Ductus Arteriosus, p 875.

TRUE

E. A transeptal approach is the one most commonly employed.
Ch. 44 Mitral Stenosis, p 878.

4

The Gastrointestinal Tract

Q *4.1. Regarding the Plain Abdominal Radiograph*

   A. The presence of more than two air-fluid levels in dilated small bowel (over 2.5 cm across) is abnormal

   B. A caecal fluid level is an abnormal finding

   C. It is unusual for the bowel calibre to be less than 5 cm in severe large bowel obstruction

   D. Normal fluid levels are usually shorter than 2.5 cm in length

   E. A "string of beads" sign caused by bubbles of gas trapped between valvulae conniventes is seen after cleansing enema administration

Q *4.2. Intrahepatic Calcification is Caused By*

   A. Chronic granulomatous disease of childhood

   B. Cavernous haemangioma

   C. Portal vein thrombosis

   D. Armillifer armillatus infestation

   E. Hepatic adenoma

A 4.1. *Regarding the Plain Abdominal Radiograph*

TRUE	*A.*
	Ch. 45 Normal Appearances, p 885.
FALSE	*B.* 18% of normal people have a caecal fluid level.
	Ch. 45 Normal Appearances, p 886.
TRUE	*C.* This is helpful when trying to distinguish between small and large bowel dilation as it is unusual for obstructed small bowel to measure more than 5 cm. An exception to this is long-standing complete obstruction.
	Ch. 45 The Distinction Between Small and Large Bowel Dilatation, p 889.
TRUE	*D.*
	Ch. 45 Small Bowel Obstruction, p 890.
FALSE	*E.* This sign is virtually diagnostic of small bowel obstruction, as it indicates dilated bowel almost completely filled with fluid. It is not seen after enemas or cathartic administration.
	Ch. 45 Small Bowel Obstruction, p 890.

A 4.2. *Intrahepatic Calcification is Caused By*

TRUE	*A.* Hepatosplenomegaly, hepatic abscesses and foci of liver calcification occur in this immunodeficiency disorder.
	Ch. 45 Abdominal Calcification, p 886.
TRUE	*B.* Phleboliths and septal calcification may occur in these tumours.
	Ch. 45 Abdominal Calcification, p 886.
TRUE	*C.* Old clot may calcify in this condition.
	Ch. 45 Abdominal Calcification, p 886.
TRUE	*D.*
	Ch. 45 Abdominal Calcification, p 886.
FALSE	*E.*
	Ch. 45 Abdominal Calcification, p 886.

Q 4.3. Causes of Pancreatic Calcification Include

A. Acute pancreatitis

B.) Gastrinoma

C. Cystic fibrosis

D. Hereditary pancreatitis

E.) Cavernous lymphangioma

Q 4.4. Causes of Adrenal Calcification in Adults Include

A. Adrenal adenoma

B. Adrenal hyperplasia

C. Wolman disease

D. Addison's disease

E. Sarcoidosis

A 4.3. *Causes of Pancreatic Calcification Include*

TRUE	A. This occurs <u>uncommonly</u> after intrapancreatic fat is broken down by pancreatic enzymes: "saponification." *Ch. 45 Pancreatic Calcification, p 887.*
TRUE	B. Calcification <u>occasionally</u> occurs in this tumour that is usually intrapancreatic and malignant. *Ch. 45 Pancreatic Calcification, p 887.*
TRUE	C. Calcific chronic pancreatitis occurs in this condition. *Ch. 45 Pancreatic Calcification, p 887.*
TRUE	D. In this pre-malignant autosomal dominant condition, large aggregations of calcification are seen on the plain abdominal film in childhood. *Ch. 45 Pancreatic Calcification, p 887.*
TRUE	E. *Ch. 45 Pancreatic Calcification, p 887.*

A 4.4. *Causes of Adrenal Calcification in Adults Include*

TRUE	A. These small (usually less than 5 cm) tumours occasionally calcify. *Ch. 45 Abdominal Calcification, p 887.*
FALSE	B. Bilateral hyperplasia is usually smooth but occasionally nodular. Calcification is not a feature. *Ch. 45 Abdominal Calcification, p 887.*
FALSE	C. This lipidosis is a cause of adrenal calcification but affected infants die within a few months of birth.
TRUE	D. Calcification is frequent when Addison's disease is due to TB of the adrenals, but this is now an uncommon cause of Addison's disease. *Ch. 45 Abdominal Calcification, p 887.*
FALSE	E. Sarcoidosis is one of a number of causes of granulomatous adrenal disease; however, unlike TB and Histoplasmosis, adrenal calcification is not a feature of this condition. *Ch. 45 Abdominal Calcification, p 887.*

Q 4.5. Small Bowel Air-Fluid Levels are Caused by

✓ A. Large bowel obstruction

✗ B. Hyperkalaemia

✓ C. Peritoneal metastases

✓ D. Gastroenteritis

✓ E. Mesenteric thrombosis

Q 4.6. Regarding Large Bowel Obstruction

✓ A. In the presence of generalized gaseous bowel distension, a left lateral decubitus radiograph may be helpful in diagnosing large bowel obstruction

✗ B. After carcinoma of the colon, volvulus is the most common cause of large bowel obstruction in western societies

✗ C. Right-sided large bowel obstruction is almost as common as left-sided obstruction

✓ D. Caecal volvulus occurs only when there is a degree of malrotation

✓ E. Sigmoid volvulus usually has a history of intermittent acute attacks over a period of time

A 4.5. *Small Bowel Air-Fluid Levels are Caused by*

TRUE

A. Established large bowel obstruction leads to small bowel obstruction and air-fluid level development.
Ch. 45 Mechanical Large Bowel Obstruction, p 893.

FALSE

B. A *low* serum potassium causes intestinal hypomotility and functional obstruction with air-fluid levels.
Ch. 45 Small Bowel Obstruction, p 890.

TRUE

C.
Ch. 45 Small Bowel Obstruction, p 890.

TRUE

D. Any cause of marked fluid accumulation in bowel lumen can produce fluid levels.
Ch. 45 Small Bowel Obstruction, p 890.

TRUE

E. Bowel ischaemia renders the gut wall more permeable to fluid ingress into the lumen. Mural thickening may accompany the clinical symptoms of sudden onset abdominal pain and bloody diarrhoea in an elderly person.
Ch. 45 Small Bowel Obstruction, p 890.

A 4.6. *Regarding Large Bowel Obstruction*

TRUE

A. This radiograph may allow the demonstration of absence of gas in the rectum, indicating large bowel obstruction instead of paralytic ileus.
Ch. 45 Mechanical Large Bowel Obstruction, p 892.

FALSE

B. *Diverticulitis* is the second commonest cause of large bowel obstruction in the USA and Great Britain.
Ch. 45 Mechanical Large Bowel Obstruction, p 892.

FALSE

C. *Left-sided* obstruction is much more the common of the two.
Ch. 45 Mechanical Large Bowel Obstruction, p 892.

TRUE

D. This is liable to occur only if the caecum and ascending colon are on a mesentery.
Ch. 45 Mechanical Large Bowel Obstruction, p 894.

TRUE

E.
Ch. 45 Mechanical Large Bowel Obstruction, p 894.

Q 4.7. *Plain Radiographic Signs Supporting a Diagnosis of Sigmoid Volvulus Include*

    A. The presence of haustra

    B. The margin of the dilated loop overlaps the soft-tissue shadow of the inferior border of the liver

    C. The dilated loop overlies dilated large bowel in the left flank

    D. The apex of the loop usually underlies the right hemidiaphragm

    E. "Shouldering" is present on a barium enema

Q 4.8. *Regarding the Radiological Features of Colitis*

    A. Normal mucosal islands seen on plain film indicate severe disease

    B. A transverse colon diameter of greater than 5.5 cm combined with the presence of normal mucosal islands is sufficient evidence to diagnose toxic megacolon

    C. The usual site of perforation in ulcerative colitis is the caecum

    D. The presence of ascites favours a diagnosis of pseudomembranous colitis

    E. The right side of the colon tends to be dilated in ischaemic colitis

A 4.7. *Plain Radiographic Signs Supporting a Diagnosis of Sigmoid Volvulus Include*

FALSE   A. Haustra are more often absent.
Ch. 45 Mechanical Large Bowel Obstruction, p 895.

TRUE   B. This is the so-called "liver overlap" sign.
Ch. 45 Mechanical Large Bowel Obstruction, p 895.

TRUE   C. This is the so-called "left flank overlap" sign and indicates that, as the descending colon is dilated, the obstruction is distal to this.
Ch. 45 Mechanical Large Bowel Obstruction, p 895.

FALSE   D. The apex of the loop usually lies underneath the *left* hemidiaphragm in sigmoid volvulus.
Ch. 45 Mechanical Large Bowel Obstruction, p 895.

TRUE   E. In chronic volvulus, shouldering may be seen due to localized thickening of bowel wall at the site of the twist.
Ch. 45 Mechanical Large Bowel Obstruction, p 895.

A 4.8. *Regarding the Radiological Features of Colitis*

TRUE   A. These represent islands of normal mucosa and their existence implies that a large area of mucosa has been ulcerated. Sometimes ulceration is so extensive that few mucosal islands remain.
Ch. 45 Mechanical Large Bowel Obstruction, p 895.

TRUE   B. Changes are seen best in the transverse colon, which is the least dependent part of the colon and thus accumulates the greatest amount of air.
Ch. 45 Mechanical Large Bowel Obstruction, p 896.

FALSE   C. The most common site of perforation is the sigmoid colon. It is usually the result of deep ulceration or toxic megacolon.
Ch. 45 Mechanical Large Bowel Obstruction, p 896.

TRUE   D.
Ch. 45 Mechanical Large Bowel Obstruction, p 896.

TRUE   E. This is because the ischaemic segment at the splenic flexure acts as an area of functional obstruction.
Ch. 45 Mechanical Large Bowel Obstruction, p 896.

Q 4.9. *Regarding the Radiology of the Acute Abdomen*

A.) Expectant treatment is the treatment of choice in pseudo-obstruction

B.) Free intraperitoneal gas is almost never seen in an acutely perforated appendix

C. Most cases of acute cholecystitis have an abnormal plain abdominal radiograph

D. False positive nonvisualization of the gall bladder using ^{99m}Tc-HIDA occurs in alcoholic liver disease

E. Paralytic ileus is commonly found in association with a leaking abdominal aortic aneurysm

Q 4.10. *Causes of Pneumoperitoneum Without Peritonitis Include*

A. Endoscopy

B.) Perforated jejunal diverticulosis

C. Therapeutic arterial embolization

D. Perforated cyst of pneumatosis intestinalis

E. Tracking of air down from a pneumomediastinum

A 4.9. *Regarding the Radiology of the Acute Abdomen*

FALSE   A. If the caecum has reached the critical diameter of 9 cm, decompression is required and caecostomy or right-sided colostomy are sometimes needed to prevent the development of ischaemic bowel and/or perforation.
Ch. 45 Pseudo-obstruction, p 897.

TRUE   B.
Ch. 45 Pneumoperitoneum, p 897.

FALSE   C. In two-thirds of cases, the plain film is normal.
Ch. 45 Acute Cholecystitis, p 901.

TRUE   D. Total parenteral nutrition (chronic fasting state) is also responsible for false positives.
Ch. 45 Acute Cholecystitis, p 901.

TRUE   E. The loops of bowel may completely obscure the signs of a leaking aneurysm on the plain radiograph.
Ch. 45 Leaking Abdominal Aortic Aneurysm, p 906.

A 4.10. *Causes of Pneumoperitoneum Without Peritonitis Include*

TRUE   A. Leakage of air through a distended stomach after endoscopic inflation can cause pneumoperitoneum without peritonitis.
Ch. 45 Pneumoperitoneum, p 899.

TRUE   B. This is the most common cause of pneumoperitoneum without peritonitis. It has a significant mortality rate.
Ch. 45 Pneumoperitoneum, p 899.

TRUE   C.
Ch. 45 Pneumoperitoneum, p 899.

TRUE   D. There is a wide spectrum of severity in this condition. An asymptomatic pneumoperitoneum may persist for months following perforation of a cyst with no apparent sequelae.
Ch. 45 Pneumoperitoneum, p 899.

TRUE   E.
Ch. 45 Pneumoperitoneum, p 899.

Q *4.11. The Following are Normal Features of the Oesophagus on a Barium Swallow*

A.) The cervical oesophagus starts at the cricopharyngeus impression—usually at C3-C4 level

B.) The post-cricoid impression is a small, posterior, web-like indentation

C. Herring-bone pattern of mucosal folds on double contrast examination

D. The A ring (tubulovestibular junction) varies in calibre during the examination

E. The mucosal gastro-oesophageal junction cannot be identified on double-contrast studies

A *4.11. The Following are Normal Features of the Oesophagus on a Barium Swallow*

FALSE

    A. The cricopharyngeal impression is usually at the C5-C6 level.
    Ch. 46 Normal Anatomy, p 909.

FALSE

    B. This is an anterior impression (as opposed to the posteriorly-placed cricopharyngeus impression) that is like a web but changes shape with swallowing.
    Ch. 46 Normal Anatomy, p 909.

TRUE

    C. This is a normal transient phenomenon.
    Ch. 46 Normal Anatomy, p 909.

TRUE

    D. This ring is visible only if the vestibule and tubular oesophagus are adequately distended.
    Ch. 46 Normal Anatomy, p 911.

FALSE

    E. This normal feature is occasionally visible as a thin, slightly radiolucent line. It is also known as the Z line, or ora serrata.
    Ch. 46 Normal Anatomy, p 911.

Q *4.12. Regarding Techniques of Examining the Oesophagus*

A. A double-contrast examination is the preferred method of detecting a web

B. A single-contrast study is the best way of demonstrating a sliding hiatus hernia

C. Oesophageal motility is best examined with the patient erect in the LAO position

D. A well-distended, single-contrast study technique is the best way of visualizing oesophageal varices

E. A normal oesophageal scintigram excludes "nutcracker" oesophagus (one with abnormally high amplitude contractions)

A 4.12. *Regarding Techniques of Examining the Oesophagus*

FALSE

A. A single-contrast study with frequent, rapid films is particularly useful for demonstrating webs, extrinsic compression and lack of distensibility from whatever cause.
Ch. 46 Barium Techniques, p 912.

TRUE

B. This is diagnosed when the B ring is more than 2 cm above the diaphragmatic impression, or by the presence of 5 or more mucosal folds seen 2 cm above the diaphragm. The B ring is also known as the transverse mucosal fold, lower oesophageal ring, Schatzki's ring and lower oesophageal diaphragm—it represents the upper margin of the gastric sling fibres.
Ch. 46 Single-Contrast Technique, p 912.

FALSE

C. Motility is best assessed when the effects of gravity have been eliminated and propagation of the barium bolus depends only on muscular function. This is best achieved in the prone RAO position.
Ch. 46 Motility Examination, p 913.

FALSE

D. Oesophageal distension compresses varices and thereby renders them less visible.
Ch. 46 Oesophageal Varices, p 926.

FALSE

E. Retained isotope in the distal oesophagus accompanied by evidence of reflux occurs in this condition. However, peristalsis may be such as to allow all the isotope to be emptied into the stomach resulting in a consequent false negative examination.
Ch. 46 Nutcracker Oesophagus, p 936.

Q *4.13. In the Investigation of Oesophagitis*

  A. Seventy to eighty percent of patients with reflux oesophagitis have demonstrable reflux on barium swallow examinations

  B. Caustic oesophagitis affects the upper third of the oesophagus most severely and becomes progressively less severe towards the cardia

  C. Herpetic oesophagitis is preceded by a flu-like prodrome

  D. Squamous carcinoma of oesophagus develops at the site of caustic strictures

  E. Candidal infection causes intramural masses

A 4.13. *In the Investigation of Oesophagitis*

FALSE

A. Less than <u>half</u> of all patients with this condition will have radiologically demonstrable reflux. Many patients require some sort of provocation (e.g., coughing, head-down tilt, a supine patient elevating the legs, an increase in abdominal pressure, etc.) to demonstrate reflux. The situation is further complicated by the observation of reflux in many asymptomatic patients.
Ch. 46 Peptic (reflux) Oesophagitis, p 914.

FALSE

B. The middle and lower thirds of the organ are the most affected, particularly at sites of relative hold-up (i.e., the aortic arch, the left main bronchus and the diaphragmatic hiatus.
Ch. 46 Chemically-Induced Oesophagitis, p 919.

TRUE

C. This occurs usually in immunosuppressed patients but sexual partners with herpetic lesions can spread it to immunocompetent individuals. Myalgia, sore throat and pyrexia may precede the oesophageal symptoms.
Ch. 46 Herpetic Oesophagitis, p 918.

TRUE

D. The incidence of oesophageal carcinoma is increased in patients with caustically induced oesophageal strictures. This classically develops after lye (sodium hydroxide) ingestion.
Ch. 46 Malignant Neoplasms, p 923.

TRUE

E. Overwhelming candida infection may result in large intramural masses composed of candidal aggregations and haemorrhage.
Ch. 46 Candidiasis, p 918.

Q 4.14. *Regarding Imaging of the Small Intestine*

    A. Mesenteric abscesses and mesenteric lymphadenopathy are CT findings in Crohn's disease

    B. A "coiled spring" appearance is a sign of coeliac disease on a barium follow through

    C. Isolated focal dilatation of a small-bowel loop is a sign of lymphoma

    D. Primary carcinoma is more common in the ileum than in the jejunum

    E. Deep ulceration occurs in 80% of cases of radiation enteritis

Q 4.15. *Regarding Imaging of the Large Bowel*

    A. Umbilication of lymphoid follicles is an abnormal finding in a childhood barium enema

    B. On evacuation proctography, the anorectal junction is seen normally above the plane of the ischial tuberosities

    C. During evacuation proctography, absence of contraction of the rectum is a cause of incomplete evacuation

    D. The major indication for anal endosonography is the assessment of proctalgia

    E. Venous intravasation of barium during an enema is a cause of liver abscess

A 4.14. Regarding Imaging of the Small Intestine

TRUE   A.
Ch. 49 Crohn's Disease, p 992.

TRUE   B. Nonobstructive intusussception commonly occurs in this condition which most characteristically causes small bowel dilatation.
Ch. 49 Coeliac Disease, p 992.

TRUE   C. This is occasionally seen owing, presumably, to loss of intestinal muscle tone as a result of lymphomatous invasion of muscle layers and neural plexi.
Ch. 49 Malignant Neoplasms, p 994.

FALSE   D. The reverse is the case. Ileal carcinoma is rare.
Ch. 49 Malignant Neoplasms, p 994.

FALSE   E. Deep ulceration is uncommon in radiation enteritis. Ulcers, when present, are typically too shallow to be appreciated radiologically.
Ch. 49 Chronic Radiation Enteritis, p 999.

A 4.15. Regarding Imaging of the Large Bowel

FALSE   A. Lymphoid nodular hyperplasia is common in children and may be prominent and extensive. Umbilication is a normal feature in this age group.
Ch. 50 Radiological Investigation, p 1012.

TRUE   B. During evacuation there is a 3 cm descent with widening of the anorectal angle from 90° to 115°.
Ch. 50 Evacuation Proctography, p 1015.

FALSE   C. The rectum does not need to contract in order for evacuation to occur. Raised intra-abdominal pressure is the major propulsive force.
Ch. 50 Evacuation Proctography, p 1015.

FALSE   D. The major indication for this technique is the demonstration of sphincter damage in faecal incontinence.
Ch. 50 Rectal and Anal Endosonography, p 1015.

TRUE   E. The potential sequelae of this rare complication are liver abscess and pulmonary embolism.
Ch. 50 Table 50.3, p 1013.

Q *4.16. Regarding the Anatomy of the Large Bowel*

    A. Both the ascending and descending colon are predominantly extraperitoneal

    B. The transverse colon distal to the hepatic flexure is supplied predominantly by the inferior mesenteric artery

    C. Absence of haustration in the proximal colon is always abnormal

    D. A post-rectal space of 15 mm or more at S4 is always abnormal

    E. Lymphoid follicles seen on a barium enema in an adult are always abnormal

A *4.16. Regarding the Anatomy of the Large Bowel*

TRUE

A. The transverse and sigmoid colons both have a mesentery, whereas the ascending and descending colons are partly extraperitoneal.
Ch. 50 Anatomy, p 1009.

FALSE

B. The superior mesenteric artery gives off a right colic–middle colic trunk that supplies the ascending and transverse colon to the level of the splenic flexure. The *descending colon* is mainly supplied by the inferior mesenteric artery.
Ch. 50 Anatomy, p 1009.

TRUE

C. There is often no haustration visible from mid-transverse colon to the rectum during a barium enema; however, haustra should always be visible in the ascending colon.
Ch. 50 Anatomy, p 1009.

FALSE

D. In the obese and elderly, up to 20 mm is within normal limits.
Ch. 50 Anatomy, p 1009.

FALSE

E. They are submucosal and cause minimal elevation and therefore no meniscus. Nodular lymphoid hyperplasia is seen as a normal variant in about 13% of adult subjects.
Ch. 50 Surface Pattern, p 1012.

Q *4.17. Concerning Large Bowel Polyps*

A. 2% of metaplastic polyps undergo malignant change per year

B. Adenomas greater than 1 cm across have an incidence of malignancy of less than 1%

C. On a double-contrast barium enema (DCBE), a ring of barium having a sharp inner edge and an unsharp outer margin indicates a polyp

D. A localized area of increased density on DCBE is a recognized sign of a polyp

E. Familial adenomatous polyposis (FAP) patients have an increased risk of desmoid tumours

A *4.17. Concerning Large Bowel Polyps*

FALSE A. These lesions are most common in the rectum and appear as sessile nodules less than 1 cm across. They have no malignant potential.
Ch. 50 Metaplastic Polyps, p 1016.

FALSE B. Only adenomas *less* than 1 cm across have this low risk of malignancy.
Ch. 50 Adenomatous Polyps, p 1016.

TRUE C.
Ch. 50 Meniscus Sign, p 1016.

TRUE D. The front and back of a polyp are coated with barium and the tumour bulk reduces the depth of air traversed by the X-ray beam. These two factors combine to give a localized area of increased density which may draw attention to an abnormality.
Ch. 50 Increased Density Sign, p 1017.

TRUE E. Gardner's syndrome is now considered as part of the spectrum of familial adenomatous polyposis. Desmoid formation (dense focal formation) is often precipitated by surgery and is a major cause of morbidity and mortality owing to recurrent local invasion and small bowel and ureteric obstruction.
Ch. 50 Familial Adenomatous Polyposis, p 1020.

Q 4.18. *Regarding Multiple Colonic Polyps*

A. The hamartomas in Peutz-Jeghers' syndrome are pre-malignant

B. Multiple colonic polyps are associated with breast cancer

C. Cronkhite-Canada syndrome is a diffuse neoplastic intestinal polyposis which is usually rapidly fatal

D. The polyps of diffuse lymphomatous polyposis of the colon tend to be larger than 5 mm diameter and umbilicated

E. In juvenile polyposis, the colonic polyps are present in infancy

A *4.18. Regarding Multiple Colonic Polyps*

FALSE
    A. The polyps are hamartomatous and are more common in the stomach and small bowel. In the large bowel they are larger, fewer, often pedunculated and may bleed. Hamartomas have no intrinsic malignant potential. There is an increased incidence of dysplasia in the overlying mucosa and an increase in upper gastrointestinal tract and extra-intestinal cancer.
Ch. 50 Peutz-Jeghers' Syndrome, p 1020.

TRUE
    B. Cowden's syndrome is a multiple (nonmalignant) hamartoma syndrome characterized by oro-cutaneous papules, multiple adenomas and malignant tumours of the breast and thyroid.
Ch. 50 Cowden's Disease, p 1021.

FALSE
    C. The polyps are not neoplastic but are due to cystic mucosal degeneration, particularly in the colon. Death occurs as a result of cachexia due to profound malabsorption.
Ch. 50 Cronkhite-Canada Syndrome, p 1021.

TRUE
    D. Umbilication of normal lymphoid follicles (maximum size 3 mm diameter) occurs in children but rarely in adults and is a useful distinguishing feature of lymphoma. The appearance may resemble aphthoid ulceration.
Ch. 50 Lymphoma, p 1024.

TRUE
    E. Polyps occur in the stomach, small bowel and colon. There is an associated increased risk of colorectal malignancy but probably not from the polyps themselves, which are hamartomas.
Ch. 50 Juvenile Polyposis, p 1020.

Q 4.19. *Regarding Gastrointestinal Endoscopy and ERCP*

- A. A barium meal is preferable to endoscopy in the assessment of the post-operative stomach

- B. Balloon dilatation of the cardia is useful in the treatment of primary achalasia

- C. When a bile duct is obstructed at ERCP, full strength 300 mgI/m1^{-1} contrast medium is required for its adequate opacification

- D. During ERCP, contrast medium should be injected until an adequate pancreatic parenchymogram is obtained

- E. In the majority of patients with gallstones and benign strictures, the bile is infected prior to ERCP

Q 4.20. *Regarding the Findings at ERCP*

- A. HIV cholangitis resembles sclerosing cholangitis

- B. A choledochocele is lined by duodenal mucosa

- C. Clonorchis sinensis causes a long, linear filling defect in the common bile duct

- D. A smooth tapering stricture of the distal bile duct within the head of the pancreas occurs in chronic pancreatitis

- E. Cholangitis is a cause of multiple contrast-filled intrahepatic cavities

A 4.19. *Regarding Gastrointestinal Endoscopy and ERCP*

FALSE
A. Endoscopy is more accurate, particularly in the assessment of the gastro-enteric anastomosis site.
Ch. 56A Endoscopy in Special Circumstances, p 1132.

TRUE
B. Although less reliable at relieving symptoms and with a high reintervention rate, balloon dilation is increasingly felt to be a viable alternative to surgical myotomy.
Ch. 56A Benign Oesophageal Strictures, p 1133.

FALSE
C. *Dilute* contrast medium is needed in order not to obscure stones.
Ch. 56A Contrast Medium, p 1135.

FALSE
D. Contrast staining of the pancreatic parenchyma should be avoided, as acute pancreatitis is a potential complication.
Ch. 56A Adequacy of Pancreatogram and Cholangiogram, p 1136.

TRUE
E. This has been shown to be the case and is an argument for using as little contrast medium as possible to complete the procedure, if biliary duct drainage is not envisaged.
Ch. 56A Adequacy of Pancreatogram and Cholangiogram, p 1136.

A 4.20. *Regarding the Findings at ERCP*

TRUE
A. Similar changes are seen as a complication of 5-Fluorouracil therapy.
Ch. 56A The Cholangiogram, p 1138.

TRUE
B. This is a rare sac-like diverticulum of the lower common bile duct. It is essentially a duodenal duplication cyst and is associated with stone formation and pancreatitis.
Ch. 56A The Cholangiogram, p 1138.

FALSE
C. It causes a small, crescentic filling defect. The worm may be seen protruding from the papilla by the endoscopist. *Ascaris lumbricoides* causes a long filling defect.
Ch. 56 The Cholangiogram, p 1138.

TRUE
D. It may be difficult to distinguish this appearance from carcinoma of the head of pancreas or a low cholangiocarcinoma.
Ch. 56A The Cholangiogram, p 1138.

TRUE
E. These are abscess cavities.
Ch. 56A The Cholangiogram, p 1138.

5

The Liver, Biliary Tract, Pancreas and Endocrine System

Q *5.1. Concerning Liver Anatomy*

    A. The middle hepatic vein drains both lobes of the liver

    B. The right hepatic vein divides the right lobe of liver into a superior and an inferior sector

    C. The left lobe of liver is divided into an anterior and a posterior sector by the left portal vein

    D. The caudate lobe receives branches from both left and right portal veins

    E. Calcification of liver parenchyma may be a normal finding in the elderly

A 5.1. Concerning Liver Anatomy

TRUE

A. This structure lies in the principal plane that divides the right from the left lobe of liver and drains both lobes.

Ch. 57 Gross Anatomy, p 1155.

FALSE

B. The right hepatic vein runs in an inferosuperior direction and divides the right lobe into anterior and posterior sectors (Segments V, VIII, VI and VII, respectively).

Ch. 57 Gross Anatomy, p 1155.

FALSE

C. By the left *hepatic* vein.

Ch. 57 Gross Anatomy, p 1156.

TRUE

D. Its hepatic venous branches drain directly into the IVC independently of the three main hepatic veins.

Ch. 57 Gross Anatomy, p 1156.

FALSE

E. The liver does not normally calcify with age. Calcification in adjacent structures such as the gall bladder, costal cartilages and blood vessels may cause confusion.

Ch. 57 Calcification, p 1158.

Q *5.2. Concerning Focal Liver Lesions*

A. Daughter cysts develop within a larger mother cyst in hydatid disease

B. A prominent air-fluid level in an intrahepatic mass implies that it is an abscess

C. "Filling in" of a lesion on delayed contrast-enhanced CT means it is almost certainly a haemangioma

D. A central, hyper reflective "punctum" surrounded by echo-poor foci is a feature of fungal abscesses

E. High-attenuation abdominal deposits may occur in angiosarcoma

A 5.2. *Concerning Focal Liver Lesions*

TRUE
    A. Hydatid disease is the only condition in which daughter cysts grow within a larger cyst. In the absence of daughter cysts, however, the lesion is indistinguishable from a simple cyst.
    Ch. 57 Hydatid Disease, p 1160.

FALSE
    B. This appearance may occur in the absence of infection, most strikingly after the therapeutic embolization of large hepatic metastases.
    Ch. 57 Gas Within the Liver, p 1159.

FALSE
    C. "Filling in" is a non-specific finding; many small, non-cystic hepatic lesions will fill-in eventually.
    Ch. 57 Haemangioma, p 1170.

TRUE
    D. The punctum is a feature said to be caused by embolization of a central arterial branch by fungal material. It is not pathognomonic.
    Ch. 57 Abscesses, p 1160.

TRUE
    E. Angiosarcomas of the liver occur after exposure to polyvinyl chloride, arsenic and Thorotrast. Thorium deposition in liver spleen and lymph nodes has a pathognomonic appearance; this radiographic appearance is, however, rarely seen nowadays as Thorotrast has not been used as a contrast agent for over 50 years.
    Ch. 57 Angiosarcoma, p 1169.

Q 5.3. *Regarding the Ultrasound Imaging of Liver Disease*

A. Regenerating nodules are usually very small and cannot be demonstrated by imaging techniques

B. Acute hepatitis and diffuse tuberculosis are causes of a "bright" liver

C. A fasting portal venous velocity of more than 12 cm per second does not occur in portal hypertension

D. High-velocity spectral traces are seen in relation to most hepatomas

E. Daughter cysts are present in 80-90% of liver hydatid cysts

Q 5.4. *Concerning Liver Scintigraphy*

A. Splenic uptake precedes hepatic uptake

B. Decreased sulphur colloid uptake by a transplanted liver is a sign of rejection

C. Eighty to 90% of an intravenous dose of ^{99m}Tc sulphur colloid is taken up by the Kupffer cells of the liver

D. Blood-pool scans are particularly useful for detecting the neovascularity of hepatic adenomas

E. Hepatoma and liver abscess can be reliably distinguished from each other by a combination of sulphur colloid scan and gallium scanning

A 5.3. *Regarding the Ultrasound Imaging of Liver Disease*

TRUE   A. Although large regenerating nodules may be visible sonographically and simulate metastases, the majority are small (2-3 mm) and undetectable on ultrasound.
Ch. 57 Diffuse Disease, p 1162.

TRUE   B. Most patients with acute hepatitis have no sonographic abnormality, though diffuse hyper reflectivity is a recognised finding.
Ch. 57 Diffuse Disease, p 1162.

FALSE   C. Although in most circumstances this value (or one greater) indicates a normal flow velocity in the presence of a portosystemic shunt (e.g., recanalization of the umbilical vein) the main portal venous flow may increase to "feed" the shunt.
Ch. 57 Diffuse Disease, p 1162.

TRUE   D. In 85% of cases, hepatoma neovascularity can be demonstrated and shown to be of high velocity.
Ch. 57 Primary Liver Tumours, p 1161.

FALSE   E. In approximately 50% of hydatid cysts, daughter cysts are evident. Their presence is pathognomonic, but their absence clearly does not rule out echinococcal infection.
Ch. 57 Hydatid Disease, p 1160.

A 5.4. *Concerning Liver Scintigraphy*

TRUE   A. The spleen takes up colloid during the arterial phase whereas normal liver uptake occurs during the portal venous phase.
Ch. 57 Liver Scintigraphy, p 1163.

TRUE   B. A "colloid shift" occurs with a relative increase in uptake by spleen and bone marrow.
Ch. 57 Abnormal Liver Scan, p 1163.

TRUE   C. This accounts for the relatively reduced uptake seen in the spleen compared to the liver on a normal scan. A bone marrow signal is not normally present.
Ch. 57 Methods, p 1163.

FALSE   D. Blood-pool scanning with labelled red cells does not demonstrate hepatic adenomas as areas of increased uptake. Haemangiomas are shown as suspected areas.
Ch. 57 Abnormal Liver Scan, p 1164.

FALSE   E. Both hepatoma and liver abscess regularly appear as photopenic areas on colloid scan and areas of increased signal on gallium scan.
Ch. 57 Abnormal Liver Scan, p 1164.

Q 5.5. *Regarding the Radiology of Hepatoma*

A. Thorotrast exposure predisposes to the development of hepatoma

B. Calcification is seen in 30-40% of hepatomas

C. Angiography plays a significant role in the initial diagnosis of hepatoma

D. Complete non-enhancement of a liver lobe on CT after intravenous contrast administration yields the "straight-line sign" that is diagnostic of portal venous occlusion

E. The presence of portal vein thrombosis makes the diagnosis of hepatoma virtually certain

A 5.5. *Regarding the Radiology of Hepatoma*

TRUE

A. Angiosarcoma is the classic tumour that occurs as a result of thorium dioxide exposure about 20-30 years previously. Hepatoma and cholangiocarcinoma are also associated with its use.

Ch. 57 Abnormal Liver Scan, p 1164.

FALSE

B. Calcification is seen in only 10% of hepatomas. It occurs considerably more frequently in cholangiocarcinoma, gall bladder carcinoma, fibrolamellar variants and in children, hepatoblastoma.

Ch. 57 Malignant Lesions, p 1168.

FALSE

C. It has little to contribute diagnostically but may be useful in pre-operative assessment.

Ch. 57 p 1181.

FALSE

D. Lobar nonenhancement occurs after intravenous contrast medium administration only when there has been complete arterial and portal venous devascularization of that lobe. On CT arterial portography (CTAP), after contrast medium has been injected into the superior mesenteric artery and scanning performed during the venous phase, nonopacification of a lobe may be demonstrated if its portal venous supply has been obliterated.

Ch. 57 Malignant Lesions and Hepatocellular Carcinoma, p 1169.

FALSE

E. Tumour *invasion* into the portal circulation is thought to be specific for hepatoma; however, thrombosis may be caused by extrinsic compression (e.g., metastatic disease).

Ch. 57 Malignant Lesions and Hepatocellular Carcinoma, p 1169.

Q 5.6. *Features of a Liver Mass in a Young Adult Suggesting Fibrolamellar Hepatoma Include*

    A. Coexistent cirrhosis

    B. A fibrous central scar

    C. Central amorphous calcification

    D. Moderately raised alpha-fetoprotein

    E. Poor definition of the edges of the mass on CT

Q 5.7. *Regarding MRI of Liver Conditions*

    A. Hepatoma is made more conspicuous by the coexistence of cirrhosis

    B. Hepatic adenomas take up magnetic iron oxide particles (MIOPs)

    C. Dilated bile ducts are rendered more visible using a STIR sequence

    D. The fibrotic central scar of Focal nodular hyperplasia is hypo-intense on T1W and T2W images in 80% of cases

    E. Haemochromatosis causes a reduction in the MR signal on all sequences.

A 5.6. *Features of a Liver Mass in a Young Adult Suggesting Fibrolamellar Hepatoma Include*

FALSE   A. There are no known underlying risk factors for the development of this tumour.
Ch. 57 Malignant Lesions, and Hepatocellular Carcinoma, p 1169.

TRUE   B. This feature occurs most regularly in fibrolamellar hepatoma and focal nodular hyperplasia.
Ch. 57 Malignant Lesions and Hepatocellular Carcinoma, p 1169.

TRUE   C. Calcification in untreated hepatoma is unusual, whereas it occurs in up to 40% of fibrolamellar variants.
Ch. 57 Malignant Lesions and Hepatocellular Carcinoma, p 1169.

FALSE   D.
Ch. 57 Malignant Lesions and Hepatocellular Carcinoma, p 1169.

FALSE   E. Fibrolamellar hepatoma is often completely or at least partially encapsulated. Contrast enhancement is variable.
Ch. 57 Malignant Lesions and Hepatocellular Carcinoma, p 1168.

A 5.7. *Regarding MRI of Liver Conditions*

FALSE   A. Both hepatoma and cirrhosis prolong T1 and T2 leading to a net loss in lesion contrast.
Ch. 57 Magnetic Resonance Imaging of the Liver, p 1175.

FALSE   B. Kupffer cells in the normal liver (and focal nodular hyperplasia) take up this intravenous contrast agent and signal strength is correspondingly reduced. This feature improves the conspicuity of lesions which do not incorporate iron oxide particles (e.g., adenomas and hepatomas).
Ch. 57 Magnetic Resonance Imaging of the Liver, p 1174.

TRUE   C. The high water content of bile gives biliary ducts a very high signal on STIR sequences. This allows their accurate distinction from portal venous radicles.
Ch. 57 Metastases, p 1175.

FALSE   D. Oedema within the scar generates hyperintensity on T_2W images in most cases.
Ch. 57 Focal Nodular Hyperplasia, p 1176.

TRUE   E.
Ch. 57 Haemachromatosis, p 1177.

Q *5.8. Regarding the Radiological Investigation of the Biliary Tract*

    A. On CT an accessory hepatic artery appears as soft tissue imme-
diately posterior to the portal vein

    B. Air seen within the biliary tree on CT indicates that adequate
biliary drainage is present

    C. A true lateral radiograph after maximal opacification of the
biliary tree is mandatory during PTC

    D. During PTC, a dilated segment II duct is the most appropriate
one to target using an ultrasound-guided approach

    E. PTC with a sheathed needle has a reduced risk of complica-
tions because a second puncture is often rendered unnecessary

Q *5.9. Causes of a Diffusely Thickened Gall Bladder Wall on Ultrasound Include*

    A. Viral Hepatitis

    B. Heart failure

    C. Cirrhosis

    D. Acalculous cholecystitis

    E. AIDS

A 5.8. *Regarding the Radiological Investigation of the Biliary Tract*

TRUE   A. Some liver surgeons request pre-operative angiography reliably to demonstrate this variant, although it is regularly seen on contrast-enhanced CT. The differential diagnosis of soft tissue in this location on unenhanced CT includes the papillary process of the caudate lobe and lymphadenopathy.
Ch. 58 Anatomical Considerations; The Vessels, p 1203.

FALSE   B. Such a finding on a plain film or CT study implies that there is a communication between the bowel lumen and the biliary tree. It does not permit quantification of the degree of that communication and is not a measure of the adequacy of biliary drainage.
Ch. 58 The Plain Abdominal Radiograph, p 1206.

TRUE   C. This is to ensure that the anterior and posterior ducts have been opacified. It is easy to miss posterior sectoral duct obstruction, if a lateral film is not routinely taken.
Ch. 58 Percutaneous Transhepatic Cholangiography, p 1210.

FALSE   D. The segment III duct lies anteriorly and is the one most appropriate to this technique.
Ch. 58 Percutaneous Transhepatic Cholangiography, p 1210.

FALSE   E. The greater diameter of a sheathed needle is felt to be responsible for the higher incidence of complications seen with such a needle in comparison with a Chiba needle.
Ch. 58 Percutaneous Transhepatic Cholangiography, p 1211.

A 5.9. *Causes of a Diffusely Thickened Gall Bladder Wall on Ultrasound Include*

TRUE   A. This is reportedly present in 80% of cases.
Ch. 58 Ultrasonography and the Gall Bladder, p 1214.

TRUE   B. Due to oedema.
Ch. 58 Ultrasonography and the Gall Bladder, p 1214.

TRUE   C. Due to fluid overload/hypoalbuminaemia.
Ch. 58 Ultrasonography and the Gall Bladder, p 1214.

TRUE   D. A helpful sign that is not always present.
Ch. 58 Ultrasonography and the Gall Bladder, p 1214.

TRUE   E. Gall bladder wall thickening is a common finding in this condition. Cytomegalovirus (CMV) and Cryptosporidium infection cause cholangitis in AIDS patients.
Ch. 58 Ultrasonography and the Gall Bladder, p 1214.

Q *5.10. Regarding Biliary Scintigraphy in Acute Cholecystitis*

A. Intestinal activity is seen within 60 minutes in 80% of normal subjects given ^{99m}Tc-HIDA

B. In acute cholecystitis, the cystic duct is almost always obstructed

C. A diagnosis of acute cholecystitis after an IV injection of ^{99m}Tc-HIDA scanning requires that the liver parenchyma and intrahepatic biliary radicles be visualized

D. In the context of non-visualization of the gall bladder, radionuclide activity seen adjacent to but outside the lumen of the common duct implies a leak

E. Pretreatment with cholecystokinin analogue is useful for the detection of chronic cholecystitis

A 5.10. *Regarding Biliary Scintigraphy in Acute Cholecystitis*

TRUE   A. Intravenous cholecystokinin can precipitate intestinal activity in the remaining 20% of normal subjects.
Ch. 58 Radionuclide Studies, p 1217.

TRUE   B. This is usually due to oedema rather than stone impaction. Visualization of the gall bladder excludes acute cholecystitis with a specificity in excess of 95%.
Ch. 58 Radionuclide Studies, p 1217.

TRUE   C. Demonstration of the liver and intrahepatic biliary radicles is required to substantiate focal pathology in the gall bladder because diffuse hepatic dysfunction may result in non-visualization of the gall bladder.
Ch. 58 Radionuclide Studies, p 1217.

FALSE   D. A variable length of cystic duct may remain patent and in communication with the common hepatic duct if calculous obstruction is located in the neck of the gall bladder. This appears as a "nubbin" of activity close to the common duct.
Ch. 58 Radionuclide Studies, p 1217.

FALSE   E. This agent, by promoting emptying, reduces the likelihood of detecting abnormal function in a chronically diseased gall bladder.
Ch. 58 Radionuclide Studies, p 1218.

Q 5.11. *Concerning the Radiology of Biliary Disease*

A. The most common enteric site of impaction of a gall stone is the duodenojejunal flexure

B. The demonstration of a dilated intrahepatic biliary tree is essential to the definitive diagnosis of obstructive jaundice

C. Multiple intra- and extra-hepatic strictures on ERCP are seen exclusively in sclerosing cholangitis

D. Chronic Ascaris lumbricoides infection is associated with bile duct cancer

E. Atrophy of a lobe of liver occurs as a sequel to portal venous obstruction by tumour

Q 5.12. *Regarding Pancreatic Pathology*

A. Fatty replacement of the pancreas occurs in cystic fibrosis

B. There is an association between multiple pancreatic cysts, von Hippel Lindau syndrome and a raised red cell count

C. At least 50% of pancreatic pseudocysts resolve spontaneously without clinical sequelae

D. Acute massive bleeding in a patient with a history of pancreatitis is almost always caused by varices secondary to splenic or mesenteric vein occlusion

E. Most pancreatic cancers are irresectable at the time of diagnosis

A 5.11. Concerning the Radiology of Biliary Disease

FALSE
A. The ileo-caecal valve, the narrowest part of the small bowel, is the most common site of stone impaction leading to gallstone obstructive ileus.
Ch. 58 Complications of Gallstones and Gall Bladder Inflammation, p 1223.

FALSE
B. Very early biliary obstruction and primary sclerosing cholangitis are included in the list of conditions in which biliary obstruction is present, but the biliary tree is not dilated.
Ch. 58 The Bile Ducts, p 1225.

FALSE
C. Extensive cholangiocarcinoma and chronic infection are capable of mimicking the appearances of sclerosing cholangitis.
Ch. 58 Primary Sclerosing Cholangitis, p 1228.

FALSE
D. A chronic inflammatory response occurs with this infection, associated with recurrent acute cholangitis and a propensity to develop granulomatous strictures. Unlike the situation obtained in Clonorchis sinensis and Opisthorchis viverrini infections, however, malignancy is not an associated sequel.
Ch. 58 Biliary Parasites, p 1231.

TRUE
E. Portal venous obstruction, biliary obstruction, or both, can cause atrophy of the related lobe or segment.
Ch. 58 Atrophy, p 1227.

A 5.12. Regarding Pancreatic Pathology

TRUE
A. This is accompanied by ductal calcification, cysts, strictures and attenuation of the main pancreatic duct.
Ch. 61 Congenital Abnormalities, p 1274.

TRUE
B. Twenty percent of patients with haemangioblastoma of the cerebellum have a raised red cell count owing to the elaboration of erythropoietin. This cerebellar tumour is associated with simple pancreatic cysts in Von Hippel Lindau disease.
Ch. 61 Congenital Abnormalities, p 1274.

TRUE
C. The symptomatic ones that fail to resolve may be drained percutaneously.
Ch. 61 Pancreatitis, p 1277.

FALSE
D. Massive bleeding secondary to pancreatitis is often the result of a ruptured arterial pseudoaneurysm.
Ch. 61 Pancreatitis, p 1277.

TRUE
E. A substantial majority at the time of diagnosis have local extension, contiguous organ invasion, distant metastases and vascular invasion, all indications of irresectability.
Ch. 61 Pancreatic Neoplasms, p 1283.

Q 5.13. Ectopic ACTH is Produced by the Following Tumours

A. Small cell tumour of the lung

B. Thymic carcinoid tumours

C. Phaeochromocytoma

D. Medullary carcinoma of the thyroid

E. Carcinosarcoma of the oesophagus

Q 5.14. Regarding the Radiology of Pituitary Tumours

A. Twenty percent of normal people have a 3 mm or greater focal area of low attenuation on CT of the pituitary

B. Eighty to 90% of microadenomas are hypointense on T1W images

C. MRI is highly accurate at detecting cavernous sinus invasion by pituitary adenoma

D. The pituitary fossa is enlarged on skull radiography in 80% of cases of both acromegaly and Cushing's syndrome

E. In young patients, the majority of craniopharyngiomas are cystic and calcified

A 5.13. *Ectopic ACTH is Produced by the Following Tumours*

TRUE A. This is the most common cause of ectopic ACTH production
Ch. 62 Radiological Techniques, p 1297.

TRUE B.
Ch. 62 Radiological Techniques, p 1297.

TRUE C.
Ch. 62 Radiological Techniques, p 1297.

TRUE D.
Ch. 62 Radiological Techniques, p 1297.

FALSE E.
Ch. 62 Radiological Techniques, p 1297.

A 5.14. *Regarding the Radiology of Pituitary Tumours*

TRUE A. An even larger number of focal abnormalities are seen in normal glands on MRI
Ch. 62 The Pituitary Gland, p 1300.

TRUE B. Thirty to 50% are also hyperintense on T2W images.
Ch. 62 Hyperpituitarism, p 1300.

FALSE C. Unfortunately, this is not the case. CT fares no better in the detection of this ominous feature.
Ch. 62 Hyperpituitarism, p 1300.

FALSE D. Correct for acromegaly. Few cases of Cushing's syndrome have an enlarged pituitary fossa.
Ch. 62 Hyperpituitarism, p 1300.

TRUE E. Calcification is common in patients under 20 years of age. A second peak occurs in the fifties when calcification is seen in approximately 50% of cases. Cysts may have a higher density than CSF on CT, owing to haemorrhage, and hyperintensity on T1W images, owing to their cholesterol content.
Ch. 62 Other Pituitary Lesions, p 1301.

Q *5.15. Regarding the Radiology of Thyroid Disorders*

    A. Both papillary and follicular thyroid carcinomas accumulate ^{131}Iodide

    B. Hyperplastic nodules are often coarsely calcified and surrounded by a hyporeflective halo on ultrasound

    C. When ectopic thyroid tissue is demonstrated thyroid tissue is rarely found in the normal site

    D. Widening of the intervertebral disc spaces occurs in juvenile myxoedema

    E. A solitary nodule within the thyroid in a thyrotoxic patient is almost always benign

Q *5.16. Regarding Thyroid Scintigraphy*

    A. Almost all thyroid cancers are cold on ^{123}Iodide scanning

    B. A rapidly growing cold nodule in Hashimoto's disease is likely to be a thyroid carcinoma

    C. Sixty to 70% of euthyroid patients with autonomous nodules become hyperthyroid within six years

    D. Hyperthyroidism rarely occurs before a nodule has reached 3 cm in diameter

    E. Hashimoto's thyroiditis regularly causes the thyroid to triple in size

A 5.15. *Regarding the Radiology of Thyroid Disorders*

TRUE   A. This is also true of their metastases that may otherwise be difficult to detect in neck, mediastinum or bone.
Ch. 62 Thyroid Disorders, p 1303.

TRUE   B. This is a typical ultrasound appearance, the non-calcified areas being isoreflective with the normal thyroid.
Ch. 62 Thyroid Disorders, p 1303.

TRUE   C.
Ch. 62 Thyroid Gland, p 1302.

TRUE   D. Other spinal features are kyphosis, flattened vertebral bodies and "bullet-shaped" vertebral bodies at L1 and L2.
Ch. 62 Thyroid Disorders, p 1302.

TRUE   E.
Ch. 62 Thyroid Disorders, p 1302.

A 5.16. *Regarding Thyroid Scintigraphy*

TRUE   A. In order for a thyroid nodule to accumulate Iodide, it requires a high degree of differentiation, which is found in few cancers.
Ch. 62 Nodules, p 1305.

FALSE   B. Lymphoma presents in this way.
Ch. 62 Nodules, p 1305.

FALSE   C. Ten to 20% become hyperthyroid, half of whom exhibit T3 toxicosis.
Ch. 62 Nodules, p 1305.

TRUE   D.
Ch. 62 Nodules, p 1305.

FALSE   E. Tender and firm enlargement to less than double the normal size is the usual outcome.
Ch. 62 Generalised Disorders, p 1305.

Q *5.17. Regarding Parathyroid Disease*

    A. Carcinoma is responsible for 25% of primary cases of hyperparathyroidism

    B. Prolonged hypocalcaemia is responsible for the development of tertiary hyperparathyroidism

    C. Generalized subperiosteal bone resorption of the phalanges may be caused by sarcoidosis

    D. The skeleton is usually normal in hypoparathyroidism

    E. Short fourth and fifth metacarpals occur in pseudo-pseudohypoparathyroidism

Q *5.18. Concerning the Thymus Gland*

    A. Diffuse thymic enlargement occurs in thyrotoxicosis

    B. Forty to 60% of thymomas have associated myasthenia gravis

    C. Forty to 60% of caucasian patients with myasthenia gravis have a thymoma

    D. In 60-80% of myasthenic patients with thymoma, the tumour can be seen on frontal chest radiography

    E. Pleural secondaries are associated with thymoma

A 5.17. *Regarding Parathyroid Disease*

FALSE   *A.* A single adenoma accounts for 80% and hyperplasia for 15%. Carcinoma causes only 4% of cases of hyperparathyroidism, the remainder being due to double adenomas.
Ch. 62 Hyperparathyroidism, p 1307.

TRUE   *B.* Parathyroid hyperplasia is a result of hypocalcaemia. However, if the duration of the hypercalcaemia is prolonged (e.g., in renal failure) an autonomous adenoma may form: this is tertiary hyperparathyroidism.
Ch. 62 Hyperparathyroidism, p 1307.

FALSE   *C.* A single phalanx may have this radiographic change in sarcoidosis but *generalized* subperiosteal bone resorption is virtually pathognomonic of hyperparathyroidism.
Ch. 62 Hyperparathyroidism, p 1307.

TRUE   *D.* The main radiological feature is soft-tissue calcification—intracerebral, periarticular and subcutaneous.
Ch. 62 Hyperparathyroidism, p 1307.

TRUE   *E.* This feature occurs with normal biochemistry in pseudo-pseudohypoparathyroidism.
Ch. 62 Hyperparathyroidism, p 1307.

A 5.18. *Concerning the Thymus Gland*

TRUE   *A.* This may be confused with lymphadenopathy on the CXR.
Ch. 62 Disorders of the Thymus, p 1310.

TRUE   *B.*
Ch. 62 Disorders of the Thymus, p 1311.

FALSE   *C.* Approximately 15% of myasthenic patients in the Western world have this tumour. Thirty-five percent of Oriental patients have a thymoma.
Ch. 62 Disorders of the Thymus, p 1311.

TRUE   *D.* If a tumour cannot be shown on CXR, it will be identified on CT as a small anterior superior mediastinal mass. CT identification is straightforward in an atrophic gland, but may be difficult in a young patient.
Ch. 62 Radiological Features of the Normal and Abnormal Thymus, p 1311.

TRUE   *E.*
Ch. 62 Radiological Features of the Normal and Abnormal Thymus, p 1311.

Q 5.19. *Regarding Pancreatic Neuroendocrine Tumours*

A. Insulinomas are virtually never extrapancreatic

B. More than 75% of patients with Gastrinomas have ulcers in atypical locations

C. Less than 10% of insulinomas are malignant

D. Glucagonoma is most often a malignant tumour that is readily visible on CT at the time of diagnosis

E. Somatostatinoma produces the clinical triad of diabetes mellitus, diarrhoea and venous thrombosis

Q 5.20. *The Following Features of Adrenal Gland Imaging are Correct*

A. The medial limb of the right adrenal is normally larger than the lateral limb

B. Calcification in the adrenal glands is usually related to Addison's disease

C. The radiological investigation of Addison's disease usually reveals glands that are normal in appearance

D. The most common radiological abnormality in non-iatrogenic adult Cushing's syndrome is bilateral adrenal hyperplasia

E. Tumours which cause Conn's syndrome are usually larger than 5 cm at the time of diagnosis

A 5.19. *Regarding Pancreatic Neuroendocrine Tumours*

TRUE A. The majority are found in the distal two thirds of the pancreas.
Ch. 62 Functioning Tumours of the Pancreas, p 1313.

FALSE B. Only 25% of patients with gastrinoma have ulcers in atypical locations.
Ch. 62 Functioning Tumours of the Pancreas, p 1313.

TRUE C. About 90% are solitary adenomas.
Ch. 62 Functioning Tumours of the Pancreas, p 1313.

TRUE D. This tumour is malignant in 60% of cases and is usually 4-7 cm in diameter at the time of diagnosis.
Ch. 62 Functioning Tumours of the Pancreas, p 1314.

FALSE E. *Glucagonoma* produces diarrhoea, diabetes mellitus, necrolytic rash, stomatitis and venous thrombosis. *Somatostatinoma* produces steatorrhoea, diabetes mellitus and gallstones by its inhibitory action on pancreatic exocrine and endocrine function and by the inhibition of gall bladder contraction.
Ch. 62 Functioning Tumours of the Pancreas, p 1314.

A 5.20. *The Following Features of Adrenal Gland Imaging are Correct*

TRUE A. Of the two posteriorly orientated limbs, the medial is the larger.
Ch. 62 The Adrenal Glands, p 1315.

FALSE B. Calcification is more often an incidental finding than an indicator of Addison's disease.
Ch. 62 Hyposecretion Disorders, p 1316.

TRUE C. As auto-immune disease is now the commonest cause of this disorder, no radiological changes are usually detectable. Occasionally, long-standing cases are seen to have atrophic glands. Enlarged glands are seen in haemorrhage and acute infection by TB, Histoplasmosis and Blastomycosis. Calcification may be seen in TB of the adrenals.
Ch. 62 Hyposecretion Disorders, p 1316.

TRUE D. The most common non-iatrogenic cause in adults is a primary hypothalamic-pituitary disorder (e.g., pituitary adenoma), which is small and does not usually enlarge the sella, associated with excessive ACTH release and consequent adrenal hyperplasia. In children the commonest non-iatrogenic cause is an adrenal carcinoma.
Ch. 62 Hypersecretion Disorders, p 1316.

FALSE E. The tumours tend to be small—typically 5-20 mm in diameter. They have a high fat content that renders them less dense than normal adrenal tissue on CT scanning.
Ch. 62 Hypersecretion Disorders, p 1316.

Q 5.21. *Regarding Phaeochromocytoma*

A. The most common extra-adrenal sites are the renal hilum and the organ of Zuckerandl

B. Calcification is present in about 10%

C. The presence of fat attenuation within an adrenal tumour strongly suggests an alternative diagnosis

D. ^{131}I-MIBG is used to localise metastatic disease

E. There is an association with angiomyolipoma

A 5.21. *Regarding Phaeochromocytoma*

TRUE

A. Ninety-five percent of these tumours are intra-abdominal, but they may occur anywhere in the sympathetic nervous system from the skull base to the bladder.
Ch. 62 Hypersecretion Disorders, p 1317.

TRUE

B. The "rule of tens" in Phaeochromocytoma is: 10% are multiple/bilateral, 10% are calcified, 10% are malignant, 10% are familial and 10% are extra-adrenal.
Ch. 62 Hypersecretion Disorders, p 1317.

TRUE

C. Fat is virtually diagnostic of a myelolipoma.
Ch. 62 Hypersecretion Disorders, p 1317.

TRUE

D. ^{123}I-MIBG is used to locate those phaeochromocytomas that are invisible on CT and MRI. Concentration of MIBG allows metastatic tumour to be selectively irradiated using ^{131}I-MIBG.
Ch. 62 Methods of Investigation, p 1318.

TRUE

E. Tuberous sclerosis is an association of both phaeochromocytoma and angiomyolipoma, as are the other neuroectodermal disorders: neurofibromatosis and Von Hippel Lindau disease. Familial phaeochromocytoma occurs also in isolation. Further associations are multiple endocrine neoplasia (MEN) types 2a and 2b.
Ch. 62 Hypersecretion Disorders, p 1316.

Q *5.22. Regarding Polycystic Ovary Syndrome*

A. Normal-sized ovaries rule out the diagnosis

B. The ovarian shape in this syndrome is spherical

C. The cysts are well demonstrated on CT

D. Unopposed chronic oestrogen stimulation of the uterus pre-disposes to endometrial carcinoma

E. About 25% of patients with the syndrome demonstrate no ovarian cysts

Q *5.23. Regarding the Radiology of the Male Reproductive System*

A. Varicocele is left-sided in about 60% of cases

B. Percutaneous embolization of the varicocele by direct puncture of the scrotal sac is the treatment of choice

C. The risk of malignancy in an undescended testis is roughly proportional to its degree of failure of descent

D. Primary impotence is due to vascular disease in 80% of cases

E. Angioplasty of the venous outflow obstruction is the treatment of choice of priapism

A 5.22. *Regarding Polycystic Ovary Syndrome*

FALSE   A. The ovaries have a normal size (and volume) in 30% of cases.
Ch. 62 Endocrine Disorders, p 1319.

TRUE   B. The ovaries lose their normal ovoid shape and become enlarged and spherical.
Ch. 62 Endocrine Disorders, p 1319.

FALSE   C. CT is unable to resolve the multiple small (5 mm or so) cysts that occur in this condition. Transvaginal ultrasound is the most sensitive diagnostic method.
Ch. 62 Endocrine Disorders, p 1320.

TRUE   D.
Ch. 62 Endocrine Disorders, p 1319.

TRUE   E. In these patients, the combination of large volume ovaries (larger than 14 ml) with the appropriate clinical signs suggests the diagnosis.
Ch. 62 Endocrine Disorders, p 1319.

A 5.23. *Regarding the Radiology of the Male Reproductive System*

FALSE   A. It is left-sided in 90%, bilateral in 10%. Isolated right-sided varicocele is very rare.
Ch. 62 Infertility, p 1320.

FALSE   B. The optimal method is transvenous embolization from a right common femoral vein approach, with placement of the catheter tip far distally in the testicular vein—ideally in the inguinal canal region.
Ch. 62 Infertility, p 1320.

TRUE   C. The most common malignancy in an undescended testis is seminoma and on average the risk of this occurring in cryptorchidism is about fifty times normal.
Ch. 62 Cryptorchidism, p 1321.

TRUE   D. Arterial dysplasia has been shown to be present in the majority of cases of primary impotence. Psychogenic factors are now thought to be less important.
Ch. 62 Impotence and Priapism, p 1321.

FALSE   E. The venous outflow type is not amenable to interventional radiological techniques. The rare high-inflow type may respond to selective transcatheter embolization of distal internal pudendal artery.
Ch. 62 Impotence and Priapism, p 1321.

6

The Genitourinary Tract

Q *6.1. Regarding the Appropriate Investigation of Urinary Tract Disorders*

    A. Ascending urethrography: posterior urethral valves

    B. Renal USS: renal scarring

    C. Transvaginal USS: visualization of the bladder neck

    D. MRI: staging of pelvic malignancy

    E. Testicular arteriography: undescended testes

A *6.1. Regarding the Appropriate Investigation of Urinary Tract Disorders*

FALSE   *A.* The method of examination for the investigation of posterior urethral valves is the *micturating cystogram*. Ascending studies will not demonstrate valves, as the latter only obstruct urinary flow when the stream is passing in the conventional direction.
Ch. 63 MCU, p 1329.

FALSE   *B.* Renal USS is notoriously inaccurate in the diagnosis of renal scarring in comparison with DMSA scans.

TRUE   *C.* Transrectal or transvaginal USS and urodynamic studies of the bladder neck are helpful in the diagnosis of bladder/bladder neck dysfunction.
Ch. 63 Ultrasound, p 1330.

TRUE   *D.* MRI is now regarded by many as the method of choice for the staging of pelvic tumours and gynaecological malignancy. MRI has little to offer in the imaging of the *upper* renal tract, though some studies suggest it may be helpful in the assessment of upper renal tract venous invasion in patients with a renal cell carcinoma.
Ch. 63 MRI, p 1331.

FALSE   *E.* The position of the origins of the testicular arteries can be extremely variable. The testicular *veins* drain to the IVC (right) and the left renal vein (left). Hence, they can be demonstrated more readily than the arteries and knowledge of their position, length and direction can be helpful in the assessment and management of patients with undescended testes.
Ch. 63 Venography, p 1332.

Q *6.2. Regarding the Intravenous Urogram*

A. Loss of the outline of a psoas muscle, which was demonstrable on a previous radiograph, is a good indicator for retroperitoneal pathology

B. A full-length, plain AXR should always include the bladder base and prostatic urethra

C. A 4-hour fluid restriction is recommended to increase the density of the pyelogram, prior to the IVU

D. A closely similar mass of iodine is found in 50 ml of omnipaque (iohexol) 350 and 60 ml of omnipaque (iohexol) 300 strength

E. The amount of iodine administered to a 70 kg patient for an IVU is approximately 21 gm

A 6.2. *Regarding the Intravenous Urogram*

FALSE A. This sign may point to retroperitoneal pathology but it is notoriously inaccurate. The psoas outline is not always visualized in normal individuals.
Ch. 63 Plain Abdominal Films, p 1327.

TRUE B. Without views of the lower tract, bladder and urethral calculi will always be missed.
Ch. 63 Plain Abdominal Films, p 1327.

FALSE C. Fluid restriction is no longer considered applicable as a patient would need to be severely dehydrated to effect any significant increase in the density of the pyelogram.
Ch. 63 Intravenous Urogram, p 1328.

TRUE D. Iohexol 350 = 350 mg/I/ml.
Therefore 50 ml of iohexol 350 = 17.5 gm of iodine.
Iohexol 300 = 300 mg I/ml.
Therefore 60 ml of iohexol 300 = 18 gm of iodine.
Ch. 63 Intravenous Urogram, p 1328.

TRUE E. 21 gm *not mgm*. A reasonable dose regime is 300 mgI/kg.
Therefore 70 kg × 300 = 21000 mg = 21 gm of iodine.
Basics.
Ch. 63 Intravenous Urogram, p 1328.

Q *6.3. Concerning the Static Renal Isotope Scan*

A. No radiopharmaceutical meets the requirements ideally necessary for a static scan

B. ^{99m}Tc DTPA is the conventional agent used for static imaging

C. After an injection of ^{99m}Tc DMSA, 50% of the isotope is secreted into the tubules in the first 3 hours

D. Images of the kidney should be obtained at 3-4 hours after the injection of ^{99m}Tc DMSA

E. SPECT (single photon emission computed tomography) may be helpful in the assessment of renal scars

A 6.3. *Concerning the Static Renal Isotope Scan*

TRUE

A. The ideal agent for a static scan should be taken up by the kidney, fixed within the renal parenchyma and not secreted.
Ch. 64 Static Renal Scan, p 1336.

FALSE

B. DTPA is a *dynamic* renal imaging agent. ^{99m}Tc DMSA (dimercaptosuccinic acid) is used for *static* imaging.
Ch. 64 Static Renal Scan, p 1336.

FALSE

C. Fifteen percent of ^{99m}Tc DMSA is excreted in the first 3 hours; of the remainder, 20% resides in the parenchyma of each kidney, principally in the proximal tubules.
Ch. 64 Static Renal Scan, p 1336.

TRUE

D. Ideally, anterior, posterior and oblique images should be obtained. Further images and delayed views may be necessary if there is any history of obstruction.
Ch. 64 Static Renal Scan, p 1336.

TRUE

E. SPECT is not routinely performed in patients with suspected renal scarring, though it may be helpful in selected cases.
Ch. 64 Static Renal Scan, p 1336.

Q 6.4. *Concerning the Dynamic Renal Scan*

A. ^{99m}Tc DTPA is handled by glomerular filtration in the same way as inulin

B. ^{99m}Tc MAG-3 is eliminated almost exclusively by tubular excretion

C. Total renal blood flow should be assessed from the first pass images

D. An indirect micturating cystogram should be performed in children under one year using ^{99m}Tc DTPA (or MAG-3) if there is a history of vesico-ureteric reflux

E. A prolonged transit of tracer, after the administration of captopril, is a typical finding in patients with renal artery stenosis

Q 6.5. *Regarding Renal Tract Investigations Undertaken with the Stated Radionuclide Tests*

A. Divided renal function: ^{99m}Tc DTPA at 2 minutes

B. Renovascular hypertension: ^{99m}Tc DTPA captopril stress test

C. Renal transit time: ^{51}Cr EDTA

D. Intrarenal distribution of function: ^{99m}Tc DMSA with or without SPECT

E. Vesico-ureteric reflux: ^{99m}Tc pertechnetate

A 6.4. *Concerning the Dynamic Renal Scan*

TRUE   A. As ^{99m}Tc DTPA is handled in the same way as inulin, it can be used for simultaneous measurement of the GFR.
Ch. 64 Dynamic Renal Scan, p 1334.

FALSE   B. ^{99m}Tc MAG-3 is excreted by both glomerular filtration and tubular excretion.
Ch. 64 Dynamic Renal Scan, p 1334.

TRUE   C.
Ch. 64 Dynamic Renal Scan, p 1334.

FALSE   D. An indirect MCUG is an excellent and quantitative method for assessing vesico-ureteric reflux. Time-activity curves are measured over the bladder, ureters and kidneys. From these data, reflux and bladder emptying rates can be calculated. This technique, however, can only be undertaken in the child that is continent; children under the age of one year require a *direct* cystogram to assess reflux or a contrast micturating cystogram.
Ch. 64 Dynamic Renal Scan, p 1334.

TRUE   E. Associated with the prolonged transit time, there is a decreased uptake of tracer. These are the typical features of functionally significant renal stenosis in most patients.
Ch. 64 Dynamic Renal Scan, p 1334.

A 6.5. *Regarding Renal Tract Investigations Undertaken with the Stated Radionuclide Tests*

TRUE   A.
Ch. 64 Table 64.1, p 1335.

TRUE   B.
Ch. 64 Table 64.1, p 1335.

FALSE   C. The correct isotope is Tc ^{99m} DTPA with deconvolution analysis.
Ch. 64 Table 64.1, p 1335.

TRUE   D.
Ch. 64 Table 64.1, p 1335.

TRUE   E.
Ch. 64 Table 64.1, p 1335.

Q *6.6 Regarding the Investigation of Urinary Incontinence*

A. During cystometrography of a patient with cystitis, no significant rise in intrinsic bladder pressure occurs during filling

B. Reversible bladder instability occurs in bladder outflow obstruction

C. Cystography allows mechanical sphincter problems to be distinguished from bladder instability

D. Stress incontinence in men suggests post-traumatic external sphincter damage

E. The "stop-test" assesses the independent working of the internal and external sphincters

A 6.6 *Regarding the Investigation of Urinary Incontinence*

TRUE   A. In a stable bladder, this is the case. Only when voluntary initiation of voiding occurs does the detrusor muscle contract.
Ch. 65 Detrusor Instability, p 1341.

TRUE   B. At least half of patients with prostatic obstruction have unstable bladders. Following prostatectomy, bladder instability often gradually resolves.
Ch. 65 Detrusor Instability, p 1342.

FALSE   C. Bladder instability requires detrusor muscle pressure measurements for its diagnosis.
Ch. 65 Urinary Incontinence, p 1343.

TRUE   D. Weakness of the female bladder neck occurs in pregnancy and childbirth, and a rise in intra-abdominal pressure above that of the urethra is all that is required to allow leakage. Stress incontinence in men is very rare in the absence of previous trauma.
Ch. 65 Urinary Incontinence, p 1343.

TRUE   E. This test normally demonstrates a rise in detrusor pressure which then falls slowly. There is also "milk-back" of urine from the urethra back into the bladder. The latter feature is deficient when the bladder neck mechanism is at fault. If both sphincters are incompetent, the patient is completely unable to prevent the leakage of urine.
Ch. 65 Urinary Incontinence, p 1343.

Q 6.7. *Concerning Changes in the Urinary Tract During Pregnancy*

    A. The ureters dilate throughout their length

    B. Dilatation is greater on the left than the right

    C. Dilation of the ureters may persist long after the pregnancy

    D. Prolonged dilatation is not associated with an increased incidence of re-infection

    E. Ovarian vein syndrome is pain in the right iliolumbar nerve ascribed to pressure from an aberrant right ovarian vein

Q 6.8. *Regarding Typical Features of Renal TB*

    A. Renal cavities that do not communicate with the collecting system

    B. Fibrotic strictures that can produce caliceal dilatation

    C. Bladder wall thickening with calcification

    D. A long-term increased risk of developing renal cell carcinoma

    E. USS is more sensitive in the detection of the early changes of this disorder than excretory urography

A 6.7. *Concerning Changes in the Urinary Tract During Pregnancy*

FALSE   A. Dilation is typically limited to the ureter above the pelvic brim.
Ch. 66 Pregnancy/Infection Dilation of the Ureter, p 1366.

FALSE   B. Dilation is typically asymmetrical and more marked on the right.
Ch. 66 Pregnancy/Infection Dilation of the Ureter, p 1366.

TRUE   C. In the great majority of these patients, there is also a history of urinary tract infection.
Ch. 66 Pregnancy/Infection Dilation of the Ureter, p 1366.

TRUE   D. Patients do complain of increased pain from the dilated system, but there is no increased incidence of re-infection.
Ch. 66 Pregnancy/Infection Dilation of the Ureter, p 1366.

FALSE   E. Ovarian vein syndrome has been described as pain and dilation of the right *ureter* caused by pressure from the dilated ovarian vein. There is extensive literature on this subject, some of which does not support the existence of the "ovarian vein syndrome" (*"The jury is still out"*).
Ch. 66 Pregnancy/Infection Dilation of the Ureter, p 1366.

A 6.8. *Regarding Typical Features of Renal TB*

FALSE   A. Cavities are the most typical lesions seen in renal TB. They do, however, communicate with the collecting system, but the communication may be narrow or difficult to demonstrate.
Ch. 66 Renal TB, p 1359.

TRUE   B. Strictures may produce widespread dilatation or localized pelvicaliceal dilation (hydrocalicosis).
Ch. 66 Renal TB, p 1359.

FALSE   C. Bladder wall thickening does occur, but it is uncommon to see calcification within it. The causes of bladder calcification include cyclophosphamide-induced cystitis, radiotherapy, schistosomiasis, TB, transitional cell carcinoma (focal) and amyloidosis.
Ch. 66 Renal TB, p 1359.

FALSE   D.

FALSE   E. USS shows the changes of advanced TB, but urography remains more sensitive even at this stage of the disease.
Ch. 66 Renal TB, p 1359.

Q 6.9. The Following are Recognised Causes of Renal Papillary Necrosis

    A. Non-steroidal anti-inflammatory drugs

    B. Medullary sponge kidney

    C. Obstetric shock

    D. Renal obstruction without infection

    E. Syphilis

Q 6.10. The Following are Signs of Papillary Necrosis on the IVU

    A. "Egg-in-a-cup" appearance

    B. Truncated calices

    C. Tracks and horns from the calices

    D. Kohler's teardrop

    E. Ring shadows in the calices

A 6.9. *The Following are Recognised Causes of Renal Papillary Necrosis*

TRUE   A. Typically phenacetin produces renal papillary necrosis, but NSAIDs and their derivatives are also associated with this disorder.
Ch. 66 Papillary Necrosis, p 1358.

FALSE   B.

FALSE   C. Obstetric shock can produce acute *cortical necrosis*. Ischaemia is important in the development of papillary necrosis, and in most, but not all, cases is a common aetiological factor.
Ch. 66 Acute Cortical Necrosis, p 1358.

FALSE   D. Obstruction *per se* does not produce papillary necrosis, though obstruction with infection can produce papillary sloughing.
Ch. 66 Papillary Necrosis, p 1358.

FALSE   E.

A 6.10. *The Following are Signs of Papillary Necrosis on the IVU*

TRUE   A.
Ch. 66 Fig. 66.10, p 1356.

FALSE   B.
Ch. 66 Fig. 66.10, p 1356.

TRUE   C.
Ch. 66 Fig. 66.10, p 1356.

FALSE   D. This normal sign is found on the AP radiograph of the hip.

TRUE   E.
Ch. 66 Fig. 66.10, p 1356.

Q *6.11. The Following are Associated with No Papillary/Caliceal Abnormality and Focal Cortical Loss as Demonstrated on IVU*

    A. Glomerulonephritis

    B. Chronic atrophic pyelonephritis

    C. Acute cortical necrosis

    D. Acute pyelonephritis

    E. Secondary amyloidosis

A 6.11. *The Following are Associated with No Papillary/Caliceal Abnormality and Focal Cortical Loss as Demonstrated on IVU*

TRUE

A. There is generalised damage to the glomeruli. The only abnormality seen on the IVU is a change in size of the kidneys that is symmetrical.
Ch. 66 Glomerulonephritis, p 1356.

FALSE

B. The other term for this disorder is focal reflux nephropathy.
Ch. 66 Table 66.1, p 1356.

TRUE

C. The majority of cases are seen in acute obstetric shock. The renal damage is more severe than in acute tubular necrosis and the changes are irreversible. The principal radiological sign is cortical calcification, which can be demonstrated as early as three weeks.
Ch. 66 Acute Cortical Necrosis, p 1356.

TRUE

D. An IVU is rarely needed in these patients. The findings include focal or diffuse renal swelling, delayed or poor pelvicaliceal system filling and in some cases there may be a dense/persistent and striated nephrogram. These findings are only demonstrated in about 25% of patients.
Ch. 66 Acute Pyelonephritis, p 1357.

TRUE

E. Secondary amyloidosis is the most common form of renal amyloid (80% occurring in patients with chronic infection).
Ch. 66 Conditions Causing General Infiltration of the Renal Parenchyma, p 1357.

Q 6.12. *Regarding Renal Tuberculosis*

    A. Most renal lesions heal spontaneously

    B. The early radiological signs are indistinguishable from renal papillary necrosis

    C. Calcification is demonstrable in 70-80% of all patients on the plain AXR (abdominal radiograph)

    D. The bladder is the second commonest site of tuberculous calcification in the urinary tract

    E. Tuberculous autonephrectomy cannot be detected during the IVU

Q 6.13. *Regarding Renal Parenchymal Disease in Adults*

    A. USS is highly specific when there is increased corticomedullary differentiation

    B. USS has a sensitivity as low as 20% in the detection of parenchymal disease

    C. USS is a good indicator of the type of renal parenchymal disease

    D. Angiography is occasionally specific for certain types of renal parenchymal disease

    E. The changes are commonly asymmetrical

A 6.12. *Regarding Renal Tuberculosis*

TRUE

A. As renal TB is acquired from blood-borne infection, bilateral disease might be expected. This is not the case, as most lesions heal spontaneously so that only one or two lesions progress to a clinical or radiological abnormality. *Ch. 66 Renal TB, p 1359.*

TRUE

B. Although this statement is true, there are some helpful differentiating features, namely: TB is unilateral (if it is bilateral it is usually asymmetrical), and it produces a very irregular appearance to the calices. *Ch. 66 Renal TB, p 1359.*

FALSE

C. Renal calcification occurs in about 30% of cases, and occurs in caseous pyonephrosis and in the renal papillae. *Ch. 66 Renal TB, p 1359.*

FALSE

D. Calcification tends to progress caudally (i.e., from kidney to ureter) (and then, very occasionally, to the bladder). (Vide infra. schistosomiasis.) *Ch. 66 Renal TB, p 1359.*

FALSE

E. Tuberculous autonephrectomy appears as a dense, lobulated, calcified mass on the plain abdominal X-ray. The kidney may demonstrate some function on the IVU. *Ch. 66 Renal TB, p 1359.*

A 6.13. *Regarding Renal Parenchymal Disease in Adults*

TRUE

A.
Ch. 66 Renal Parenchymal Disease, p 1351.

TRUE

B.
Ch. 66 Renal Parenchymal Disease, p 1351.

FALSE

C.
Ch. 66 Renal Parenchymal Disease, p 1351.

TRUE

D. Polyarteritis nodosa is demonstrated by the presence of multiple small aneurysms of the intra-renal arteries. *Ch. 66 Renal Parenchymal Disease, p 1351.*

FALSE

E.
Ch. 66 Renal Parenchymal Disease, p 1351.

Q 6.14. *Concerning a Duplex or Partially Duplex Kidney*

    A. A bifid renal pelvis is present in no more than 1% of the population

    B. Minor ureteric duplication is present in about 20% of patients with duplex kidneys

    C. Partial duplication is associated with a hypertrophied column of Bertin

    D. A bifid renal system may have a similar appearance to renal TB

    E. Contralateral renal agenesis is an associated finding

Q 6.15. *Regarding Normal Intravenous Urography*

    A. A nephrogram may still be present 6 hours after the injection of contrast medium

    B. The renal length is between 11 and 16 cm in adults

    C. The left kidney is longer than the right by up to 2 cm

    D. The kidneys can move up to 6 cm between the phases of respiration

    E. A papillary blush

A 6.14. *Concerning a Duplex or Partially Duplex Kidney*

FALSE   A. Bifid renal pelves are demonstrated in 10% of IVUs.
Ch. 66 Excretion Urography, p 1352.

FALSE   B. 4%.
Ch. 66 Excretion Urography, p 1352.

TRUE   C. The duplex renal pseudo-tumour.
Ch. 66 Excretion Urography, p 1352.

TRUE   D. There is occasionally a "cut-off" in the mid-pole of the kidney that should not be mistaken for renal TB or a tumour.
Ch. 66 Excretion Urography, p 1352.

FALSE   E. No association.

A 6.15. *Regarding Normal Intravenous Urography*

TRUE   A. This occurs in about 1/3 of all patients, particularly when high doses are used.
Ch. 66 Excretion Urography, p 1352.

TRUE   B. The range of the size of the kidneys is wide. This measurement is only an approximation as other factors including magnification and angulation will affect the apparent size.
Ch. 66 Excretion Urography, p 1352.

TRUE   C.
Ch. 66 Excretion Urography, p 1352.

TRUE   D. A similar change in position can be demonstrated between the supine/erect positions.
Ch. 66 Excretion Urography, p 1352.

TRUE   E. This is commonly found in association with low osmolality contrast media and can be distinguished from medullary sponge kidney by the absence of the streaks or pools of contrast medium that occur in the latter.
Ch. 66 Excretion Urography, p 1352.

Q 6.16. *Regarding Intravenous Urography*

A. When the kidneys and ureters are obscured by bowel gas on the plain radiograph, a tomograph is essential

B. Tomograms should always be obtained prior to the injection of contrast medium, when the renal outlines cannot be visualized

C. The thickness of the renal substance is readily assessed on the routine IVU film series

D. The normal renal substance appears to be thicker at the poles on excretion urography

E. The notches of fetal lobation always lie between the papillae

Q 6.17. *Normal Imaging Features of the Kidney Include*

A. Lower echogenicity of the renal pyramids than the renal cortex on USS

B. Bright spots at the apices of the renal pyramids on USS

C. A lower limit of normal renal length of 9 cm as demonstrated on USS

D. Corticomedullary differentiation on the unenhanced CT scan

E. Increased contrast enhancement of a renal pseudotumour in comparison with the normal renal parenchymal enhancement

A 6.16. *Regarding Intravenous Urography*

TRUE
A. If the kidneys are not visualized, fine calculi can be missed. The failure to detect small calculi is the most common error in diagnosis on the IVU.
Ch. 66 Plain Film of the Abdomen, p 1352.

FALSE
B. The renal outlines are satisfactorily delineated after the injection of contrast medium; tomography, for the sole purpose of assessing the renal outlines, provides little useful information and only adds to the radiation dose received by the patient.
Ch. 66 Plain Film of the Abdomen, p 1352.

TRUE
C. The renal substance thickness is judged to be the distance from the surface of the kidney to the tips of the renal papillae.
Ch. 66 Excretion Urography, p 1352.

TRUE
D. This is a urographic artefact caused by the obliquity of the kidney.
Ch. 66 Excretion Urography, p 1353.

FALSE
E. This is not always so on intravenous urography.
Ch. 66 Excretion Urography, p 1353.

A 6.17. *Normal Imaging Features of the Kidney Include*

TRUE
A.
Ch. 66 Ultrasonography, p 1354.

FALSE
B. The bright spots represent the arcuate arteries that lie at the *bases* of the renal pyramids.
Ch. 66 Ultrasonography, p 1354.

TRUE
C. This length corresponds to an IVU length of 11-11.5 cm.
Ch. 66 Ultrasonography, p 1354.

FALSE
D. This is demonstrated only after intravenous contrast medium administration at about 1 minute.
Ch. 66 Computed Tomography, p 1355.

FALSE
E. All renal tissue has the same enhancement characteristics: this is a useful method for distinguishing between tumour and pseudotumour.
Ch. 66 Computed Tomography, p 1355.

Q 6.18. *Regarding Focal Reflux Nephropathy (FRN)*

A. The great majority of affected patients develop this condition in early adult life

B. The condition is usually progressive in adult life, when urinary infection is not controlled

C. A common clinical presentation in adult life is with hypertension

D. The urogram demonstrates renal scars as areas of focal loss of renal parenchyma with underlying renal deformity

E. Focal renal scars are commoner in the right kidney than the left kidney

Q 6.19. *Regarding Urinary Schistosomiasis*

A. It is very common on the west coast of Africa

B. It is caused by the ova descending from the kidney in the ureter and embedding in the bladder

C. The intermediate host is the snail

D. The worms incite a severe local inflammatory reaction

E. The calcified baldder is small and rigid and its function is impaired

A 6.18. *Regarding Focal Reflux Nephropathy (FRN)*

FALSE
    A. FRN usually develops in childhood as a consequence of reflux. A small number of cases develop in adult life in association with a neurogenic bladder.
Ch. 66 FRN, p 1363.

FALSE
    B. After childhood, the disease remains stable even with repeated urinary tract infections.
Ch. 66 FRN, p 1363.

TRUE
    C. Hypertension and infection are the most common modes of radiological and clinical presentation.
Ch. 66 FRN, p 1363.

TRUE
    D. These findings may involve the whole or part of the kidney.
Ch. 66 FRN, p 1363.

TRUE
    E. The upper poles are the most common region to be affected.
Ch. 66 FRN, p 1363.

A 6.19. *Regarding Urinary Schistosomiasis*

FALSE
    A. East Africa, the southern shores of the Mediterranean, Arabia and Asia.
Ch. 66 Bilharzia, p 1364.

FALSE
    B. The ova are deposited, via the vesical venous plexus, into the base of the bladder by the female worm.
Ch. 66 Bilharzia, p 1364.

TRUE
    C. The miracidia mature within the *ova* and escape into water. In the snail's liver, they mature into cercaria which enter man via the skin.
Ch. 66 Bilharzia, p 1364.

FALSE
    D. The worms are benign. The ova produce a severe reaction that produces oedema, inflammation and stricture formation.
Ch. 66 Bilharzia, p 1364.

FALSE
    E. The calcification lies within the submucosa and not the muscle, hence the bladder is not rigid and not functionally impaired.
Ch. 66 Bilharzia, p 1364.

Q *6.20. Regarding Fungal Infections of the Urinary Tract*

     A. *Candida albicans* is the most frequent fungal infection in diabetic patients

     B. The most common appearance is that of a fungus ball

     C. *Candida albicans* is a gas-forming organism

     D. Fungal infections may induce papillary necrosis

     E. *Candida albicans* can produce an echo-poor ball on USS, which may be indistinguishable from normal urine in the bladder

Q *6.21. Concerning Xanthogranulomatous Pyelonephritis (XGP)*

     A. There is a strong association with Pseudomonas infection

     B. In adults the focal form is commoner than the general form

     C. The diffuse general form is invariably associated with urinary obstruction

     D. CT demonstrates rounded, low-attenuation areas of soft-tissue density within the renal substance

     E. Breach of the renal capsule and extension into the perirenal spaces is more suggestive of a malignant renal neoplasm than XGP

A 6.20. *Regarding Fungal Infections of the Urinary Tract*

TRUE   *A.*
                Ch. 66 Fungal Infections, p 1365.

TRUE   *B.* The appearances are that of a round, shaggy, and sometimes laminated ball of fungus in the pelvis or bladder.
                Ch. 66 Fungal Infections, p 1365.

TRUE   *C.* Infection may produce air in the collecting system or bladder.
                Ch. 66 Fungal Infections, p 1365.

TRUE   *D.*
                Ch. 66 Fungal Infections, p 1365.

FALSE   *E.* The USS findings of Candida are those of a discrete echogenic ball.
                Ch. 66 Fungal Infections, p 1365.

A 6.21. *Concerning Xanthogranulomatous Pyelonephritis (XGP)*

FALSE   *A.* XGP is associated with Proteus infection and calculus disease.
                Ch. 66 XGP, p 1365.

FALSE   *B.* There are two forms of XGP: the focal form and the general form. The focal form of XGP produces an inflammatory reaction and can be indistinguishable from a renal tumour. This is the rarer form.
                Ch. 66 XGP, p 1365.

FALSE   *C.* XGP is seen in patients with calculus disease in the majority of cases. Obstruction is generally present, but not invariably so, and it is not a diagnostic feature of the disease.
                Ch. 66 XGP, p 1365.

TRUE   *D.* These are due to lipid within foam cells.
                Ch. 66 XGP, p 1365.

FALSE   *E.* The peri-renal spread is a major feature of XGP and may cause fistulae to the skin or neighbouring areas.
                Ch. 66 XGP, p 1365.

Q 6.22. *Regarding Urinary Tract Infections*

    A. Emphysematous pyelonephritis is often fatal

    B. Squamous metaplasia is replacement of the normal transitional epithelium by squamous epithelium, which may become keratinized

    C. Leukoplakia occurs on normal transitional cell epithelium

    D. Malakoplakia is a granulomatous infection

    E. There is a 60-70% association between pyeloureteritis cystica and urinary tract infections

Q 6.23. *Regarding the Plain Film Findings of Renal Masses*

    A. Renal Cell Carcinoma contains visible calcification in more than 30% of cases

    B. A fatty lucency within the renal contour is diagnostic of a renal lipoma

    C. Central calcification within a renal mass is suggestive of a benign aetiology

    D. Peripheral calcification is more likely to indicate a benign than a malignant lesion

    E. Xanthogranulomatous pyelonephritis does not occur in the absence of renal calculi

A 6.22. *Regarding Urinary Tract Infections*

TRUE   A. This disease is most frequently seen in diabetic patients. The most common gas-forming organisms are *Candida albicans* and *E. coli*.
Ch. 66 Emphysematous Pyelonephritis and Emphysematous Cystitis, p 1366.

TRUE   B. It is associated with recurrent UTIs and urinary stones.
Ch. 66 Squamous Metaplasia, Leukoplakia and Cholesteatoma, p 1366.

FALSE   C. Leukoplakia consists of areas of sharply-defined white patches on areas of squamous metaplasia. It tends to occur in the renal pelvis.
Ch. 66 Squamous Metaplasia, Leukoplakia and Cholesteatoma, p 1366.

TRUE   D. Malakoplakia is a rare granulomatous infection involving women with *E. coli* infections. It commonly affects the bladder and lower urinary tract.
Ch. 66 Malakoplakia, p 1366.

FALSE   E. The association between pyeloureteritis cystica and urinary tract infections is not close. The former disorder is characterized by cysts in the submucosa of the renal pelvis and ureter.
Ch. 66 Pyeloureteritis Cystica, p 1366.

A 6.23. *Regarding the Plain Film Findings of Renal Masses*

FALSE   A. This is present in only 10% of cases.
Ch. 67 Plain Abdominal Radiography, p 1371.

FALSE   B. Renal lipomas are much rarer than angiomyolipomas, which also contain fat. The latter are not uncommonly seen as areas of fat density on the plain film.
Ch. 67 Plain Abdominal Radiography, p 1371.

FALSE   C. This feature is highly suggestive of malignancy and about 87% of calcified renal tumour masses are malignant.
Ch. 67 Plain Abdominal Radiography, p 1371.

TRUE   D. Only about 20-30% of renal lesions with peripheral calcification are malignant.
Ch. 67 Plain Abdominal Radiography, p 1371.

FALSE   E. Calculi are present in 75% of cases of xanthogranulomatous pyelonephritis, but their absence does not exclude the diagnosis.
Ch. 67 Inflammatory Masses, p 1379.

Q 6.24. *Regarding the Features of Renal Cystic Masses*

A. The collecting system of a multicystic dysplastic kidney does not opacify during intravenous urography

B. Hepatic involvement in multicystic dysplastic kidney is usually confined to a single lobe

C. Multilocular renal cyst (benign cystic nephroma) has a characteristic honeycomb appearance on CT and Ultrasound, and requires no further follow-up

D. Hydatid disease commonly affects the kidney

E. Peripelvic cysts are of lymphatic origin and may be confused with hydronephrosis on ultrasound.

Q 6.25. *Concerning Inflammatory Masses of the Kidney*

A. Acute focal pyelonephritis appears on CT as a streaky, poorly enhancing mass with increased density on unenhanced images

B. Calculi are more commonly associated with renal abscesses than with xanthogranulomatous pyelonephritis

C. Xanthogranulomatous pyelonephritis closely mimics renal cell carcinoma in many cases

D. Malacoplakia more commonly affects the bladder than the kidneys

E. Malacoplakia is a vascular mass at angiography

A 6.24. *Regarding the Features of Renal Cystic Masses*

TRUE
    A. This is a congenital unilateral non-functioning kidney in which the renal parenchyma appears as a cluster of cysts.
Ch. 67 Multicystic Renal Dysplasia, p 1378.

FALSE
    B. The liver is not involved in this condition.
Ch. 67 Multicystic Renal Dysplasia, p 1378.

FALSE
    C. Well-defined cysts separated by echogenic septa are seen in this mass. Although it is considered benign, sarcomatous change in the septa occurs, and the lesion may be locally aggressive. Surgical excision is usually recommended.
Ch. 67 Multiocular Renal Cysts, p 1378.

FALSE
    D. Even in endemic areas, hydatid disease of the kidney is uncommon.
Ch. 67 Hydatid Cysts of the Kidney, p 1378.

TRUE
    E. These cysts track along infundibula, and careful examination is required to demonstrate the fact that they do not communicate with the renal pelvis.
Ch. 67 Parapelvic and Peripelvic Cysts, p 1377.

A 6.25. *Concerning Inflammatory Masses of the Kidney*

TRUE
    A. There may be a hyperdense haemorrhagic component. The poor enhancement represents the poor function of the affected segment.
Ch. 67 Acute Focal Pyelonephritis, p 1379.

FALSE
    B. Calculi occur in 75% of cases of xanthogranulomatous pyelonephritis. The association with renal abscess is considerably weaker.
Ch. 67 Renal Abscesses, p 1379.

TRUE
    C. There may simply be a nonspecific focal renal mass with no obvious fat density or calculous disease. The histology may even be similar. The foam cells of xanthogranulomatous pyelonephritis resemble hypernephroma cells unless a fat stain is used. Both imaging and histology may confuse xanthogranulomatous pyelonephritis with hypernephroma.
Ch. 67 Xanthogranulomatous Pyelonenephritis, p 1379.

TRUE
    D. Multiple noncalcified intrarenal masses may also occur in this condition, which is considered to be caused by the incomplete digestion of *E. coli* by macrophages.
Ch. 67 Malacoplakia, p 1379.

FALSE
    E.
Ch. 67 Malacoplakia, p 1379.

Q 6.26. *The Following Statements Apply to Angiomyolipomas*

A. Angiomyolipomas contain smooth muscle

B. Adenoma sebaceum is present in 60-70% of patients with this tumour

C. They often present with flank pain, a renal mass and haematuria

D. They are usually solitary

E. They may be seen as hyper-reflective masses on ultrasound

Q 6.27. *Regarding Patients with Urothelial Tumours*

A. Eighty-five to 90% of patients present with haematuria

B. Haematuria often precedes silent obstruction

C. Urgency and frequency may be the only presenting features in about 10% of patients

D. In general, the role of the radiologist is to diagnose upper-tract tumours, and the endoscopist to diagnose lower-tract (i.e., bladder) tumours

E. If a bladder tumour is diagnosed at cystoscopy then an IVU is not necessary

A 6.26. *The Following Statements Apply to Angiomyolipomas*

TRUE *A.* They are hamartomas which have no malignant potential and contain muscle, fat and abnormal vascularity.
Ch. 67 Angiomyolipomas, p 1381.

FALSE *B.* About 20% of patients with this tumour have tuberous sclerosis and these patients may have adenoma sebaceum.
Ch. 67 Angiomyolipomas, p 1381.

TRUE *C.* This is because angiomyolipomas are prone to spontaneous haemorrhage.
Ch. 67 Angiomyolipomas, p 1381.

TRUE *D.* Except in the case of Tuberous sclerosis. In the latter the tumours are often multiple and bilateral and are seen in association with renal cysts.
Ch. 67 Angiomyolipomas, p 1381.

TRUE *E.* A focal hyper-reflective mass on ultrasound is highly suggestive of the diagnosis though the mass may be iso-echoic or even sonolucent.
Ch. 67 Angiomyolipomas, p 1382.

A 6.27. *Regarding Patients with Urothelial Tumours*

TRUE *A.* Of these, 15% have associated dysuria and frequency.
Ch. 68 Clinical Presentation, p 1398.

TRUE *B.*
Ch. 68 Clinical Presentation, p 1398.

TRUE *C.*
Ch. 68 Clinical Presentation, p 1398.

TRUE *D.* This is somewhat simplistic. However, the endoscopist can directly visualize and biopsy lesions in the bladder but cannot assess the ureters and pelves routinely. (Most patients now undergo outpatient flexible cystoscopy.)
Ch. 68 Diagnosis: The Role of Radiology, p 1399.

FALSE *E.* Urothelial tumours are multiple in 20% of patients and further lesions should always be sought.
Ch. 68 Diagnosis: The Role of Radiology, p 1399.

Q 6.28. *Regarding the Frequency of Urothelial Tumours*

    A. Bladder tumours are about five times more common than renal pelvic tumours

    B. Simultaneous bilateral ureteric tumours occur in approximately 1/1000 patients with urothelial malignancy

    C. Five percent of patients will have multiple lesions

    D. Ten percent of patients with renal pelvic urothelial tumours will develop bladder tumours in less than 15 months

    E. About 20% of affected patients have carcinoma in situ

Q 6.29. *The Following Are More Commonly Associated with Upper Renal Tract Urothelial Tumours than Bladder Tumours*

    A. Finnish nephrosis

    B. Phenacetin abuse

    C. Cyclophosphamide

    D. Balkan nephropathy

    E. Medullary sponge kidney

A 6.28. *Regarding the Frequency of Urothelial Tumours*

FALSE   A. The ratio is 64 bladder: 1 pelvic tumour.
Ch. 68 Pathology and Aetiology, p 1398.

FALSE   B. The true incidence is about 1% (i.e., 1/100).
Ch. 68 Pathology and Aetiology, p 1398.

FALSE   C. Twenty percent of patients with upper-tract or bladder tumours will have multiple lesions at presentation.
Ch. 68 Pathology and Aetiology, p 1398.

FALSE   D. The true incidence is 50%.
Ch. 68 Pathology and Aetiology, p 1398.

FALSE   E. Eighty percent of patients have papillary tumours, 20% have solid tumours and 3% have carcinoma in situ.
Ch. 68 Pathology and Aetiology, p 1398.

A 6.29. *The Following Are More Commonly Associated with Upper Renal Tract Urothelial Tumours than Bladder Tumours*

FALSE   A. This is an intrauterine renal disorder that is associated with raised amniotic AFP.

TRUE   B. These tend to be highly aggressive tumours.
Ch. 68 Pathology and Aetiology, p 1398.

FALSE   C. Cyclophosphamide, cyclamates and saccharine promote the formation of *bladder* tumours.
Ch. 68 Pathology and Aetiology, p 1398.

TRUE   D. The aetiology of this disorder is thought to be infective, possibly a fungus or virus. There is a high incidence of noninvasive well-differentiated papillary tumours of which 90% are in the upper tract and 10% are bilateral.
Ch. 68 Pathology and Aetiology, p 1398.

FALSE   E. No such association.

Q 6.30. *Concerning Urothelial Tumours*

    A. The vast majority are squamous cell tumours

    B. The ureter is the second most common site for urothelial tumours

    C. Most tumours of the bladder are due to environmental aromatic amine exposure

    D. Only 5–10% of bladder tumours are attributable to smoking

    E. Hairdressers have a higher incidence of bladder cancer than the general population

Q 6.31. *Concerning Urinary Calculi*

    A. Calcium oxalate and phosphate stones are more common in males than females

    B. Peanuts and spinach increase the urinary secretion of oxalate.

    C. Triple phosphate stones are seen in over 50% of patients with hyperphosphatasia

    D. Struvite stones are commoner in women than men

    E. Cystinosis is associated with the excessive excretion of dibasic amino acids

A 6.30. Concerning Urothelial Tumours

FALSE   A. Over 90% of tumours of urothelium are *transitional* cell tumours.
Ch. 68 Pathology and Aetiology, p 1398.

FALSE   B. The ureter is the least common site; the bladder and renal pelvis are the most common sites.
Ch. 68 Pathology and Aetiology, p 1398.

TRUE   C. Most urothelial tumours can now be attributed to environmental exposure to aromatic amines. The known carcinogens have now been banned.
Ch. 68 Pathology and Aetiology, p 1398.

FALSE   D. Current data suggest that 30–40% of urothelial tumours are directly due to smoking.
Ch. 68 Pathology and Aetiology, p 1398.

TRUE   E. Certain trades including tailors, printers, leather workers and hairdressers have a higher incidence of bladder cancer. No carcinogen(s) has yet been identified in these groups of patients.
Ch. 68 Pathology and Aetiology, p 1398.

A 6.31. Concerning Urinary Calculi

TRUE   A.
Ch. 68 Structure and Aetiology, p 1391.

TRUE   B. Tea, rhubarb and chocolate also increase the urinary secretion of oxalate.
Ch. 68 Structure and Aetiology, p 1391.

FALSE   C. Hyperphosphatasia is a cause of dense bones in children and can produce skeletal changes similar to those seen in Paget's disease.

TRUE   D. They represent 20% of all renal calculi.
Ch. 68 Structure and Aetiology, p 1391.

FALSE   E. Cystinuria is an inherited defect characterized by failure of absorption of cystine, ornithine, arginine and lysine.
Ch. 68 Structure and Aetiology, p 1391.

Q *6.32. Well-Recognised Associations of Renal Calculi Include*

        A. Previous nephrectomy

        B. Caliceal cysts

        C. Malrotation of the kidneys

        D. Congenital hepatic fibrosis (CHF)

        E. Ureteroceles

Q *6.33. The Following Can Usually be Demonstrated on the Plain Abdominal Radiograph*

        A. Cystine stones

        B. Xanthine stones

        C. Sloughed papillae

        D. Urate stones

        E. Oxalate stones

A 6.32. *Well-Recognised Associations of Renal Calculi Include*

FALSE   *A.*
Ch. 68 Anatomical Causes of Calculi, p 1393.

TRUE   *B.*
Ch. 68 Anatomical Causes of Calculi, p 1393.

TRUE   *C.* This may produce stasis and increased infection rates that are associated with urinary calculi.
Ch. 68 Anatomical Causes of Calculi, p 1393.

TRUE   *D.* CHF is associated with renal tubular ectasia and medullary sponge kidneys.
Ch. 68 Anatomical Causes of Calculi, p 1393.

TRUE   *E.* Again, producing stasis and infection.
Ch. 68 Anatomical Causes of Calculi, p 1393.

A 6.33. *The Following Can Usually be Demonstrated on the Plain Abdominal Radiograph*

TRUE   *A.* Cystine stones are radio-opaque but tend to be less radio-dense than the ribs or transverse processes and have a ground glass appearance.
Ch. 68 Imaging, p 1393.

FALSE   *B.* Pure xanthine stones tend to be radiolucent.

FALSE   *C.* Papillae can only be demonstrated when calcified. They tend to be triangular with a ring of calcium when calcified.
Ch. 68 Imaging, p 1393.

FALSE   *D.* Classically radiolucent.
Ch. 68 Imaging, p 1393.

TRUE   *E.* Oxalate stones are often denser than bone.
Ch. 68 Imaging, p 1393.

Q 6.34. *Regarding Renal Tract Calculi*

___

    A. About 10% of renal tract stones occur as a result of primary hyperparathyroidism

    B. Urinary calculi are usually an admixture of organic and inorganic complexes

    C. The nidus of the stone may have a different chemical composition to the main bulk of the stone

    D. About 50% of stone formers may expect a recurrence in their lifetime

    E. The ingestion of large amounts of protein and purine account for the high incidence of stone disease in the USA

Q 6.35. *The Following Infections are Associated with Nominated Types of Urinary Stones*

___

    A. Klebsiella and magnesium ammonium phosphate stones

    B. *E. coli* and magnesium ammonium phosphate stones

    C. Pseudomonas pyocaneae and magnesium ammonium phosphate stones

    D. Campylobacter and uric acid stones

    E. *Streptococcus faecalis* and calcium phosphate stones

A 6.34. *Regarding Renal Tract Calculi*

TRUE A. Over 80% of renal tract calculi are labelled as idiopathic. Early detection and treatment are necessary to prevent inevitable renal tract damage.
Ch. 68 Urinary Calculi, p 1391.

TRUE B. Most stones contain a small amount of organic matrix.
Ch. 68 Structure and Aetiology, p 1391.

TRUE C. A calcium phosphate stone may be at the centre of an oxalate stone. It is the composition of the urine that determines the main bulk of the stone.
Ch. 68 Structure and Aetiology, p 1391.

TRUE D.
Ch. 68 Structure and Aetiology, p 1391.

TRUE E. Other factors include a hot climate, sunshine (elevated vitamin D), dehydration and antacids: in fact, most causes of hypercalcaemia.
Ch. 68 Structure and Aetiology, p 1391.

A 6.35. *The Following Infections Are Associated with Nominated Types of Urinary Stones*

TRUE A.
Ch. 68 Structure and Aetiology, p 1391.

TRUE B.
Ch. 68 Structure and Aetiology, p 1391.

TRUE C.
Ch. 68 Structure and Aetiology, p 1391.

FALSE D.
Ch. 68 Structure and Aetiology, p 1391.

FALSE E.
Ch. 68 Structure and Aetiology, p 1391.

Q 6.36. *The Following Are Well-Recognised Causes of Medullary Nephrocalcinosis*

        A. Secondary hyperparathyroidism

        B. Osteoporosis

        C. Myelomatosis

        D. Ellis-van Creveld Syndrome

        E. Sarcoidosis

Q 6.37. *The Following Produce Cortical Nephrocalcinosis*

        A. Nephrotic syndrome due to glomerulonephritis

        B. Obstetric shock

        C. Nail patella syndrome

        D. Paget's disease

        E. Oxalosis

A 6.36. The Following Are Well-Recognised Causes of Medullary Nephrocalcinosis

TRUE A. Both primary and secondary hyperparathyroidism can produce nephrocalcinosis.
Ch. 68 Medullary Nephrocalcinosis, p 1395.

TRUE B. A rare cause.
Ch. 68 Table 68.1, p 1392.

TRUE C.
Ch. 68 Table 68.1, p 1392.

TRUE D. There are many causes of nephrocalcinosis, many of them obscure. An extensive, but not exhaustive, list can be found in Reeder and Felson's Gamuts in radiology.

TRUE E.
Ch. 68 Table 68.1, p 1392.

A 6.37. The Following Produce Cortical Nephrocalcinosis

TRUE A. Albright coined the term "nephrocalcinosis" in 1934. This refers to the deposition of calcium salts within the *substance* of the kidney, whereas the term "nephrolithiasis" is calculus formation within the *collecting* system of the kidney.
Ch. 68 Cortical Nephrocalcinosis, p 1395.

TRUE B. Any cause of acute cortical necrosis.
Ch. 66 Acute Cortical Necrosis, p 1396.

FALSE C. This syndrome is associated with hypoplasia or absence of the nails and patellae, palpable iliac horns, hereditary nephropathy (with medullary nephrocalcinosis) short stature and foot abnormalities. The "gold medal" candidates may be shown a radiograph demonstrating radial head subluxation/dislocation, which is a commonly associated finding.

FALSE D. Paget's disease is associated with medullary nephrocalcinosis.

TRUE E. Oxalosis, mercury poisoning, renal vein thrombosis, drug therapy and hereditary nephritis can all produce renal cortical calcification.

Q 6.38. *Regarding Medullary Sponge Kidney (MSK)*

     A. A localized and diffuse form may exist

     B. The affected kidney is often smaller than the non-affected one

     C. Up to 25% of patients with renal calculi have medullary sponge kidney (MSK)

     D. There is an association with cystic bronchiectasis

     E. Most patients eventually lose function in the affected kidney

Q 6.39. *Concerning Obstruction in the Urinary Tract*

     A. Hydronephrosis implies at least a degree of obstruction

     B. The degree of dilation of the collecting system is a useful guide to the severity of the obstruction

     C. Primary megaureter occurs in the absence of anatomical or functional obstruction

     D. If the 15 minute IVU film fails to show an opacified collecting system, the next film should be taken about 1 hour later.

     E. A urinoma, if present in urinary obstruction, opacifies during an IVU in the majority of cases

A 6.38. *Regarding Medullary Sponge Kidney (MSK)*

TRUE   A. The disorder may be asymmetrical. The radiographic features include cystic dilations of the collecting tubules, producing a characteristic beaded pattern on the IVU.
Ch. 68 Medullary Sponge Kidney, p 1396.

FALSE   B. The affected kidney is usually *larger* than its counterpart: there is an association with ipsilateral hemihypertrophy of the body.
Ch. 68 Medullary Sponge Kidney, p 1396.

TRUE   C. MSK is vastly under-diagnosed according to Yendt.
Ch. 68 Medullary Sponge Kidney, p 1396.

FALSE   D. The most common associations are *congenital hepatic fibrosis* and *hemihypertrophy.*
Ch. 68 Medullary Sponge Kidney, p 1396.

FALSE   E. Only a small proportion of patients lose function.
Ch. 68 Medullary Sponge Kidney, p 1396.

A 6.39. *Concerning Obstruction in the Urinary Tract*

FALSE   A. Hydronephrosis (dilation of the renal pelvis and calices) may occur in the absence of obstruction. A good example of this is severe vesico-ureteric reflux that produces nonobstructive hydronephrosis.
Ch. 69 Hydronephrosis, p 1408.

FALSE   B. It is wrong to assume that mild dilatation of the collecting system reflects mild obstruction. Some patients with acute complete obstruction have no evidence of dilatation in the first 24-48 hours after the onset of obstruction.
Ch. 69 Hydronephrosis, p 1408.

TRUE   C. The abnormality here is nondistensibility of a normal calibre, juxtavesical segment, which fails to transmit peristalsis. It may be non-obstructive and reflux is usually absent.
Ch. 69 Primary Megaureter, p 1419.

FALSE   D. At least 2 hours should be allowed to elapse in order to avoid unnecessary radiographs.
Ch. 69 Delayed Contrast Excretion, p 1410.

FALSE   E. Opacification is seen in only about one third of cases of urinoma. Typically the kidney is displaced anteriorly and superolaterally by the collection of extravasated urine within Gerota's fascia.
Ch. 69 Urinoma, p 1411.

Q *6.40. Regarding CT in Urinary Tract Obstruction*

    A. "Stranding" of peripelvic fat by contrast medium is a recognized sign of obstruction

    B. A prolonged cortico-medullary nephrogram occurs in obstruction

    C. Modern CT is more sensitive for stone detection than a plain abdominal radiograph

    D. Non-contrast enhanced CT rivals the IVU in the assessment of acute obstruction

    E. It is the most useful test for the assessment of a transplant kidney

A 6.40. *Regarding CT in Urinary Tract Obstruction*

TRUE
 A. Stranding of the peripelvic and periureteric fat is a reliable sign of obstruction.
 Ch. 69 Computed Tomography, p 1416.

TRUE
 B. The cortical-medullary nephrogram, seen transiently on an IVU, is prolonged on CT. A reverse cortical-medullary nephrogram is seen when progressive contrast medium accumulation occurs in the medullary pyramids to the extent that they are denser than the cortex.
 Ch. 69 Computed Tomography, p 1416.

TRUE
 C. Many "non-radiopaque" calculi have a high attenuation on CT and are readily visible. Helical scanning is important as it eliminates interslice gaps and ensures that stones lying between adjacent slices are not missed.
 Ch. 69 Computed Tomography, p 1416.

TRUE
 D. Non-contrast-enhanced helical CT has been shown to be a rapid and cost-effective way of diagnosing obstructing stones in hospitals which have a 24-hour CT service.
 Ch. 69 Computed Tomography, p 1416.

FALSE
 E. Ultrasound can detect minimal pelvicaliceal dilatation in a transplant kidney owing to the proximity of the transducer to the parenchyma.
 Ch. 69 Ultrasonography, p 1415.

Q 6.41. *The Following are Associated with Congenital Ureteric Obstruction*

    A. Circumcaval ureter

    B. Primary megaureter

    C. Bladder diverticulum

    D. Hydrometrocolpos

    E. Multicystic dysplastic kidney

Q 6.42. *Regarding Uroradiology*

    A. A radiographic calcific focus below the level of the ischial spines is too low to be intraureteric

    B. A patient with acute renal colic should empty the bladder before an IVU

    C. Nearly 50% of ureteric transitional cell carcinomas produce a stricture rather than a filling defect

    D. In hydronephrosis of pregnancy the ureters below the pelvic brim tend to be spared

    E. Ureteric intussusception is caused by fibroepithelial polyps

A 6.41. The Following are Associated with Congenital Ureteric Obstruction

TRUE   A. Usually on the right side.
Ch. 69 Congenital Ureteric Obstructions, p 1420.

TRUE   B. This abnormality may be obstructive or nonobstructive.
Ch. 69 Congenital Ureteric Obstructions, p 1420.

TRUE   C.
Ch. 69 Congenital Ureteric Obstruction, p 1420.

TRUE   D. This condition may be congenital or acquired. When caused by a congenital anomaly, it may present in the newborn period (e.g., if there is an abnormal single perineal orifice for the bladder and vagina) ($\pm$ rectum). Hydronephrosis is an association of the infantile type. Imperforate hymen and other causes of vaginal obstruction may not present with hydrometrocolpos until menarche.
Ch. 69 Congenital Ureteric Obstructions, p 1422.

TRUE   E. In this condition, extrarenal obstruction occurs early in fetal life and leads to renal dysplasia. Pathology on the contralateral side is common and includes PUJ obstruction and ureteric; anomalies.
Ch. 69 Congenital Ureteric Obstruction, p 1420.

A 6.42. Regarding Uroradiology

FALSE   A. This "rule" is very unreliable, particularly in women.
Ch. 69 Acquired Ureteric Obstructions—Intraluminal, p 1421.

FALSE   B. If a small stone is impacted in the distal ureter, it may be obscured early on by contrast medium accumulation in the bladder. A distended bladder may act as a window through which a stone can be visualized, because the intravesical contrast medium is diluted.
Ch. 69 Acquired Ureteric Obstructions—Intraluminal, p 1421.

FALSE   C. Only 5% of transitional cell carcinomas present as a stricture without an intraluminal filling defect. It may be impossible to distinguish between this type of tumour and other causes of a stricture (e.g., previous stone passage, instrumentation, etc.).
Ch. 69, Acquired Ureteric Obstructions—Intraluminal, p 1421.

TRUE   D. Most pregnant women develop at least some evidence of urinary tract obstruction by the third trimester. In most subjects, this is predominantly right-sided and tends to disappear within a few weeks of delivery.
Ch. 69 Hydronephrosis of Pregnancy, p 1423.

TRUE   E. This tumour is the most common benign neoplastic cause of ureteric obstruction and appears as a long smooth mobile intraluminal filling defect. It tends to present in young adults as flank pain.
Ch. 69 Urothelial Tumours, p 1422.

Q 6.43. *Regarding Posterior Urethral Valves*

    A. The diagnosis is suspected when fetal bladder distension is accompanied by intra-uterine polyhydramnios

    B. The detection and treatment of this disorder in utero permits salvage of renal function

    C. The diagnosis in most patients is made prenatally

    D. The condition rarely presents in adulthood

    E. May be mimicked by massive vesico-ureteric reflux

Q 6.44. *There is an Association Between the Following Disorders*

    A. Bladder agenesis: absence of the urethra

    B. Dwarf bladder: achondroplasia

    C. Hutch diverticulum: bladder outflow obstruction

    D. Bladder extrophy: cleidocranial dysostosis

    E. Double bladder: penis didelphys

A 6.43. *Regarding Posterior Urethral Valves*

FALSE   A. *Oligohydramnios* is a consequence of bladder outflow obstruction.
Ch. 69 Posterior Urethral Valves, p 1424.

FALSE   B. If obstruction occurs early in gestation, irreversible renal dysplasia results.
Ch. 69 Posterior Urethral Valves, p 1424.

FALSE   C. Only a minority of these lesions are picked up on the prenatal ultrasound scan. The condition may be clinically silent, leading to delay in diagnosis and severe renal damage. More commonly, palpable kidneys and/or symptoms of urinary tract infection and obstruction allow the diagnosis to be made after birth and sometimes before serious renal damage has developed.
Ch. 69 Posterior Urethral Valves, p 1424.

TRUE   D. Although very unusual, an adult presentation is well recognized.
Ch. 69 Posterior Urethral Valves, p 1424.

TRUE   E. A distended bladder and bilateral hydroureteronephrosis may occur in both these conditions.
Ch. 69 Posterior Urethral Valves, p 1424.

A 6.44. *There is an Association Between the Following Disorders*

TRUE   A. This condition is generally incompatible with life.
Ch. 70 Congenital Abnormalities, p 1429.

FALSE   B. Dwarf bladder (bladder hypoplasia) is associated with other anomalies of the urinary tract (not, as its name implies, skeletal dwarfism).
Ch. 70 Congenital Abnormalities, p 1429.

FALSE   C. Hutch diverticula are congenital diverticula and are not thought to be secondary to outflow obstruction.
Ch. 70 Congenital Abnormalities, p 1429.

FALSE   D. Both disorders demonstrate separation of the pubic bones, but the bladder is normal in cleidocranial dysostosis.
Ch. 70 Congenital Abnormalities, p 1429.

TRUE   E.
Ch. 70 Fig. 70.5, p 1429.

Q 6.45. *The Following are Appropriate to the Normal Bladder*

    A. The optimum spin-echo sequence for demonstration of the bladder wall is a T2-weighted image

    B. The chemical shift artefact is best demonstrated on T2-weighted images

    C. The position of the chemical shift can be varied by alterations in the direction of the phase and frequency gradients

    D. A 6 mm thick bladder wall shown on ultrasound

    E. On CT the outer wall of the bladder is generally well delineated by perivesical fat

Q 6.46. *Regarding Cross-Sectional Imaging for Prostatic Carcinoma*

    A. CT is recommended for routine tumour staging

    B. CT is recommended for the assessment of co-existent disease

    C. CT is not recommended in patients with advanced disease

    D. A CT scan should include the abdomen when no nodal enlargement is demonstrated in the pelvis

    E. Normal nodes as demonstrated by CT and MRI do not warrant surgical excision when an open therapeutic procedure is undertaken

A 6.45. *The Following are Appropriate to the Normal Bladder*

TRUE   A. There is a considerable difference in the relaxation times of urine and the bladder wall on a T2-weighted sequence. The bladder wall is of lower intensity than the urine.
Ch. 70 Radiological Evaluation, p 1427.

TRUE   B.
Ch. 70 Fig. 70.4, p 1428.

TRUE   C. This effect can be useful when examining the bladder wall.
Ch. 70 Radiological Evaluation, p 1427.

TRUE   D. The bladder wall can appear thickened in the half-full state or following micturition. Assessment of wall thickness should be made with a full bladder.
Ch. 70 Radiological Imaging, p 1428.

TRUE   E.
Ch. 70 Radiological Imaging, p 1428.

A 6.46. *Regarding Cross-Sectional Imaging for Prostatic Carcinoma*

FALSE   A. CT is insensitive and nonspecific for carcinoma of the prostate.
Ch. 70 Tumours of the Prostate, p 1443.

FALSE   B. CT is not cost-effective in screening for comorbid disease in the newly diagnosed case.
Ch. 70 Tumours of the Prostate, p 1443.

FALSE   C. CT is extremely useful when assessing lymphadenopathy.
Ch. 70 Tumours of the Prostate, p 1443.

FALSE   D. If no nodes are demonstrated in the pelvic scan, the scan need not proceed proximal to the aortic bifurcation.
Ch. 70 Tumours of the Prostate, p 1443.

FALSE   E. Neither the internal anatomy of lymph nodes nor tumour cell infiltration can be assessed by CT or MR. The normal size of a node does not preclude malignant infiltration.
Ch. 70 Tumours of the Prostate, p 1443.

Q 6.47. *Regarding the Imaging of Prostatic Carcinoma*

A. Advanced tumours are often difficult to detect on transrectal ultrasound (TRUS)

B. A serum PSA (prostatic specific antigen) and digital examination are more sensitive than TRUS

C. TRUS should be used to assess the site of the lesion prior to excision biopsy

D. The staging of prostatic cancer is either by the TNM or the Jewitt classification

E. TRUS is as accurate as MRI in staging

Q 6.48. *Concerning Prostatic Carcinoma*

A. Prostatic carcinoma is the commonest male cancer

B. About 10% of carcinomas develop in the central zone of the gland

C. Over 95% of carcinomas are squamous cell in type

D. The clinical staging of prostatic carcinoma is relatively accurate in comparison to imaging

E. An area of hypoechogenicity within the prostate is pathognomonic of prostatic carcinoma on TRUS

A 6.47. *Regarding the Imaging of Prostatic Carcinoma*

TRUE   A. This is because the whole of the peripheral zone may be replaced by tumour.
Ch. 70 Tumours of the Prostate, p 1444.

TRUE   B. Furthermore, they are cheaper.
Ch. 70 Tumours of the Prostate, p 1444.

FALSE   C. The role of TRUS is to locate the tumour, biopsy the tumour and sample the rest of the gland. An excision biopsy is when the whole lesion is excised.
Ch. 70 Tumours of the Prostate, p 1443.

TRUE   D.
Ch. 70 Table 70.2, p 1446.

TRUE   E.
Ch. 70 Tumours of the Prostate, p 1443.

A 6.48. *Concerning Prostatic Carcinoma*

TRUE   A. Thirty percent of men at 50 years and 90% of men at 90 years have carcinoma at autopsy.
Ch. 70 Tumours of the Prostate, p 1443.

TRUE   B. Twenty percent originate in the transitional zone and 70% in the peripheral zone.
Ch. 70 Tumours of the Prostate, p 1443.

FALSE   C. Most are adenocarcinomas; occasionally sarcomas develop.
Ch. 70 Tumours of the Prostate, p 1443.

FALSE   D. It is believed that 72% of patients staged clinically are understaged.
Ch. 70 Tumours of the Prostate, p 1443.

FALSE   E. Prostatic carcinoma is hypoechoic, but many other disorders can produce similar findings.
Ch. 70 Tumours of the Prostate, p 1444.

Q 6.49. *Regarding Tumours of the Prostate*

A. Benign prostatic hypertrophy (BPH) occurs in the central zone and tends to compress the urethra

B. An enlarged prostate pushes the trigone upwards to produce the "fish hook" deformity of the lower ureters

C. The PSA (prostate specific antigen) levels parallel the size of the prostate gland

D. TRUS may demonstrate well-defined or poorly defined nodules and variable echo characteristics

E. MRI is now capable of distinguishing BPH from carcinoma

Q 6.50. *Concerning Inflammation and Infection of the Prostate*

A. Chronic prostatitis is believed to be due to noninfective congestion that subsequently becomes secondarily infected

B. A prostatic abscess begins in the central zone and tends to spread to the peripheral zone

C. Non-specific prostatitis is believed to be caused by a mycobacterium

D. Radiological examination is usually of little help

E. Early calcification on CT is the hallmark of a chronic prostatic abscess

A 6.49. *Regarding Tumours of the Prostate*

FALSE A. BPH is predominantly a transitional zone disorder. Histologically, the changes are predominantly glandular and, less commonly, interstitial.
Ch. 70 Tumours of the Prostate, p 1443.

TRUE B. Otherwise known as the "J" deformity.
Ch. 70 Fig. 70.47, p 1444.

TRUE C. This should be borne in mind when the patient has a very large gland, and only mildly elevated PSA levels could be misdiagnosed as a cancer.
Ch. 70 Tumours of the Prostate, p 1444.

TRUE D. A surgical capsule may be seen between the central and peripheral zones.
Ch. 70 Tumours of the Prostate, p 1444.

FALSE E. The appearances are so varied that no such distinction can be made.
Ch. 70 Tumours of the Prostate, p 1444.

A 6.50. *Concerning Inflammation and Infection of the Prostate*

TRUE A. *Acute* prostatitis is primarily due to infection by gonococcal, staphylococcal, streptococcal and coliform bacteria.
Ch. 70 Infectious Processes of the Prostate, p 1442.

FALSE B. The converse. Immunocompromised and AIDS patients are particularly likely to develop a prostatic abscess.
Ch. 70 Infectious Processes of the Prostate, p 1442.

FALSE C. Non-specific prostatitis is due to the escape of prostatic contents and bacterial products or urine into the prostate.
Ch. 70 Infectious Processes of the Prostate, p 1442.

TRUE D. A plain film or IVU may well be helpful in the search for the primary cause (e.g., TB, schistosomiasis). The diagnosis is usually based upon history and examination.
Ch. 70 Infectious Processes of the Prostate, p 1442.

FALSE E. Prostatic abscesses tend not to calcify.

Q *6.51. The Following are Normal MRI Features of the Prostate*

    A. T1-weighted images demonstrate the zonal anatomy

    B. T2-weighted images demonstrate the zonal regions in 70% of patients over the age of 35 years

    C. When the transitional zone is demonstrated on T2-weighted images it has a heterogeneous high signal

    D. The seminal vesicles are of high signal intensity on T2-weighted images

    E. The levator ani muscles exhibit a higher signal intensity than the peripheral zone

Q *6.52. Concerning the Radiological Evaluation of the Prostate Gland*

    A. Transabdominal US demonstrates the zonal anatomy

    B. TRUS (transrectal ultrasound scanning) demonstrates the peripheral zone and its hypoechogenic structure

    C. Corpora amylacea are echogenic, calcific foci that are present between the transitional and peripheral zones

    D. The ductus deferens lies between the seminal vesicles and the prostate on the sagittal view (TRUS)

    E. On the sagittal view of a TRUS, the differentiation between the central zone and the peripheral zone is seldom seen

A 6.51. The Following are Normal MRI Features of the Prostate

FALSE   A. The prostate has an intermediate homogeneous intensity on T1-weighted images.
Ch. 70 Normal Anatomy, p 1427.

FALSE   B. T2-weighted images demonstrate the zonal anatomy in only 35% of patients over the age of 35 years.
Ch. 70 Normal Anatomy, p 1427.

FALSE   C. The transitional zone is of uniformly low signal intensity.
Ch. 70 Normal Anatomy, p 1427.

TRUE   D.
Ch. 70 Fig. 70.42, p 1441.

FALSE   E. The levator ani muscles are of lower signal intensity irrespective of the sequence employed.
Ch. 70 Normal Anatomy, p 1427.

A 6.52. Concerning the Radiological Evaluation of the Prostate Gland

FALSE   A. Transabdominal US demonstrates the prostate as a uniform low level echogenic mass at the base of the bladder with no differentiation into prostatic zones.
Ch. 70 Radiological Evaluation, p 1438.

FALSE   B. The peripheral zone has a medium to high echogenic signal in comparison with the rest of the gland.
Ch. 70 Radiological Evaluation, p 1438.

FALSE   C.
Ch. 70 Radiological Evaluation, p 1438.

TRUE   D.
Ch. 70 Radiological Evaluation, p 1438.

TRUE   E.
Ch. 70 Radiological Evaluation, p 1438.

Q 6.53. *Concerning the Normal Prostate Gland*

A. Denonvilliers' fascia separates the prostate gland from the rectum

B. A lobular anatomical arrangement only exists in the fetal gland

C. The transitional zone of the prostate only occupies about 5% of the gland

D. The volume of the central zone is larger in younger people

E. The neurovascular bundles are demonstrated antero-lateral to the peripheral zone

Q 6.54. *Monitoring Response to Therapy in Patients with Bladder Tumours*

A. Periodic IVUs are recommended

B. MRI, using contrast medium and a variety of sequences, can reliably distinguish between radiation changes and tumour recurrence

C. CT and MRI are very helpful in differentiating between non-specific granulation tissue and local recurrence

D. The typical changes demonstrated on MRI after radiotherapy include abnormal signal intensity of the outer muscle wall on T2-weighted images and mural enhancement (after i/v contrast administration) on T1-weighted images

E. Radiation changes to the bowel are usually demonstrated within one month of treatment

A 6.53. *Concerning the Normal Prostate Gland*

TRUE
   A. This is a double layer of fascia between the two organs.
    Ch. 70 Normal Anatomy, p 1427.

TRUE
   B. The adult gland is a complex structure of glandular and nonglandular tissue, the latter being divided into three zones.
    Ch. 70 Normal Anatomy, p 1427.

TRUE
   C. The remainder of the gland is occupied by the peripheral zone (70%) and the central zone (25%).
    Ch. 70 Normal Anatomy, p 1427.

TRUE
   D. The zonal anatomy changes with age. The central zone gradually decreases in size with age, whereas the transitional zone tends to increase in size giving rise to BPH.
    Ch. 70 Normal Anatomy, p 1427.

FALSE
   E. They are demonstrated postero-laterally and are the commonest site for extra-capsular extension of carcinoma.
    Ch. 70 Normal Anatomy, p 1427.

A 6.54. *Monitoring Response to Therapy in Patients with Bladder Tumours*

TRUE
   A. There is a significant incidence of further lesions in the upper tract as well as the bladder; therefore, careful monitoring is necessary.
    Ch. 70 Tumours of the Bladder, p 1432.

FALSE
   B. Unfortunately this is not true.
    Ch. 70 Tumours of the Bladder, p 1432.

FALSE
   C. Any new local mass could be either. In these circumstances, biopsy is essential.
    Ch. 70 Tumours of the Bladder, p 1432.

TRUE
   D.
    Ch. 70 Tumours of the Bladder, p 1432.

FALSE
   E. Radiation changes may take many months or even years to develop.
    Ch. 70 Tumours of the Bladder, p 1432.

Q 6.55. *Assessing Bladder Tumours*

    A. Large doses of i/v contrast medium are recommended to show tumour enhancement on CT

    B. Pelvic nodes exceeding 15 mm in their trans-axial diameter should be assumed to be malignant

    C. The accuracy for assessing lymphadenopathy varies between 65 and 85%

    D. A coronal plane of imaging (MRI) is recommended for the assessment of vaginal or uterine extension

    E. MR imaging is not significantly better than CT in the accuracy of its staging

Q 6.56. *Concerning Radiological Assessment of Bladder Tumours*

    A. The IVU and cystogram are still useful in the staging of bladder carcinoma

    B. Transurethral and transrectal USS have staging accuracies of 75-95%

    C. The major role of CT is to stage the bladder tumour

    D. Angiography plays an important role in preoperative assessment

    E. Loss of the fat plane between the seminal vesicles and the bladder invariably suggests tumour invasion

A 6.55. Assessing Bladder Tumours

FALSE   A. Large doses of contrast medium accumulate in the bladder and obscure small tumours, or produce artefacts that degrade the image.
Ch. 70 Tumours of the Bladder, p 1432.

TRUE   B. All nodes > 10 mm in their trans-axial diameter should be suspected of being malignant.
Ch. 70 Tumours of the Bladder, p 1432.

TRUE   C. The CT staging accuracy varies from 42-92% with an accuracy of 65-85% in the assessment of perivesical spread.
Ch. 70 Tumours of the Bladder, p 1432.

FALSE   D. A sagittal plane of imaging is needed for the evaluation of uterine or vaginal invasion. Furthermore, this plane of imaging is extremely useful for evaluation of the seminal vesicles.
Ch. 70 Tumours of the Bladder, p 1432.

TRUE   E. The accuracy of staging for both modalities is similar. The slight advantage of MRI is its ability to assess the dome of the bladder in the sagittal and coronal planes.
Ch. 70 Tumours of the Bladder, p 1432.

A 6.56. Concerning Radiological Assessment of Bladder Tumours

FALSE   A. They only demonstrate filling defects and do not assess wall invasion or tumour extension.
Ch. 70 Tumours of the Bladder, p 1432.

TRUE   B. Transabdominal USS is not very accurate and is of limited value as some areas of the bladder are not easily visualized.
Ch. 70 Tumours of the Bladder, p 1432.

TRUE   C. The reliability of CT in diagnosing the early stages of bladder cancer is poor. The higher the stage of the tumour, the greater the accuracy and the modality is useful for the assessment of perivesical spread, lymphadenopathy and distant metastases.
Ch. 70 Tumours of the Bladder, p 1432.

FALSE   D.
Ch. 70 Tumours of the Bladder, p 1432.

FALSE   E. This sign should always be interpreted with caution as the normal seminal vesicular angle may be lost if the rectum is over-distended or if the patient is scanned in the prone position.
Ch. 70 Tumours of the Bladder, p 1432.

Q 6.57. Imaging Criteria Used in the Staging of Bladder Tumours

    A. CT cannot differentiate T1 to T3b tumours

    B. T1 to T3a tumours are best demonstrated using a SE T1-weighted MRI sequence

    C. A T3b tumour is easily demonstrable on a T1-weighted image sequence

    D. Pelvic lymph node(s) of 12 mm in their trans-axial diameter would not be regarded as significant using MRI criteria

    E. Tis (carcinoma in situ; TMN staging) is demonstrated on T2-weighted images as an area of reduced signal intensity after gadolinium contrast enhancement

Q 6.58. Concerning Tumours of the Bladder

    A. Ten percent of bladder tumours arise from a non-epithelial source

    B. Adenocarcinoma is the least common epithelial bladder tumour

    C. All epithelial tumours are malignant

    D. A T3a tumour has breached the bladder muscle

    E. A T2 tumour is limited by the lamina propria

A *6.57.* *Imaging Criteria Used in the Staging of Bladder Tumours*

FALSE   A. CT cannot differentiate T1 to T3a tumours. Learn the local staging of bladder carcinoma from "G and A" 3rd Ed.
Ch. 70 Table 70.1, p 1428.

FALSE   B. T1 to T3a tumours are diagnosed when the tumour is confined to the bladder wall. The outer region of bladder is low signal intensity on T2-weighted images.
Ch. 70 Table 70.1, p 1428.

TRUE   C. The low signal from the tumour is accentuated by the bright signal from the fat.
Ch. 70 Table 70.1, p 1428.

FALSE   D. The MRI and CT criteria are the same: nodal enlargement of >10 mm is significant.
Ch. 70 Table 70.1, p 1428.

FALSE   E.
Ch. 70 Table 70.1, p 1428.

A *6.58.* *Concerning Tumours of the Bladder*

TRUE   A. These include leiomyoma, fibroma and their malignant counterparts.
Ch. 70 Tumours of the Bladder, p 1432.

TRUE   B. The incidence is as follows; adenocarcinoma (1%), squamous carcinoma (1.5-10%), and transitional cell carcinoma accounts for the rest (approximately 90%).
Ch. 70 Tumours of the Bladder, p 1432.

TRUE   C.
Ch. 70 Tumours of the Bladder, p 1432.

FALSE   D. A *T3b* breaches the muscle and enters the perivesical fat or peritoneum.
Ch. 70 Fig. 70.15, p 1432.

FALSE   E. A T2 tumour has superficially invaded the muscular wall.
Ch. 70 Table 70.1, p 1433.

Q 6.59. *Concerning Bladder Trauma*

A. Intra-peritoneal bladder rupture results in the accumulation of contrast medium around the dome of the bladder

B. Extra-peritoneal bladder rupture results in streaks of contrast medium spreading laterally across the bony pelvis

C. Elliptical extravasation of contrast medium around the bladder suggests subserosal rupture

D. Rapid onset of peritonitis, within 6 hours, following intraperitoneal rupture

E. All forms of bladder rupture require major surgical intervention

Q 6.60. *Regarding the Radiology of the Renal Vasculature*

A. The posterior branch of the renal artery is the predominant supply to the upper pole

B. Multiple renal arteries are best referred to as accessory arteries as they provide a collateral supply to the kidney in disease states

C. Simple cysts are often outlined by a ring of fine veins in the venous phase of angiography

D. Angiomyolipoma is a hypervascular tumour which may be mistaken for renal-cell carcinoma on angiography

E. Less than 10% of renal-cell carcinomas are hypovascular

A   6.59. *Concerning Bladder Trauma*

TRUE   A. Contrast medium can also be seen to accumulate around bowel loops.
            Ch. 70 Trauma, p 1431.

TRUE   B.
            Ch. 70 Trauma, p 1431.

TRUE   C. This is an extremely rare form of bladder rupture.
            Ch. 70 Trauma, p 1431.

FALSE   D. The clinical signs of bladder rupture may not be apparent for up to 24 hours; if, therefore, bladder rupture is suspected in cases of pelvic trauma, a cystogram is performed.

FALSE   E. Small tears or damage (e.g., surgical instrumentation) may only require drainage.
            Ch. 70 Trauma, p 1431.

A   6.60. *Regarding the Radiology of the Renal Vasculature*

TRUE   A. The anterior branch is the predominant supply to the lower pole.
            Ch. 71 Conventional (film) arteriography and intra-arterial DSA, p 1454.

FALSE   B. All renal arteries are end-arteries (i.e., they supply only their own portion of the kidney, which is likely to become ischaemic if they are damaged).
            Ch. 71 Congenital Lesions, p 1455.

TRUE   C. They have no pathological circulation, appearing as filling defects in the nephrogram phase, and may have thin veins spread around them in the venous phase.
            Ch. 71 Tumours and Cysts, p 1455.

TRUE   D. The vascular pattern is often bizarre and may feature aneurysms and arteriovenous shunts.
            Ch. 71 Benign Tumours, p 1456.

TRUE   E.
            Ch. 71 Malignant Tumours, p 1457.

Q 6.61. *Regarding the Radiology of Renal Vascular Disease*

A. In established renal artery stenosis a collateral circulation often develops from the intercostal arteries

B. Most (noniatrogenic) renal aneurysms are intrarenal

C. An increasingly dense nephrogram is sometimes seen in renal vein thrombosis

D. The "cortical rim" sign on CT indicates acute cortical necrosis

E. Subcapsular renal haematoma is a cause of non-function

Q 6.62. *Features Suggestive of Renal Artery Stenosis (RAS) on Radionuclide Imaging Include*

A. Decreased perfusion on first-pass images

B. Decreased relative function

C. Reduced intrarenal transit time

D. Radionuclide tracer appearing in the collecting system only after 5 minutes

E. Increase in renal blood flow in the contralateral kidney after captopril administration

A *6.61. Regarding the Radiology of Renal Vascular Disease*

TRUE   A. Capsular collaterals may arise from intercostals and adrenal arteries. The internal iliac and gonadal vessels collateralize via peri-ureteric channels. The main collaterals are the first three lumbar arteries.
Ch. 71 Renal Artery Stenosis, p 1458.

FALSE   B. Most are extrarenal and secondary to atheroma. Fibromuscular dysplasia is also associated with aneurysm formation. The majority of *post-traumatic* pseudoaneurysms are intrarenal, including those resulting from renal biopsy.
Ch. 71 Renal Aneurysms, p 1458.

TRUE   C. This may rarely occur, sometimes with striations.
Ch. 71 Renal Vein Thrombosis, p 1463.

FALSE   D. In the presence of acute renal *infarction*, collateral vessels to the renal capsule generate a high-attenuation rim to the kidney following the administration of contrast medium
Ch. 71 Renal Infarction, p 1462.

TRUE   E. The renal capsule is bound down so tightly that a subcapsular haematoma can cause a rise in intrarenal pressure. This diminishes the vascular supply leading to renal nonfunction and, occasionally, malignant hypertension.
Ch. 71 Subcapsular Haematoma, p 1461.

A *6.62. Features Suggestive of Renal Artery Stenosis (RAS) on Radionuclide Imaging Include*

TRUE   A.
Ch. 71 Identification of RAS, p 1466.

TRUE   B. Defined as less than 45% of the total bilateral renal uptake. This sign is reliable only in unilateral disease.
Ch. 71 Identification of RAS, p 1466.

FALSE   C. Intrarenal transit time is increased.
Ch. 71 Identification of RAS, p 1466.

TRUE   D.
Ch. 71 Identification of RAS, p 1466.

TRUE   E.
Ch. 71 Identification of RAS, p 1466.

Q *6.63. Concerning the Radiology of Renovascular Hypertension*

A. Magnetic Resonance Imaging (MRI) better demonstrates the changes of fibromuscular dysplasia than those of atheromatous renal artery stenosis

B. If bilateral renal artery stenoses are present, percutaneous renal angioplasty should ideally be performed on both sides during a single procedure.

C. Balloon dilation of fibromuscular hyperplasia is rarely of sustained benefit to the patient

D. Balloon dilation of ostial stenoses is associated with an early reintervention rate

E. Screening for renovascular hypertension with Doppler ultrasound has a sensitivity of 90%

A 6.63. *Concerning the Radiology of Renovascular Hypertension*

FALSE

A. MRA of the renal arteries is not very successful and only the proximal 3–4 cm is reliably visualized. As fibromuscular dysplasia typically affects the distal two thirds of the renal artery, MRA is not good at diagnosing this condition.

Ch. 71 Magnetic Resonance Angiography, p 1468.

TRUE

B. This is not only more convenient but also prevents a successful reduction in blood pressure remitting from a unilateral intervention from causing a damaging reduction in blood flow to the contralateral (untreated) kidney.

Ch. 71 The Radiological Treatment of Renovascular Hypertension Technique, p 1473.

FALSE

C. Considerable and sustained improvement is seen in the majority of cases. This is probably the treatment of choice.

Ch. 71 The Radiological Treatment of Renovascular Hypertension, p 1474.

TRUE

D. These stenoses are atheromatous, and the plaque is contiguous with aortic atheroma. One theory is that balloon dilation of the ostium merely squeezes the atheroma out into the aorta, only for it to return soon afterwards. This is the argument that is put forward as grounds for the primary stenting of ostial stenosis.

Ch. 71 The Radiological Treatment of Renovascular Hypertension, p 1473.

FALSE

E. This is unfortunately not the case. The success rate is compromised by difficulty in identifying the renal arteries, the presence of multiple renal arteries and the wide variation in normal peak systolic velocity values. The sensitivity is at best, 70%.

Ch. 71 Duplex and Colour Doppler, p 1468.

Q *6.64. Regarding Injury to the Genitourinary Tract*

    A. Significant renal injury is present in 25% of patients with microscopic haematuria after blunt abdominal trauma

    B. Normal urinalysis effectively excludes significant renal injury

    C. Ultrasound is the investigation of choice in the initial assessment of renal damage in the multiple trauma patient

    D. Most bladder ruptures are extraperitoneal

    E. The most common urethral injuries are posterior in location

A 6.64. *Regarding Injury to the Genitourinary Tract*

FALSE   A. Significant renal injury will be found in only 1–2% of patients with microscopic haematuria, as opposed to 25% of patients with *gross* haematuria. *Ch. 72 Assessment, p 1478.*

FALSE   B. A kidney which has had severe injury (e.g., avulsion of its vascular pedicle) is unable to contribute any urine for urinalysis. *Ch. 72 Assessment, p 1478.*

FALSE   C. Ultrasound gives no indication of renal function and may reveal no abnormality in the presence of a renal arterial occlusion caused by traumatic subintimal thrombus. *Computed Tomography* is the investigation of choice in the initial assessment of the multiple trauma patient. *Ch. 72 Imaging, p 1479.*

TRUE   D. Extraperitoneal rupture occurs in at least 80% of cases. Flame-shaped strands of contrast medium are seen in the perivesical space anterior and lateral to the bladder on cystography. A "bladder within bladder" appearance may be seen on ultrasound. *Ch. 72 Classification, p 1485.*

TRUE   E. These occur in association with fractures of the pelvic rami. Complete tearing allows the prostate and bladder to ascend into the peritoneal cavity. *Ch. 72 Posterior Urethra, p 1486.*

Q 6.65. *Regarding Imaging of the Kidney in Renal Failure*

    A. Demonstration of a dilated pelvicalyceal system implies the presence of obstruction

    B. Ultrasound is the method of choice for excluding obstruction of the renal pelvis in polycystic kidney disease

    C. High dose urography uses about 60 mg of Iodine per kg of patient weight

    D. Obstructive renal failure is ruled out when collecting system dilation is not identified on ultrasound, CT, antegrade or retrograde pyelography

    E. High-dose urography should not be used to diagnose obstruction if a definite nephrogram has not been identified on standard dose urography

Q 6.66. *An Increasingly Dense Nephrogram on IV Urography is Seen in*

    A. Acute obstruction

    B. Acute tubular necrosis (ATN) complicating underlying glomerular disease

    C. Acute cortical necrosis

    D. Renal ischaemia

    E. Acute suppurative pyelonephritis

A *6.65. Regarding Imaging of the Kidney in Renal Failure*

FALSE

A. Distension or apparent distension of the pelvicaliceal system has many causes other than obstruction; these include residual post-obstructive dilation, infection, clubbed calices in reflux nephropathy, a well-filled system in a well hydrated subject, extrarenal pelvis and a large major calix.
Ch. 73 Ultrasonography, p 1492.

FALSE

B. Multiple cysts and polycystic kidney disease pose particular problems when obstruction is suspected. It is frequently impossible to diagnose obstruction in the presence of these disorders.
Ch. 73 Ultrasonography, p 1492.

FALSE

C. A normal IVU uses about 300 mgI/kg. High dose urography employs twice this amount (i.e., 600 mgI/kg).
Ch. 73 High Dose Urography, p 1492.

FALSE

D. It has been well established that dilation of the collecting system may not occur in the presence of obstruction in certain instances. These include very low urine output and certain infiltrative processes in the retroperitoneum that inhibit pelviureteric dilation (e.g., retroperitoneal fibrosis).
Ch. 73 Diagnosis of the Cause of Renal Failure: Further Procedures, p 1494.

TRUE

E.
Ch. 73 High Dose Urography, p 1492.

A *6.66. An Increasingly Dense Nephrogram on IV Urography is Seen in*

TRUE

A.
Ch. 73 Nonobstructed Kidneys, p 1495.

TRUE

B. ATN alone generally causes an immediate persistent nephrogram, but in the presence of glomerular disease, an increase in radio-density over time may be seen.
Ch. 73 Nonobstructed Kidneys, p 1495.

FALSE

C.
Ch. 73 Nonobstructed Kidneys, p 1495.

TRUE

D.
Ch. 73 Nonobstructed Kidneys, p 1495.

TRUE

E. This occasionally causes an increasingly dense nephrogram.
Ch. 73 Nonobstructed Kidneys, p 1495.

Q 6.67. *Regarding the Radiology of Renal Transplantation*

A. During donor arteriography, renal arteries tend to fill earlier than lumbar arteries

B. Routine selective renal arteriography is mandatory in all donors to rule out the presence of supernumerary renal arteries

C. During evaluation of the transplant kidney, isotope uptake between 80 and 180 seconds after injection is an index of renal function

D. Reduced corticomedullary differentiation on MRI of the transplant kidney is specific for acute rejection

E. Identification of a dilated collecting system in a transplant kidney is an indication for urgent nephrostomy

A *6.67. Regarding the Radiology of Renal Transplantation*

TRUE   A. This can be a helpful distinguishing feature. A further clue is that the lumbar arteries have a characteristic bend where they curve backwards around the vertebral body.
Ch. 73 Vascular Studies, p 1497.

FALSE   B. There is a very small but unacceptable risk of damaging a normal kidney during selective angiography. This should be reserved for those cases in which there is doubt about the number of renal arteries supplying the kidney to be donated.
Ch. 73 Vascular Studies, p 1497.

TRUE   C. This period reflects early glomerular filtration and is an indicator of renal function.
Ch. 73 Radionuclide Imaging, p 1498.

FALSE   D. Like an increased resistivity index, reduced corticomedullary differentiation on MRI is non-specific and occurs in several conditions, notably acute rejection, cyclosporin nephrotoxicity and ATN.
Ch. 73 Magnetic Resonance Imaging, p 1503.

FALSE   E. Minor degrees of dilatation can occur normally in a transplant kidney. Transplant ureteric reflux can cause dilatation without obstruction. On the other hand, an increase in the size of the collecting system accompanied by deteriorating function requires urgent investigation.
Ch. 73 Urological Complications, p. 1503.

Q 6.68. *Concerning Radiological Assessment of Renal Transplant Complications*

    A. The most common perinephric collection is a urinoma

    B. Transplant renal arterial occlusion cannot be distinguished from acute rejection by radionuclide imaging

    C. Radionuclide scans reliably differentiate between transplant renal artery stenosis and chronic rejection

    D. Renal vein thrombosis causes retrograde arterial flow during diastole on Doppler ultrasound of the transplant artery

    E. A post-transplant biopsy renal arteriovenous fistula causes a perivascular colour mosaic on Doppler ultrasound

Q 6.69. *Concerning the Paediatric IVU Examination of the Urinary Tract*

    A. The plain film is to be avoided as part of the normal IVU

    B. Three ml/Kg of iohexol 300 would be an appropriate dose in the neonate

    C. A 35 degree "angled-up" view centred over the xiphisternum is necessary to give good anatomical detail of the upper-pole calices

    D. An IVU is not recommended below the age of 3 months

    E. Normal renal outlines preclude the need for DMSA

A 6.68. Concerning Radiological Assessment of Renal Transplant Complications

FALSE

A. The most common collection is a lymphocele, which often contains septa, but may be indistinguishable from a urinoma.
Ch. 73 Fluid Collections, p 1504.

TRUE

B. Nonperfusion occurs in both conditions and, when present, warrants further investigation with Doppler ultrasound and/or angiography.
Ch. 73 Vascular Complications, p 1506.

FALSE

C.
Ch. 73 Vascular Complications, p. 1506.

TRUE

D. Renal vein thrombosis causes retrograde arterial flow during diastole on Doppler ultrasound of the transplant artery.
Ch. 73 Renal Vein Thrombosis, p. 1510.

TRUE

E. This is caused by pulsatile vibration of the renal parenchyma and the associated turbulent blood flow.
Ch. 73 Haemorrhage and Arteriovenous Fistulae, p 1507.

A 6.69. Concerning the Paediatric IVU Examination of the Urinary Tract

FALSE

A. The same criteria apply to the child as to the adult. The plain film is necessary to assess nephrocalcinosis and to detect renal tract stones that could easily be missed after the administration of contrast medium.
Ch. 74 Plain Film and IVU, p 1515.

TRUE

B. Children need a higher dose than adults owing to the relatively poor function of the immature kidney.
Ch. 74 Plain Film and IVU, p 1515.

FALSE

C. The correct view is a 35 degree *angled-down* view. It is extremely useful, especially in the assessment of the upper-pole calices in a duplex system.
Ch. 74 Plain Film and IVU, p 1515.

FALSE

D. An IVU is contraindicated in children under the age of 48 hours, as the normal kidneys tend not to be visualized.
Ch. 74 Plain Film and IVU, p 1515.

FALSE

E. Furthermore, the IVU will not give an accurate assessment of differential function.
Ch. 74 Plain Film and IVU, p 1515.

Q 6.70. *Calcification on the Plain AXR is Demonstrated in Over 50% of the Following Abdominal Tumours of Childhood*

    A. Neuroblastoma

    B. Rhabdomyosarcoma

    C. Renal-cell carcinoma of childhood

    D. Mesoblastic nephroma

    E. Nephroblastomatosis

Q 6.71. *Concerning Neuroblastoma*

    A. Over 50% of such tumours arise in the abdomen

    B. Most patients present with metastases

    C. Some patients present with the "doll's eye syndrome"

    D. The ^{99m}Tc MDP bone scan is normal in stage 4s

    E. Urinary 5-HIAA levels are helpful in the diagnosis

A 6.70. *Calcification on the Plain AXR is Demonstrated in Over 50% of the Following Abdominal Tumours of Childhood*

TRUE A. This is a finely stippled or amorphous type of calcification.
Ch. 74 Neroblastoma, p 1547.

FALSE B. Calcification is not usually present.
Ch. 74 Rhabdomyosarcoma, p 1548.

FALSE C. Calcification is seen in approximately 25% of cases.

FALSE D.

FALSE E.

A 6.71. *Concerning Neuroblastoma*

TRUE A. Neuroblastoma is the commonest extra-cranial solid malignancy to occur in the early years of life. Over two thirds of the intra-abdominal tumours occur in the adrenal glands.
Ch. 74 Neuroblastoma, p 1547.

TRUE B. This is the most common form of presentation.
Ch. 74 Neuroblastoma, p 1547.

FALSE C. The *dancing eye* syndrome.
Ch. 74 Neuroblastoma, p 1547.

TRUE D. Stage 4s is defined as localized primary tumour. Stage (1 or 2) with metastatic disease in one or more of the following; liver, skin or marrow.
Ch. 74 Neuroblastoma, p 1547.

FALSE E. The urinary levels of VMA and HVA are elevated in the latter stages of the disease (i.e., 2b to 4s).
Ch. 74 Neuroblastoma, p 1547.

Q   6.72. *Concerning Wilms' Tumour*

A. There is a peak age at 1 year

B. Bilateral tumours occur in 20% of patients

C. Forty to 50% of patients present with haematuria

D. Tumour calcification on the AXR is present in up to 50% of patients

E. MRI has significantly improved tumour staging and is now the imaging modality of choice

Q   6.73. *Concerning Hypertension in Children*

A. Renal pathology is the cause in over 90% of children over one year old

B. Essential hypertension generally shows borderline readings

C. If the USS demonstrates a small kidney, a ^{99m}Tc DMSA scan and an MCU are indicated

D. An Iodine-123 MIBG scan should be carried out in suspected cases of phaeochromocytoma

E. There is an association with neurofibromatosis

A 6.72. *Concerning Wilms' Tumour*

FALSE   A. The peak age is 3-4 years.
Ch. 74 Renal tumours, p 1544.

FALSE   B. Only 5% of patients have bilateral tumours. It is nevertheless, imperative that both kidneys are fully assessed prior to therapy.
Ch. 74 Renal tumours, p 1544.

FALSE   C. The incidence of haematuria is 15%. Hypertension may occasionally be present.
Ch. 74 Renal tumours, p 1544.

FALSE   D. Only 20% of patients demonstrate calcification on the plain abdominal radiograph.
Ch. 74 Renal tumours, p 1544.

FALSE   E. MRI has not changed the staging or improved treatment protocols to date.
Ch. 74 Renal tumours, p 1544.

A 6.73. *Concerning Hypertension in Children*

TRUE   A. The younger the child, especially <1 year old, and the more severe the hypertension, the more likely it is that the hypertension is secondary rather than primary hypertension.
Ch. 74 Hypertension, p 1544.

TRUE   B. These patients generally have a good family history.
Ch. 74 Hypertension, p 1544.

TRUE   C. The ^{99m}Tc DMSA scan is necessary to assess function and an MCUG to look for VUR. If these examinations are normal, an IVU is recommended.
Ch. 74 Hypertension, p 1544.

TRUE   D. A CT scan should be undertaken in the region of increased tracer uptake. Many phaeochromocytomas in children are extra-adrenal in location.
Ch. 74 Hypertension, p 1544.

TRUE   E.
Ch. 74 Hypertension, p 1544.

Q 6.74. *The Following Statements are True in Respect of Vesico-Ureteric Reflux (VUR)*

    A. Damage to the kidney is usually present at the time of the first UTI

    B. VUR is familial

    C. Renal damage is seen in 30% of children without UTI following the antenatal diagnosis of non-obstructed hydronephrosis

    D. Pyelonephritic scars are the commonest cause of hypertension in children

    E. A normal MCUG

Q 6.75. *Concerning Abdominal Masses in the Neonate*

    A. The most common abdominal mass in an apparently healthy neonate is a Wilms' tumour

    B. Mesoblastic nephroma is the commonest solid renal mass in the neonate

    C. Urgent surgery is required for most cases of multicystic dysplastic kidneys

    D. A mesoblastic nephroma is benign

    E. Myelolipomas are demonstrated in patients with tuberose sclerosis

A 6.74. *The Following Statements are True in Respect of Vesico-Ureteric Reflux (VUR)*

TRUE   A. Scarring usually occurs within the first year of life and possibly within the first 6 months.
       Ch. 74 Infection, p 1541.

TRUE   B.
       Ch. 74 Infection, p 1541.

TRUE   C. Infection is not always the cause of scarring.
       Ch.l 74 Infection, p 1541.

TRUE   D. There is a 10% risk of a scarred kidney leading to hypertension.
       Ch. 74 Neonatal Infection, p 1541.

TRUE   E. VUR may be intermittent.
       Ch. 74 Infection, p 1541.

A 6.75. *Concerning Abdominal Masses in the Neonate*

FALSE   A. The most common renal mass is a multicystic dysplastic kidney.
       Ch. 74 The Neonate, p 1539.

TRUE   B. The mean age at diagnosis is 3 1/2 months. A mesoblastic nephroma may demonstrate some renal function.

FALSE   C. Surgery is only indicated when the patient is symptomatic from the mass effect.
       Ch. 74 The Neonate, p 1539.

FALSE   D. A mesoblastic nephroma requires complete excision as tumour spillage may produce a recurrence.
       Ch. 74 The Neonate, p 1539.

FALSE   E. The renal features of tuberose sclerosis, apart from cysts, include *angiomyolipomas*. Myelolipomas are found in the adrenal glands of adults.

Q 6.76. *The Following are Features of the Prune Belly Syndrome (PBS)*

      A. Undescended testes

      B. Renal dysplasia

      C. The disorder is unique to males.

      D. The upper ureters are disproportionately dilated in comparison with the lower ureters.

      E. A posterior urethral valve on MCUG is pathognomonic of this condition.

Q 6.77. *Concerning Megaureter in Children*

      A. Secondary megaureter is more common than primary megaureter

      B. Electron microscopy demonstrates an aganglionic distal segment

      C. Girls are more frequently affected than boys

      D. Vesico-ureteric reflux often co-exists with megaureter

      E. Surgery is always the treatment of choice

A 6.76. *The Following are Features of the Prune Belly Syndrome (PBS)*

TRUE   A. The features of this syndrome are undescended testes, absence of the anterior abdominal wall, dysplastic kidneys, "sigmoid" lower ureters and prostatic hypoplasia.
Ch. 74 Bladder Anomalies, p 1535.

TRUE   B. An absent abdominal wall muscle makes the PBS.
Ch. 74 Bladder Anomalies, p 1535.

FALSE   C. PBS does occur in females, but very rarely.
Ch. 74 Bladder Anomalies, p 1535.

FALSE   D. The converse.
Ch. 74 Bladder Anomalies, p 1535.

FALSE   E. There is often a wide posterior urethra with *no* PUV or thickened bladder wall.
Ch. 74 Bladder Anomalies, p 1535.

A 6.77. *Concerning Megaureter in Children*

FALSE   A. Secondary causes are rarely found in paediatrics; they include tumours and calculi.
Ch. 74 Renal, Pelvic and Ureteric Anomalies, p 1529.

FALSE   B. Electron microscopy demonstrates abnormal muscle fibres, with fibrosis in the lower ureter where it enters the bladder.
Ch. 74 Renal, Pelvic and Ureteric Anomalies, p 1529.

FALSE   C. The opposite.
Ch. 74 Renal, Pelvic and Ureteric Anomalies, p 1529.

TRUE   D. As this disorder is more common in boys, a micturating cystourethrogram (MCUG) is necessary to assess for reflux and examine the posterior urethra.
Ch. 74 Renal, Pelvic and Ureteric Anomalies, p 1529.

FALSE   E. There is much dispute amongst paediatric urologists, especially in patients in whom vesico-ureteric reflux is present, as to the correct management of these children.
Ch. 74 Renal, Pelvic and Ureteric Anomalies, p 1529.

Q 6.78. Concerning Renal Tract Duplication

A. The Weigert-Meyer law explains the inverse relationship between the insertion of the ureters and the position of the renal segment they drain

B. A simple ureterocele can be demonstrated in the upper moiety ureter of a duplex kidney

C. Dilatation in the upper moiety of a duplex system is most likely to be due to ureteric obstruction

D. Reflux tends to occur more frequently in the lower-pole moiety ureter

E. PUJ obstruction tends to occur in the upper moiety

Q 6.79. The Following are Associated with Renal Cysts

A. Tuberose sclerosis

B. Dysplastic kidney

C. Turner's syndrome

D. Megacalicosis

E. Zellweger syndrome

A 6.78. *Concerning Renal Tract Duplication*

TRUE	A.
	Ch. 74 Renal, Pelvic and Ureteric Anomalies, p 1529.
FALSE	B. Simple ureterocetes tend to occur in nonduplex systems (i.e., are orthotopic). The ureterocele in a duplex system is ectopic (i.e., not simple). *Ch. 74 Renal, Pelvic and Ureteric Anomalies, p 1529.*
TRUE	C. Obstruction tends to occur at the vesico-ureteric junction where there may be a congenital stenosis, a ureterocele stenosis or a stone. *Ch. 74 Renal, Pelvic and Ureteric Anomalies, p 1529.*
TRUE	D. See above. *Ch. 74 Renal, Pelvic and Ureteric Anomalies, p 1529.*
FALSE	E. Pelviureteric junction obstruction tends to occur in the *lower-pole moiety*. It is an uncommon finding in a duplex system. *Ch. 74 Renal, Pelvic and Ureteric Anomalies, p 1529.*

A 6.79. *The Following are Associated with Renal Cysts*

TRUE	A.
	Ch. 74 Polycystic Renal Disease, p 1527.
FALSE	B. Dysplastic kidney(s), per se, are not associated with cysts. *Ch. 74 Polycystic Renal Anomalies, p 1524.*
TRUE	C.
	Ch. 74 Renal Pelvis and Ureteric Anomalies, p 1524.
FALSE	D.
	Ch. 74 Renal Pelvis and Ureteric Anomalies, p 1529.
TRUE	E.
	Ch. 74 Renal Pelvis and Ureteric Anomalies, p 1524.

Q *6.80. Regarding Routine Indications for a Micturating Cystogram*

    A. A urinary tract infection in a child under the age of 1 year

    B. The follow-up of vesico-ureteric reflux

    C. The screening of girls with UTI

    D. The demonstration of a thick-walled bladder on USS

    E. The investigation of children with renal failure of unknown cause

Q *6.81. Concerning the Dynamic Radionuclide Scan*

    A. The blood-flow phase occurs between 30 and 60 seconds

    B. The blood-flow phase can be used to estimate the percentage of cardiac output to the kidneys

    C. A renal curve falling to less than 75% of its maximum value would be considered "normal drainage"

    D. A poor response to a diuretic stimulus may be normal in children with a full bladder

    E. A ^{57}Cr-DTPA scan is the best method for the assessment of differential renal function

A 6.80. *Regarding Routine Indications for a Micturating Cystogram*

TRUE   A. This is irrespective of sex.
Ch. 74 MCUG, p 1517.

FALSE   B. A radionuclide scan is recommended for follow-up, as it entails a much lower radiation dose than a micturating cystourethrogram, and it is a qualitative and quantitative examination.
Ch. 74 MCUG, p 1517.

FALSE   C. As above, the radiation dose is significantly lower.
Ch. 74 MCUG, p 1517.

TRUE   D. A thick-walled bladder suggests hypertrophy that may be secondary to outflow obstruction. In males posterior urethral valves are the commonest type of outflow obstruction.
Ch. 74 MCUG, p 1517.

TRUE   E.
Ch. 74 MCUG, p 1517.

A 6.81. *Concerning the Dynamic Radionuclide Scan*

FALSE   A. The blood-flow phase is the earliest phase (0-15 seconds), followed by the uptake and the transit/drainage phases.
Ch. 74 Radionuclide Scans, p 1520.

TRUE   B. This can be estimated if the initial sequences are acquired rapidly.
Ch. 74 Radionuclide Scans, p 1520.

TRUE   C. Normal drainage can also be defined as 50% fall of its maximum over 20 minutes.
Ch. 74 Radionuclide Scans, p 1520.

TRUE   D. A poor response may also be demonstrated in children with poor renal function and grossly dilated collecting systems.
Ch. 74 Radionuclide Scans, p 1520.

FALSE   E.

Q 6.82. *The Indications, in Children, for a Static Renal Scan Include*

    A. The acute phase of a renal infection

    B. Assessment of the "wet girl" with a normal ultrasound scan and intravenous urogram

    C. Estimating the degree of reflux

    D. The estimation of differential renal function when there is gross dilation of the collecting systems

    E. The assessment of protein loss in patients with the nephrotic syndrome

Q 6.83. *Concerning the Embryology of the Urinary Tract*

    A. The pronephros eventually develops into the renal tubules

    B. The mesonephric duct develops from the pronephric duct

    C. The paramesonephric duct forms the ductus deferens

    D. The Müllerian ducts are the primitive precursors of the Fallopian tubes

    E. The ureteric bud develops as a dorsomedial outgrowth from the caudal aspect of the mesonephric duct

A 6.82. *The Indications, in Children, for a Static Renal Scan Include*

TRUE   A. A ^{99m}Tc DMSA scan is ideal for assessing renal involvement in the acute phase.
Ch. 74 Radionuclide Scans, p 1520.

TRUE   B. ^{99m}Tc DMSA may be the only way of detecting an occult duplex kidney.
Ch. 74 Radionuclide Scans, p 1520.

FALSE   C. Reflux can be estimated by an MCUG scan, a ^{99m}Tc DTPA (and ^{99m}Tc MAG-3 by an indirect radioisotope cystogram) or by a direct isotope cystogram. Reflux *cannot* be assessed by static scanning.
Ch. 74 Radionuclide Scans, p 1520.

TRUE   D. Static scanning is the best technique in this situation and may also be useful in chronic renal failure.
Ch. 74 Radionuclide Scans, p 1520.

FALSE   E. Although ^{99m}Tc DMSA is bound to protein, it is not used in the assessment of the nephrotic syndrome.
Ch. 74 Radionuclide Scans, p 1520.

A 6.83. *Concerning the Embryology of the Urinary Tract*

FALSE   A. Although the pronephros is important in the development of the metanephros, it is formed at 3 weeks and resorbed by the 4th week "in utero."
Ch. 74 Embryology, p 1529.

FALSE   B. The other way around.
Ch. 74 Embryology, p 1529.

FALSE   C. The mesonephric duct forms the Wolffian duct, which in turn develops into the ductus deferens.
Ch. 74 Embryology, p 1529.

FALSE   D. The Müllerian ducts develop to form the lower urethra, a small portion of the vagina and the vestibule.
Ch. 74 Embryology, p 1529.

TRUE   E. The ureteric bud unites with the metanephric blastema to form the metanephros and thus forms the primitive kidney.
Ch. 74 Embryology, p 1529.

Q *6.84. Regarding Congenital Renal Anomalies*

    A. The incidence of unilateral renal agenesis is between 1/1000 and 1/2000

    B. A thoracic kidney can present as a posterior mediastinal mass

    C. A horse-shoe kidney is always associated with malrotation of the kidneys

    D. Horse-shoe kidneys are associated with an increased risk of neuroblastoma

    E. There is an increased incidence of vesico-ureteric reflux in the crossed kidney in patients with crossed, fused, renal ectopia

Q *6.85. Regarding Typical Features of Renal Dysplasia*

    A. Large kidney(s)

    B. Large cortical cysts

    C. Localized lower pole dysplasia

    D. There is an increased incidence of PUJ obstruction

    E. An association with Meckel's diverticulum

A 6.84. *Regarding Congenital Renal Anomalies*

TRUE
A. This is only an estimate, as the true incidence is difficult to ascertain. In some cases, multicystic kidneys may resorb at 6-24 months of fetal life, thus, presenting as renal agenesis.
Ch. 74 Renal Anomalies, p 1524.

TRUE
B. Thoracic kidneys are often associated with diaphragmatic eventration. Almost all ectopic kidneys take their blood supply from their final position, hence a thoracic kidney will tend to be supplied from the thoracic aorta.
Ch. 74 Renal Anomalies, p 1524.

TRUE
C. This is a characteristic feature of a horse-shoe kidney. The ureters pass anteriorly over the lower poles of the kidney.
Ch. 74 Renal Anomalies, p 1524.

FALSE
D. *Wilms' tumour*; renal stones and PUJ obstruction are more frequent in patients with a horse-shoe kidney.
Ch. 74 Renal Anomalies, p 1524.

TRUE
E. The importance of this condition is that there is also an increased incidence of PUJ obstruction.
Ch. 74 Renal Anomalies, p 1524.

A 6.85. *Regarding Typical Features of Renal Dysplasia*

FALSE
A. The kidney is generally small.
Ch. 74 Renal Anomalies, p 1524.

FALSE
B. US shows loss of the normal corticomedullary differentiation and small (1-2 mm) transonic areas suggestive of tiny cortical cysts.
Ch. 74 Renal Anomalies, p 1524.

FALSE
C. When dysplasia is localized, it may be demonstrated in the upper pole: the Usk-Upmark Kidney.
Ch. 74 Renal Anomalies, p 1524.

FALSE
D. The most common associated renal tract disorder is VUR.
Ch. 74 Renal Anomalies, p 1524.

FALSE
E. Renal dysplasia is associated with the Meckel *syndrome*, the Beckwith-Weidemann syndrome and the Lawrence-Moon-Biedl syndrome.
Ch. 74 Renal Anomalies, p 1524.

Q *6.86. Regarding Features of Multicystic Dysplastic Kidney*

    A. Ureteric atresia

    B. A normal or small-sized kidney

    C. A large cyst situated near the renal hilum

    D. Fifty percent of patients have either a stenosis in the upper third of the opposite ureter or a PUJ obstruction

    E. Hemihypertrophy

Q *6.87. Concerning Polycystic Renal Disease*

    A. There is a significant number of children in whom the differentiation between the dominant and recessive forms is impossible

    B. Hepatic fibrosis is always associated with autosomal recessive polycystic disease (ARPD)

    C. ARPD is generally associated with a family history

    D. Potassium loss is a common complication in children with ARPD

    E. Autosomal dominant polycystic disease (ADPD) presents in infancy in 30-40% of cases

A 6.86. *Regarding Features of Multicystic Dysplastic Kidney*

TRUE   A. This is characteristic of this disorder.
Ch. 74 Renal Anomalies, p 1524.

TRUE   B. Although the kidney is often large and contains many cysts, it may be normal in size or even small.
Ch. 74 Renal Anomalies, p 1524.

FALSE   C. A large cyst is often demonstrated over the *lateral* aspect of the kidney. This feature enables MDK to be differentiated from PUJ obstruction on USS.
Ch. 74 Renal Anomalies, p 1524.

TRUE   D. If the USS of the opposite kidney is normal at birth, an IVU or a dynamic renal scan may be necessary at 3 months of age.
Ch. 74 Renal Anomalies, p 1524.

FALSE   E.
Ch. 74 Renal Anomalies, p 1524.

A 6.87. *Concerning Polycystic Renal Disease*

TRUE   A. Although doubt may exist in some cases, careful attention to the antenatal USS (including the liver) may help to resolve these diagnostic difficulties.
Ch. 74 Polycystic Renal Disease, p 1527.

FALSE   B. ARPD is always associated with hepatic fibrosis, with or without biliary ectasia (similar to that seen in Caroli's disease). The *converse* is not always true.
Ch. 74 Polycystic Renal Disease, p 1527.

FALSE   C. Clinically, there is no family history. Children present with bilateral abdominal masses or haematemesis in adolescence.
Ch. 74 Polycystic Renal Disease, p 1527.

FALSE   D. During the first month of life, *sodium* loss is a common complication. Irreversible renal failure is not common.
Ch. 74 Polycystic Renal Disease, p 1527.

FALSE   E. ADPD has been described in infancy but presentation at this age is extremely rare.
Ch. 74 Polycystic Renal Disease, p 1527.

Q *6.88. Regarding Posterior Urethral Valves (PUV)*

    A. The commonest presentation is with UTI and septicaemia

    B. Type 1 urethral valves are associated with renal dysplasia

    C. Functional renal studies are necessary to assess the renal tract prior to surgery

    D. There is an association with the prune belly syndrome

    E. There is an association with Turner's syndrome

A *6.88. Regarding Posterior Urethral Valves (PUV)*

FALSE   A. This is an extremely rare mode of presentation. The diagnosis is usually made in early infancy or during the antenatal period of ultrasound scanning. Bilateral hydronephrosis and a full bladder are demonstrated. The findings are associated with progressive olgohydramnios which may require in utero drainage.
Ch. 74 Urethral Anomalies, p 1537.

FALSE   B. There are three types of urethral valves. The most common is type 1, in which two folds, at the level of the verumontanum, have a central slit-like orifice. Type 3 valves have a narrow pinpoint orifice and are associated with renal dysplasia and minimal renal tract dilation.
Ch. 74 Urethral Anomalies, p 1537.

FALSE   C. A dynamic scan is recommended 3-4 weeks following surgical ablation of the valve, after correction of any metabolic imbalance.
Ch. 74 Urethral Anomalies, p 1537.

FALSE   D. The posterior urethra is dilated in patients with PBS, but this is due to prostatic hypoplasia and laxity of the ligaments around the base of the bladder.
Ch. 74 Bladder Anomalies, p 1537.

FALSE   E. PUVs occur in males; Turner's syndrome occurs in females.
Ch. 74 Urethral Anomalies, p 1537.

Q 6.89. The Following Statements are True in the Neonate/Infant

A. The blood flow to the kidney at birth and in the neonatal period is predominantly to the cortical regions

B. The GFR increases three-fold during an infant's first year of life

C. Sodium reabsorption, in the neonate, is predominantly in the proximal tubule

D. There is a small extracellular fluid space

E. During the first week of life radionuclide imaging reaches acceptable levels of accuracy

A *6.89. The Following Statements are True in the Neonate/Infant*

FALSE

A. Blood flow is predominantly to the juxtamedullary regions; this effect is produced by the high vascular resistance of the kidney during this developmental period.
Ch. 74 The Neonate, p 1539.

TRUE

B. The kidney is fully mature at about the time of puberty.
Ch. 74 The Neonate, p 1539.

FALSE

C. Sodium reabsorption occurs predominantly in the distal tubule owing to the poor development of the proximal tubule. Proximal tubular function can be assessed by para amino hippurate. Adult function is achieved by two years of age.
Ch. 74 The Neonate, p 1539.

FALSE

D. The converse. Infants and neonates have a large volume of distribution that is due to their large extracellular fluid space.
Ch. 74 The Neonate, p 1539.

FALSE

E. Below 4 weeks of age, most radionuclide imaging is of relatively poor quality. If there is any doubt as to the sensitivity, specificity or accuracy of a study, a repeat scan at about 3 months is recommended.
Ch. 74 The Neonate, p 1539.

Q *6.90. Regarding Percutaneous Nephrostomy*

    A. Puncture of an upper-pole calix is preferred as this facilitates wire manipulation into the ureter

    B. Passage through the maximum available depth of renal parenchyma is preferred in order to maximise stability of the nephrostomy drain

    C. Renal pseudoaneurysms caused by central punctures are best treated by transcatheter embolisation

    D. Percutaneous nephrostomy should be performed in all cases of malignant ureteric obstruction to avoid death from renal failure

    E. Percutaneous nephrostomy should not be performed on horseshoe kidneys

A 6.90. *Regarding Percutaneous Nephrostomy*

FALSE

    A. A lower-pole calix is the preferred target, because an intercostal approach (with the risk of pneumothorax) is very seldom necessary to gain access to this site, and because the risk of bleeding is less owing to the orientation of interlobar arteries.

    Ch. 75 Percutaneous Needle Nephrostomy, p 1552.

FALSE

    B. The *minimum* depth of renal parenchyma is traversed during puncture of a lower-pole calix. This reduces the risk of bleeding from an interlobar artery.

    Ch. 75 Percutaneous Needle Nephrostomy, p 1552.

TRUE

    C. Superselective transcatheter embolization using a 3Fr co-axial catheter and microcoils is the treatment of choice for these lesions.

    Ch. 75 Percutaneous Needle Nephrostomy, p 1552.

FALSE

    D. The technique is generally best reserved for patients who have treatable disease. Nephrostomy may prevent painless early death from obstructive renal failure but may allow the malignancy to invade the sacral plexus and cause intractable pain; therefore, it is not recommended.

    Ch. 75 Percutaneous Needle Nephrostomy, p 1552.

FALSE

    E. Malrotated and horseshoe kidneys are not contraindications to this procedure.

    Ch. 75 Trocar or Seldinger Technique, p 1553.

Q 6.91. *Regarding Interventional Uroradiology and Lithotripsy*

    A. Dilation of a track to 30 Fr is performed during percutaneous nephrolithotomy

    B. Balloon dilation of the prostatic urethra is now the treatment of choice for obstruction caused by non-calcified prostate glands

    C. Extracorporeal shock wave lithotripsy (ESWL) using ultrasound requires general or epidural anaesthetic

    D. Stones in the lower one-third of the ureter are often amenable to treatment by extracorporeal shock wave lithotripsy

    E. Impacted upper ureteric stones are best treated in situ by ESWL

A *6.91. Regarding Interventional Uroradiology and Lithotripsy*

TRUE   A. This allows the nephroscope to be inserted percutaneously, and small stones can be grasped and removed. Larger stones can be subjected to disintegration methods.
Ch. 75 Percutaneous Nephrolithotomy, p 1554.

FALSE   B. Only a slight and transient benefit occurs in most patients.
Ch. 75 Balloon Dilation of the Prostate, p 1564.

FALSE   C. The second generation ultrasound machines create multiple shock waves, which travel through soft tissue via many different paths, and the patient experiences no pain.
Ch. 75 Extracorporeal Shock Wave Lithotripsy, p 1567.

TRUE   D. If such stones lie below the ischial spines they can be localized easily and subjected to ESWL. Above the ischial spine level, treatment by ureteroscopic laser fragmentation is used.
Ch. 75 Lower Third Stones, p 1567.

FALSE   E. Ureteric stones pose focusing difficulties for ESWL. The simplest way to manage them is to attempt to disimpact them by flushing them back into the renal pelvis using a retrograde catheter. A double-J stent is then inserted to prevent re-entry into the ureter and ESWL is performed.
Ch. 75 Upper Third Stones, p 1567.

7

The Skeletal System

Q *7.1. The Following are Features of a Neuropathic Fracture*

    A. Bony destruction

    B. Dislocation

    C. Disorganization

    D. Decreased bony density

    E. Bony debris

Q *7.2. Regarding Stress Fractures of Bone*

    A. Plain radiographs, at the time of presentation, demonstrate the lesion in most cases

    B. A subtle periosteal reaction or a transverse linear band of sclerosis is not demonstrated for at least one month

    C. A bone scan is positive in no more than 20% of patients immediately after the injury

    D. If the fracture occurs in normal bone it is termed an insufficiency fracture

    E. March fractures can occur anywhere in the metacarpals

A 7.1. *The Following are Features of a Neuropathic Fracture*

TRUE   *A.*

   Ch. 76 General Considerations, p 1574.

TRUE   *B.*

   Ch. 76 General Considerations, p 1574.

TRUE   *C.*

   Ch. 76 General Considerations, p 1574.

FALSE   *D.* There is usually an *increase* in bone density manifest by sclerosis and hetero-topic bone formation.
   Ch. 76 General Considerations, p 1574.

TRUE   *E.* The neuropathic fracture can be represented by the "5Ds" (listed in this question).
   Ch. 76 General Considerations, p 1574.

A 7.2. *Regarding Stress Fractures of Bone*

FALSE   *A.* Most are not seen at the initial presentation.
   Ch. 76 General Considerations, p 1574.

FALSE   *B.* The signs of a stress fracture are generally seen about 1-2 weeks after the injury.
   Ch. 76 General Considerations, p 1574.

FALSE   *C.* The bone scan is nearly always immediately positive in patients, at the time of injury.
   Ch. 76 General Considerations, p 1574.

FALSE   *D.* A stress fracture in normal bone is a "fatigue" fracture; in abnormal bone it is termed an "insufficiency" fracture.
   Ch. 76 General Considerations, p 1574.

FALSE   *E.* March fractures were described in the *feet* of soldiers, not in the hands.
   Ch. 76 General Considerations, p 1574.

Q 7.3. *The Following Muscles and Bony Sites Are Associated in Avulsion Fractures*

A. Sartorius and anterior inferior iliac spine

B. The reflected head of rectus femoris and the anterior inferior iliac spine

C. The hamstrings and the ischial spine

D. Adductor avulsion and the inferior pubic ramus

E. Iliopsoas and the lesser femoral trochanter

Q 7.4. *Concerning Fractures of the Pelvis and Sacrum*

A. Bilateral disruption of the sacroiliac ligaments without dislocation is often not associated with a fracture

B. Vertical shear forces on the pelvis produce the Malgaigne complex

C. Urethral injury is uncommon with straddle injuries

D. Judet's views are recommended for pubic rami fractures

E. A lateral sacral and coccygeal view is recommended if a coccyx fracture is clinically suspected

A 7.3. *The Following Muscles and Bony Sites Are Associated in Avulsion Fractures*

FALSE   A. Anterior *superior* iliac spine.
Ch. 76 The Pelvis, p 1576.

FALSE   B. The *straight* head.
Ch. 76 The Pelvis, p 1576.

FALSE   C. The ischial *tuberosity*.
Ch. 76 The Pelvis, p 1576.

FALSE   D. The inferior *ischial* ramus.
Ch. 76 The Pelvis, p 1576.

TRUE   E.
Ch. 76 The Pelvis, p 1576.

A 7.4. *Concerning Fractures of the Pelvis and Sacrum*

TRUE   A. This type of injury is produced by anterior-posterior compression of the pelvis on disruption of the sacro-iliac joints and the public symphysis: the so-called "open book" appearance.
Ch. 76 The Pelvis, p 1576.

TRUE   B. This injury results in a fracture of the medial ilium or sacrum and is seen in conjunction with fractures of the superior and inferior pubic rami on the ipsilateral side.
Ch. 76 The Pelvis, p 1576.

FALSE   C.
Ch. 76 The Pelvis, p 1576.

FALSE   D. Judet's views demonstrate the anterior and posterior pelvic columns.
Ch. 76 The Pelvis, p 1576.

FALSE   E. Guidelines for the use of X-rays. Royal College of Radiologists.
Ch. 76 The Pelvis, p 1576.

Q 7.5. *Regarding Injuries to the Shoulder*

A. Most dislocations of the glenohumeral joint are anterior

B. A Hill-Sachs fracture occurs in 20% of patients with an anterior shoulder dislocation

C. The presence of the Hill-Sachs lesion and the Bankhart lesion imply recurrent dislocation

D. A posterior dislocation fixes the humerus in external rotation

E. The "trough sign" is a vertical sclerotic density paralleling the medial cortex of the humeral head after a posterior dislocation

Q 7.6. *Concerning Fractures of the Upper Limb*

A. A grade II acromioclavicular injury represents complete disruption of the acromioclavicular ligaments and partial disruption of the coracoclavicular ligaments

B. Neer's classification is used to classify fractures of the proximal humerus

C. The anterior fat pad sign ("sail sign"), at the elbow joint, signifies a fracture even without any history of injury

D. The Monteggia injury is a fracture of the proximal ulna and a dislocation of the radial head

E. A Galeazzi injury is a fracture of the distal ulna with distal radial dislocation

A 7.5. *Regarding Injuries to the Shoulder*

TRUE   *A.* Ninety percent are anterior dislocations.
Ch. 76 The Shoulder, p 1584.

TRUE   *B.* This is an indentation fracture of the postero-superior aspect of the humeral head.
Ch. 76 The Shoulder, p 1584.

FALSE   *C.* These fractures were previously thought to signify recurrent dislocation, but either or both may be found after the first dislocation.
Ch. 76 The Shoulder, p 1584.

FALSE   *D.* Posterior dislocations produce the light bulb sign—this is the appearance of the humeral head when it is in *internal* rotation.
Ch. 76 The Shoulder, p 1584.

TRUE   *E.* This is an impaction fracture analogous to the Hill-Sachs deformity produced by an anterior dislocation.
Ch. 76 The Shoulder, p 1584.

A 7.6. *Concerning Fractures of the Upper Limb*

TRUE   *A.* A Grade I injury consists of widening of acromioclavicular joint with partial disruption of the acromioclavicular ligaments. A Grade III injury consists of complete disruption of both the acromioclavicular ligaments and the coracoclavicular ligaments. These injuries produce marked upward subluxation of the clavicle on the plain radiographs.
Ch. 76 Acromioclavicular Injury, p 1588.

TRUE   *B.* This classification is important as it has a bearing on the management of these fractures.

FALSE   *C.* A displaced anterior fat pad indicates a joint effusion and may therefore occur in the absence of a fracture. Nevertheless, it is often seen in fractures, especially of the *radial head*. The *posterior fat pad* sign is strongly indicative of a fracture. The fat pad signs may be negative even when there has been extensive trauma to elbow and this may signify severe capsular disruption.
Ch. 76 The Elbow, p 1888.

TRUE   *D.*
Ch. 76 The Forearm, p 1591.

FALSE   *E.* This injury is a distal radial fracture with distal ulnar dislocation.
Ch. 76 The Forearm, p 1591.

Q 7.7. *Eponyms Associated with the Injuries Described*

A. Colles' fracture: a fracture of the distal radius

B. Hutchinson's fracture: an isolated fracture of the distal radial styloid

C. Mitchell's fracture: a fracture of the distal ulnar styloid

D. Smith's fracture: a wrist fracture in which there is volar angulation of the distal radial fragment

E. Barton's fracture: a displaced fracture of the volar lip of the distal radius without involvement of the dorsal lip

Q 7.8. *Regarding Fractures of the Scaphoid*

A. Scaphoid injuries account for about 75% of all carpal fractures

B. A fracture across the waist of the scaphoid may render its distal pole avascular

C. The avascular segment of the scaphoid generally appears dense on CT

D. Rupture of the scapholunate ligament is accompanied by a scaphoid fracture in over 80% of cases

E. Scaphoid fractures are the most common injury in the wrist in children under 10 years old

A 7.7. *Eponyms Associated with the Injuries Described*

TRUE   A. But not the complete description. The term Colles' fracture is best avoided as everyone knows more about a Colles' fracture than you do. Just describe the fracture and you "won't go wrong."
Ch. 76 Wrist, p 1592.

TRUE   B. Or the chauffeur's crank handle fracture.
Ch. 76 Wrist, p 1592.

FALSE   C.

TRUE   D. Or the reverse Colles' fracture.
Ch. 76 Wrist, p 1592.

TRUE   E. It is even possible to get a reversed Barton's fracture.
Ch. 76 Wrist, p 1592.

A 7.8. *Regarding Fractures of the Scaphoid*

TRUE   A. "The scaphoid is the most expensive bone in the body," said O. Craig, referring to the medico-legal consequences of missing a scaphoid fracture.

FALSE   B. The blood supply to the scaphoid is via the distal pole (from the recurrent artery to the scaphoid). Hence, a fracture across the waist can render the *proximal* portion avascular.
Ch. 76 Wrist, p 1592.

TRUE   C. This appearance is due to a combination of surrounding bone disuse, osteoporosis and sclerosis in the avascular bone produced by fat necrosis.
Ch. 76 Wrist, p 1592.

FALSE   D. This type of ligament disruption produces widening between the scaphoid and the lunate—the so-called Terry Thomas sign.
Ch. 76 Wrist, p 1592.

FALSE   E. Scaphoid fractures are more frequently seen in young adults.

Q 7.9. *Concerning Injuries to the Lower Limb*

    A. Dislocations of the hip joint are most frequently posterior

    B. Lateral tibial plateau fractures are more common than medial tibial plateau fractures

    C. The Segond fracture is an avulsion of the lateral collateral ligament of the knee associated with a disruption of the posterior cruciate ligament

    D. A bipartite patella is bilateral in less than 50% of individuals

    E. The extension of an intermediate or high MRI signal to the capsular margin suggests a meniscal tear

Q 7.10. *Concerning the Hip*

    A. A frog lateral view requires the femora to be abducted and externally rotated

    B. The Garden classification is used for trochanteric fractures

    C. A subcapital fracture is more likely to produce AVN (avascular necrosis) of the femoral head than a basal fracture

    D. There is a significant risk of AVN with intertrochanteric fractures

    E. An isolated fracture of the lesser trochanter should be regarded as an uncommon injury in the elderly and warrants further investigation

A 7.9. *Concerning Injuries to the Lower Limb*

TRUE
A. These injuries are often associated with a fracture of the posterior lip of the acetabulum; the resulting fragment of bone can produce sciatic nerve damage.
Ch. 76 The Hip, p 1597.

TRUE
B. There is a complicated system of classification of tibial plateaux fractures. Suffice to say that the most common injury is produced by a valgus force leading to lateral tibial plateau fractures.
Ch. 76 The Hip, p 1597.

FALSE
C. This fracture is associated (80%) with a disruption of the *anterior* cruciate ligament.
Ch. 76 The Knee, p 1602.

FALSE
D. A bipartite patella is a normal variant in which a separate ossific fragment posterolateral segment is demonstrated bilaterally in 80% of affected individuals.
Ch. 76 The Knee, p 1602.

FALSE
E. Such a signal is frequently seen and is not regarded as abnormal. It represents the normal intrameniscal vascular structures.
Ch. 76 The Knee, p 1602.

A 7.10. *Concerning the Hip*

TRUE
A. This view is useful for the demonstration of a slipped upper femoral epiphysis.
Ch. 76 The Hip, p 1597.

FALSE
B. The Garden classification is used for *femoral neck* fractures. The importance of this system of classification is that the surgical management is based upon it.
Ch. 76 The Hip, p 1592.

TRUE
C. This is because of the anatomy of the blood supply of the femoral neck.
Ch. 76 The Hip, p 1592.

FALSE
D. Intertrochanteric fractures rarely disrupt the blood supply to the femoral head.
Ch. 76 The Hip, p 1592.

TRUE
E. Fractures of the *greater* trochanter are common injuries in the elderly, but fractures of the *lesser* trochanter are uncommon and should be viewed with suspicion. Many of these injuries are associated with metastases; therefore, a cause should be sought.
Ch. 76 The Hip, p 1592.

Q 7.11. The Following Eponyms and Fractures are Associated

A. Bennett's fracture: fracture at the first carpometacarpal joint

B. Rolando's fracture: comminuted fracture of the proximal portion of the first metacarpal

C. Gamekeeper's thumb: disruption of the radial collateral ligament of the thumb

D. Skier's thumb: fracture of the first metacarpal

E. Mallet finger: fracture of the distal phalanx due to a direct blow

Q 7.12. Concerning Fractures of the Lower Limb

A. An inversion injury may result in a fracture of the medial malleolus with a fracture of the proximal shaft of the fibula

B. The pylon fracture describes an injury to the dome of the talus by a direct blow from the distal tibia

C. A fracture of the *neck* of the talus may produce osteonecrosis (AVN) of the dome

D. A Boehler's angle, of the os calcis, of 35 degrees is abnormal

E. Osteochondral fractures of the talar dome are best demonstrated on the lateral view

A 7.11. *The Following Eponyms and Fractures are Associated*

TRUE   A. Such a fracture is unstable as the distal fragment is distracted by the unopposed abductor pollicis longus.
Ch. 76 The Hand, p 1596.

TRUE   B.
Ch. 76 The Hand, p 1596.

FALSE   C. No. The *ulnar* collateral ligament.
Ch. 76 The Hand, p 1596.

FALSE   D. This is the "modern" equivalent of the gamekeeper's thumb. Perhaps the injury has now gone upmarket or gamekeeping has become more lucrative.
Ch. 76 The Hand, p 1596.

FALSE   E. This injury is due to a rupture of the distal insertion of the extensor tendon at the base of the distal phalanx.
Ch. 76 The Hand, p 1596.

A 7.12. *Concerning Fractures of the Lower Limb*

FALSE   A. The described fracture results from an *eversion* injury with the disruption of the interosseous ligament. This fracture complex is referred to as the Masonneuve fracture.
Ch. 76 The Ankle, p 1605.

TRUE   B.
Ch. 76 The Ankle, p 1605.

TRUE   C. The talus has no muscle attachments. Most of the blood supply enters through the distal portion of the bone; hence, a fracture may result in AVN of the proximal portion.
Ch. 76 The Hindfoot, p 1607.

FALSE   D. Boehler's angle has a normal range of 28-40 degrees. A fracture of the calcaneum will tend to reduce or even reverse Boehler's angle.
Ch. 76 The Hindfoot, p 1607.

FALSE   E. MRI is necessary to elucidate these injuries
Ch. 76 The Hindfoot, p 1607.

Q 7.13. Regarding Injuries to the Foot

A. The Lisfranc fracture dislocation is associated with a fracture at the base of the second metatarsal

B. A march fracture most commonly occurs in the first metatarsal

C. Freiberg's infraction occurs in the first metatarsal head

D. The Jones' fracture is situated transversely across the base of the fifth metatarsal

E. Fractures of the phalanges require prolonged immobilization

Q 7.14. Concerning Fractures of the Spine

A. Compression fractures usually involve the superior vertebral endplate and do not disrupt the inferior endplate

B. The most common sites for fracture dislocation are the lower cervical spine and the thoracolumbar junction

C. Fractures of the posterior elements do not commonly occur without accompanying fractures of the vertebral bodies

D. A gap in the neural arch of C1 may be a normal variant

E. The cervicodorsal junction must be demonstrated at all costs in cases of suspected traumatic damage

A 7.13. *Regarding Injuries to the Foot*

TRUE   A. Lisfranc fractures are either homolateral (in which all the metatarsals are shifted laterally) or divergent (in which the first metatarsal is shifted medially).
Ch. 76 The Mid- and Forefoot, p 1608.

FALSE   B. Usually the second to fourth metatarsal.
Ch. 76 The Mid- and Forefoot, p 1608.

FALSE   C. This injury is a flattening of the *second* metatarsal head due to abnormal stresses.
Ch. 76 The Mid- and Forefoot, p 1608.

TRUE   D. This must be distinguished from the normal apophysis, which is parallel to the long axis of the bone.
Ch. 76 The Mid- and Hindfoot, p 1608.

FALSE   E. Most phalangeal fractures are insignificant and therefore require analgesia and mobilization.

A 7.14. *Concerning Fractures of the Spine*

TRUE   A. These are commonly caused by flexion injuries.
Ch. 76 The Spine, p 1609.

TRUE   B. There is often an associated anterior wedged compression fracture of the lower vertebral body and fractures of the posterior vertebral elements.
Ch. 76 The Spine, p 1609.

TRUE   C. The exceptions to this rule are fractures to the transverse processes of the lumbar spine and the neural arches of C1 and C2.
Ch. 76 The Spine, p 1609.

TRUE   D. Whether there is a gap or fracture of the posterior arch of C1 or C2, the lesion is stable.
Ch. 76 The Spine, p 1609.

TRUE   E. Failure to demonstrate this region can be catastrophic for the patient (and for the Defence Unions).

Q 7.15. *The Following Fractures of the Spine are Stable*

    A. Clay shoveller's fracture

    B. Flexion teardrop fracture

    C. Isolated posterior arch of C1 fracture

    D. Unilateral facet dislocation

    E. Bilateral facet dislocation

Q 7.16. *Features That Distinguish Unifacetal Dislocation and Anterior Subluxation from a Hyper-Extension Fracture Dislocation in Spinal Injury*

    A. Anterior subluxation is solely a soft-tissue injury

    B. Absence of fracture

    C. Subluxation of only the facet joints

    D. Anterior displacement of the entire vertebra

    E. Neurological symptoms

A *7.15. The Following Fractures of the Spine are Stable*

TRUE	*A.*
	Ch. 76 The Spine, p 1609.
FALSE	*B.*
	Ch. 76 The Spine, p 1609.
TRUE	*C.*
	Ch. 76 The Spine, p 1609.
TRUE	*D.*
	Ch. 76 The Spine, p 1609.
FALSE	*E.*
	Ch. 76 The Spine, p 1609.

A *7.16. Features That Distinguish Unifacetal Dislocation and Anterior Subluxation from a Hyper-Extension Fracture Dislocation in Spinal Injury*

TRUE	*A.*
	Ch. 76 The Spine, p 1609.
TRUE	*B.*
	Ch. 76 The Spine, p 1609.
TRUE	*C.*
	Ch. 76 The Spine, p 1609.
TRUE	*D.*
	Ch. 76 The Spine, p 1609.
FALSE	*E.* Both injuries can produce neurological symptoms and therefore this sign is not helpful.

Q *7.17. Regarding Cervical Fractures*

  A. The Jefferson fracture is a burst posterior and anterior arch of the axis

  B. The hangman's fracture is a traumatic spondylolisthesis of the axis

  C. Plain film tomography remains the best method for the assessment of fractures of the dens

  D. An extension teardrop fracture has a high association with a hangman's fracture

  E. The flexion teardrop fractures are usually stable

Q *7.18. Concerning Tumours of the Bone*

  A. A vertebral haemangioma has a low signal on T1-weighted images and T2-weighted images owing to the presence of moving blood

  B. Angiography of patients with Gorham's disease (vanishing bone disease) demonstrates the arteriovenous malformation

  C. An intraosseous lipoma usually arises in the medulla of bone

  D. A brown tumour of bone has similar histology to a giant-cell tumour

  E. Synovial osteochondromatosis changes to a synovioma in 1-5% of cases

A *7.17. Regarding Cervical Fractures*

FALSE
A. The *atlas*.
Ch. 76 The Atlas, p 1614.

TRUE
B. This fracture should be called the hangee's fracture, as most hangmen do not hang themselves.
Ch. 76 The Axis, p 1614.

TRUE
C. Dens fractures may lie in the plane of cut of a CT scan and can be missed.
Ch. 76 The Axis, p 1614.

TRUE
D. The teardrop fracture, per se, is not associated with any neurological defect. It is, however, found in association with a hangman's fracture, which must be excluded.
Ch. 76 The Spine, p 1614.

FALSE
E. The flexion teardrop is a triangular fragment of bone at the antero-inferior portion of the vertebral body. There is, however, posterior displacement of the vertebral body, diastasis of the interfacetal joints and disruption of the posterior ligamentous complex. It is usually associated with neurological injury.
Ch. 76 The Teardrop Fracture, p 1618.

A *7.18. Concerning Tumours of the Bone*

FALSE
A. A vertebral haemangioma has a high *fat* content; therefore, the lesion appears "bright" on both MRI sequences.
Ch. 77 Angiomas, p 1652.

FALSE
B. Histologically, the bone is replaced by angiomatous tissue, but no angiomas or arteriovenous malformations can be demonstrated angiographically.
Ch. 77 Gorham's Disease, p 1654.

TRUE
C. This lesion may produce cortical scalloping and trabeculation of bone; it may resemble a cyst.
Ch. 77 Lipoma, p 1654.

TRUE
D.
Ch. 77 Brown Tumour of Hyperparathyroidism, p 1656.

FALSE
E. Synovial chondromatosis rarely undergoes malignant change; when it does, it becomes a synovial chondrosarcoma.
Ch. 77 Synovial Chondromatosis, p 1657.

Q *7.19. Regarding Fibrous Tumours of the Bone*

    A. Disregarding the size of the lesions, the histological and plain-film findings of fibrous cortical defects and non-ossifying fibromata are identical

    B. Non-ossifying fibromas are associated with tuberose sclerosis

    C. The radiological appearances of a benign fibrous histiocytoma closely resemble those of a giant-cell tumour

    D. Bufkin tumours (post traumatic cortical desmoid) have malignant potential

    E. Desmoplastic fibromas are predominantly medullary lesions

Q *7.20. Concerning Benign Osteoid Tumours of the Bone*

    A. The nidus of an osteoid osteoma does not generally exceed 5 mm in diameter

    B. The pain of an osteoblastoma is usually relieved by aspirin

    C. Forty to 50% of osteoblastomas are found in the spine

    D. Osteoid osteomas may involve adjoining bones

    E. There is a recurrence rate for osteoblastomas, after curettage or excision, of 70-80%

A *7.19. Regarding Fibrous Tumours of the Bone*

TRUE   A. When uncomplicated, a non-ossifying fibroma is a larger lesion than a fibrous cortical defect. When large enough, it may produce a pathological fracture.
Ch. 77 Non-ossifying Fibroma, p 1649.

FALSE   B. Multiple non-ossifying fibromas are associated with *type 1 neurofibromatosis*.
Ch. 77 Non-ossifying Fibroma, p 1649.

TRUE   C. Histologically, the lesion resembles a giant-cell tumour, and some pathologists believe it to be a senescent form of the latter.
Ch. 77 Benign Fibrous Histiocytoma, p 1651.

FALSE   D. These benign lesions result from avulsive stress at the insertion of the distal fibres of the adductor magnus muscle at the medial metaphysis of the distal femur. They heal without treatment.
Ch. 77 Post-traumatic Cortical Desmoid, p 1651.

FALSE   E. This very rare tumour occurs within the periosteum. Two patterns are seen resembling, respectively, either a fibrosarcoma or an expanding trabeculated lesion.
Ch. 77 Desmoplastic Fibroma, p 1651.

A *7.20. Concerning Benign Osteoid Tumours of the Bone*

TRUE   A. An arbitrary size definition of the diameter of the nidus of an osteoid osteoma is less than 10 mm, although most do not exceed 5 mm.
Ch. 77 Osteoid Osteoma, p 1639.

FALSE   B. This is one way in which an osteoblastoma can be differentiated from an *osteoid osteoma*, the pain of the latter being relieved by aspirin.
Ch. 77 Osteoblastomas, p 1640.

TRUE   C. The majority of these involve the vertebral arch and may produce a painful scoliosis.
Ch. 77 Osteoblastomas, p 1640.

FALSE   D. This is a recognized feature of *osteoblastoma*.
Ch. 77 Osteoblastomas, p 1640.

FALSE   E. The recurrence rate is reported to be 10%.
Ch. 77 Osteoblastomas, p 1640.

Q 7.21. *Concerning Cysts of the Bone*

  A. Solitary bone cysts occur most commonly in the proximal humerus and the proximal femur

  B. Approximately one third of aneurysmal bone cysts are secondary to a preceding benign or malignant lesion

  C. Aneurysmal bone cysts are classically in the epiphysis of a child

  D. The giant cells of the giant-cell tumour possess malignant potential

  E. Most giant-cell tumours occur after the fusion of the epiphyses of the long bones

Q 7.22. *Concerning the General Characteristics of Bone Tumours*

  A. Metastases are the most common malignant tumours of bone in patients over the age of 45 years

  B. Primary bone tumours are rare in children below the age of 5 years

  C. A giant-cell tumour does not metastasize

  D. The pattern of growth of the primary tumour is assessed by the Lodwick pattern

  E. Endosteal cortical scalloping suggests a benign lesion

A 7.21. *Concerning Cysts of the Bone*

TRUE   A. Most cases present in children. Radiologically they may not be unilocular. Very occasionally a fragment of cortex may come to lie within the cyst to produce the "falling fragment" sign.
Ch. 77 Solitary Bone Cysts, p 1643.

TRUE   B. It is unusual to demonstrate the primary bone lesion radiologically.
Ch. 77 Aneurysmal Bone Cyst, p 1645.

FALSE   C. No. The metaphysis.
Ch. 77 Aneurysmal Bone Cyst, p 1645.

FALSE   D. Although giant-cell tumours of bone do have malignant potential, it is the *stromal cells* of the tumour that have the malignant potential.
Ch. 77 Giant-Cell Tumour, p 1646.

TRUE   E. Eighty percent of patients are between 18 and 45 years; the tumour is rare under the age of 16 years.
Ch. 77 Giant-Cell Tumour, p 1646.

A 7.22. *Concerning the General Characteristics of Bone Tumours*

TRUE   A. Even if the tumour looks like a classical primary bone tumour, it is more likely to be a metastasis.
Ch. 77 General Characteristics of Bone Tumours, p 1630.

TRUE   B. The most common bone tumours in the first decade are neuroblastoma and leukaemia.
Ch. 77 General Characteristics of Bone Tumours, p 1630.

FALSE   C. Occasionally, histologically "benign" tumours do metastasize; these include giant-cell tumours and chondroblastomas.
Ch. 77 General Characteristics of Bone Tumours, p 1630.

TRUE   D. Lodwick I   Sharp geographical zone of transition
Lodwick II   Moth-eaten destruction
Lodwick III   Permeative destruction
Ch. 77 General Characteristics of Bone Tumours, p 1630.

FALSE   E. Scalloping suggests slow growth that can also occur in malignant tumours (e.g., chondrosarcoma).
Ch. 77 General Characteristics of Bone Tumours, p 1630.

Q 7.23. *Regarding Benign Tumours of the Bone*

    A. Maffucci's syndrome comprises enchondromata and haemangiomas

    B. Sixty percent of chondromas of the hands and feet present with fractures

    C. Ollier's disease is autosomally dominant in most cases

    D. Bizarre parosteal osteochondromatous proliferation (BPOP) occurs mainly in the long bones

    E. The incidence of malignant degeneration in diaphyseal aclasis is in the order of 1%

Q 7.24. *Concerning Benign Tumours of the Bone*

    A. The most common site for a chondroblastoma is the metaphysis of a long bone

    B. Chondroblastomas tend to occur in the immature skeleton

    C. More than 75% of chondromyxoid fibromas occur in the proximal tibia

    D. Five percent of chondromyxoid fibromas undergo malignant transformation

    E. Painful osteoid osteomas are usually demonstrable on plain radiography

A 7.23. *Regarding Benign Tumours of the Bone*

TRUE A.
  Ch. 77 Chondroma, p 1633.

TRUE B. These occur in the second to fourth decades with a range of 10-80 years.
  Ch. 77 Chondroma, p 1633.

FALSE C. A sporadic disorder.
  Ch. 77 Multiple Chondromas, p 1634.

FALSE D. The lesions are commonly isolated and arise in relationship to the small bones of the hands and feet.
  Ch. 77 BPOP, p 1634.

TRUE E. Malignant degeneration occurs in 1% of osteochondromas in isolation. These benign tumours change into chondrosarcoma.
  Ch. 77 Osteochondroma, p 1635.

A 7.24. *Concerning Benign Tumours of the Bone*

FALSE A. The lesion is usually located in the *epiphysis*.
  Ch. 77 Chondroblastoma, p 1635.

TRUE B. The incidence of chondroblastomas falls dramatically in adult life, and the tumour is rare after the age of 30 years.
  Ch. 77 Chondroblastoma, p 1635.

FALSE C. Although the proximal tibia is the most common site, only 25% of lesions occur in this position.
  Ch. 77 Chondromyxoid Fibroma, p 1637.

FALSE D. Malignant change is virtually unknown in patients with chondromyxoid fibroma.
  Ch. 77 Chondromyxoid Fibroma, p 1637.

FALSE E. The absence of significant plain film changes in the early stages of this disorder often results in the diagnosis being delayed for between 6 months and several years.
  Ch. 77 Osteoid Osteoma, p 1639.

Q 7.25. *Regarding the Diagnosis of Metastatic Disease of Bone*

    A. Bony metastases are rarely demonstrated by conventional radiography when less than 2 cm in diameter

    B. A blastic metastasis is produced as a result of tumour laying down bone

    C. MRI is more sensitive than scintigraphy and more specific than radiography

    D. MRI high-signal return can be expected on STIR images

    E. Uterine carcinoma produces bony metastases more commonly than does thyroid carcinoma

Q 7.26. *Concerning the General Features of Bony Metastases*

    A. Ten percent of bony metastases are solitary at presentation

    B. Imaging is usually able to demonstrate pulmonary lesions when bony metastases are present

    C. Clinically, skeletal metastases are present in 20-30% of all patients with carcinoma

    D. Bony metastases from carcinoma of the pancreas are seen more commonly than those from hypernephroma

    E. Fifty percent of metastases to the hands and feet are due to carcinoma of the lung

A 7.25. *Regarding the Diagnosis of Metastatic Disease of Bone*

TRUE	A.	Most bony metastases are within the medulla of the bone and expand to destroy the medulla and the cortex. Lytic metastases are not well demonstrated below 20 mm in diameter, and even larger lesions can be missed when the bone is osteopenic, especially in the bony pelvis. *Ch. 78 Diagnosis of Metastatic Disease in Bone, p 1663.*
FALSE	B.	A blastic response is due to the production of new bone by local osteoblasts, not metastatic tumour cells. *Ch. 78 Diagnosis of Metastatic Disease in Bone, p 1663.*
FALSE	C.	The other way around in both cases. *Ch. 78 Diagnosis of Metastatic Disease in Bone, p 1663.*
TRUE	D.	*Ch. 78 Diagnosis of Metastatic Disease in Bone, p 1663.*
TRUE	E.	*Ch. 78 Table 78.2, p 1663.*

A 7.26. *Concerning the General Features of Bony Metastases*

TRUE	A.	A solitary bone metastasis is more common than a primary bone lesion. *Ch. 78 Metastatic Neoplasia of Bone, p 1661.*
TRUE	B.	There are exceptions to the rule (e.g., paradoxical embolism, retrograde venous embolism [via Batson's plexus]) or the trans-pulmonary passage of tumour micro-emboli. *Ch. 78 Metastatic Neoplasia of Bone, p 1661.*
TRUE	C.	*Ch. 78 Metastatic Neoplasia of Bone, p 1661.*
TRUE	D.	Although hypernephroma metastasizes to bone more readily than pancreatic carcinoma, the latter disease is much more common. *Ch. 78 Metastatic Neoplasia of Bone, p 1661.*
TRUE	E.	In the remainder, there is a tendency for carcinoma arising in the subdiaphragmatic viscera to involve the foot rather than the hand. *Ch. 77 Bony Metastases, p 1662.*

Q *7.27. The Nominated Primary Tumour Sites Are Associated with the Stated Radiological Features*

    A. Breast carcinoma: predominantly osteoblastic or mixed lesions

    B. Thyroid carcinoma: expansile lytic lesions of bone

    C. Bladder carcinoma: predilection for the leg bones and pelvis

    D. Pancreatic carcinoma: blastic vertebral metastases

    E. Melanoma: osteoblastic metastases

Q *7.28. The Following Features Favour the Diagnosis of Bony Metastases Rather Than a Primary Malignancy of Bone*

    A. Diaphyseal location in long bone

    B. Bony expansion

    C. Soft-tissue mass

    D. Bone lesions in patients below the age of 1 year

    E. Vertebral pedicle involvement

A *7.27. The Nominated Primary Tumour Sites Are Associated with the Stated Radiological Features*

FALSE   A. Most lesions are *osteolytic*. Nevertheless, the most common cause of an osteoblastic bone lesion (in a female) is breast carcinoma.
Ch. 78 Breast, p 1663.

TRUE   B.
Ch. 78 Thyroid, p 1664.

TRUE   C.
Ch. 78 Bladder, p 1665.

TRUE   D.
Ch. 78 Pancreas, p 1665.

FALSE   E. Predominantly lytic and occasionally expansile.
Ch. 78 Melanoma, p 1665.

A *7.28. The Following Features Favour the Diagnosis of Bony Metastases Rather Than a Primary Malignancy of Bone*

TRUE   A.
Ch. 78 Table 78.3, p 1664.

FALSE   B. Although some metastases expand bone, most do not.
Ch. 78 Table 78.3, p 1664.

FALSE   C. This is generally associated with primary bone tumours.
Ch. 78 Table 78.3, p 1664.

FALSE   D.
Ch. 78 Table 78.3, p 1664.

TRUE   E.
Ch. 78 Table 78.3, p 1664.

Q *7.29. Concerning the Investigation of Metastatic Bone Disease*

      A. A skeletal survey is recommended to establish the diagnosis of metastases in all patients with a known primary carcinoma

      B. The site of the primary tumour is not found in 1-5% of patients

      C. Gd-DTPA-enhanced MRI can, in most instances, distinguish between benign and malignant bone lesions

      D. The metastases from Ewing's sarcoma tend to resemble those of leukaemia on plain radiography in children

      E. Medulloblastoma only metastasizes after surgery

Q *7.30. Regarding the General Features of Primary Bone Tumours*

      A. When an osteosarcoma of a long bone is diagnosed, without any evidence of pulmonary metastases, the patient has a greater than 60% chance of a 5-year survival

      B. MRI is preferable to CT for initial staging

      C. CT should be undertaken to assess for pulmonary metastases in all patients with malignant bone tumours

      D. MRI has a sensitivity of 80-90% in the assessment of tumour recurrence

      E. CT may be of value in the follow-up of patients with primary bone tumours

A 7.29. *Concerning the Investigation of Metastatic Bone Disease*

FALSE

A. Radiography is only recommended in symptomatic regions or regions that are positive on a radionuclide bone scan.
Ch. 78 Management of the Investigation of Metastatic Disease by the Radiologist, p 1666.

FALSE

B. The primary site is not established in as many as 15-20% of patients.
Ch. 78 Skeletal Scintigraphy, p 1666.

TRUE

C. Malignant tumours of bone (primary and secondary) obtain their arterial supply from their host tissues. Enhancement occurs early (within 2 minutes); benign and infective lesions do not enhance so quickly.
Ch. 78 Skeletal Scintigraphy, p 1666.

TRUE

D. The metastases from a Ewing's tumour can also resemble those of neuroblastoma.
Ch. 78 Metastatic Bone Disease in Children, p 1666.

FALSE

E. While this is generally the case, many reports exist to suggest it is not invariably so.
Ch. 78 Metastatic Bone Disease in Children, p 1666.

A 7.30. *Regarding the General Features of Primary Bone Tumours*

TRUE

A. Hence the importance of accurate staging.
Ch. 78 Primary Malignant Neoplasms of Bone, p 1666.

TRUE

B. MRI gives more information about the contiguous soft tissues and the extent of the tumour and bone marrow involvement than CT.
Ch. 78 Primary Malignant Neoplasms of Bone, p 1666.

TRUE

C. To miss a single pulmonary metastasis would significantly alter the staging, treatment and prognosis.

TRUE

D. Recurrence is best demonstrated as a high signal on T2W images.
Ch. 78 Primary Malignant Neoplasms of Bone, p 1666.

TRUE

E. Most cases should be followed up with MRI, but in some instances, CT may be of value. CT remains the investigation of choice for the investigation of pulmonary metastases.

Q *7.31. Concerning Bone Tumours of Chondroid Origin*

    A. Secondary chondrosarcomas may develop in chondromyxoid fibroma

    B. Chondrosarcoma may dedifferentiate into osteosarcoma

    C. The peak age incidence is below 25 years

    D. The most common site for chondrosarcoma is the distal femur

    E. Most calcified chondroid tumours, especially in the elderly, are inactive

Q *7.32. Concerning the Radiology of Chondrosarcoma*

    A. Plain radiology permits reasonable assessment of the medullary spread of this tumour

    B. Most chondrosarcomas have a hypervascular blood supply

    C. An enhancing rim around the tumour, as demonstrated by CT or MRI, suggests a good prognosis

    D. More than 75% of lesions demonstrate a periosteal reaction on plain radiography

    E. An osteochondroma with a cartilage cap thicker than 20 mm is likely to be malignant

A 7.31. *Concerning Bone Tumours of Chondroid Origin*

TRUE   *A.* Other lesions which may undergo sarcomatous change include enchondroma, osteochondroma and chondroblastoma.
Ch. 78 Chondrosarcoma, p 1667.

FALSE   *B.* These tumours may dedifferentiate into malignant fibrous histocytoma or fibrosarcoma.
Ch. 78 Chondrosarcoma, p 1667.

FALSE   *C.* Peak age incidence is 50 years. Over half the patients are over 40 years.
Ch. 78 Chondrosarcoma, p 1667.

FALSE   *D.* The commonest sites are the pelvis and *proximal* femora.
Ch. 78 Fig. 78.9, p 1668.

FALSE   *E.* The majority are active but benign; when malignant, they are usually grade I chondrosarcomas that only need observation.
Ch. 78 Chondroid Tumours, p 1667.

A 7.32. *Concerning the Radiology of Chondrosarcoma*

FALSE   *A.* This is even untrue for lesions with a well-defined zone of transition.
Ch. 78 Chondrosarcoma, p 1667.

FALSE   *B.* The tumours are mainly avascular; hence, they enhance poorly with contrast medium.
Ch. 78 Chondrosarcoma, p 1667.

FALSE   *C.* Such enhancement suggests dedifferentiation into a MFH (malignant fibrous histiocytoma) or fibrosarcoma.
Ch. 78 Chondrosarcoma, p 1667.

FALSE   *D.* Only about half of the patients exhibit a periosteal reaction on plain radiography.
Ch. 78 Chondrosarcoma, p 1667.

TRUE   *E.* Most osteochondromata have caps less than 5 mm.
Ch. 78 Chondrosarcoma, p 1667.

Q 7.33. *Concerning Osteosarcoma*

    A. It is the most common malignant lesion of bone

    B. It can only arise in bone

    C. It is uncommon under the age of 10 years

    D. When the jaw is affected, it carries a poor prognosis

    E. Systemic symptoms are uncommon

Q 7.34. *The Typical Features of Osteosarcoma Are*

    A. Equal sex incidence

    B. Seventy-five percent of lesions are found in the distal femur and the proximal tibia

    C. The tumour is often highly vascular

    D. Enzyme cytochemistry of the tumour cells demonstrates no alkaline phosphatase

    E. Soft-tissue extension of the tumour occurs early in the disease

A 7.33. *Concerning Osteosarcoma*

FALSE   A. It is second in incidence to multiple myeloma.
Ch. 78 Osteosarcoma, p 1671.

FALSE   B. Soft-tissue osteosarcomas have been recorded.
Ch. 78 Osteosarcoma, p 1671.

TRUE   C. Eighty percent of patients are under the age of 30 years, but most of these are older than 10 years.
Ch. 78 Osteosarcoma, p 1671.

FALSE   D. When the tumour arises in the jaw, the prognosis is better than when it occurs elsewhere in the skeleton.
Ch. 78 Osteosarcoma, p 1671.

FALSE   E. Systemic symptoms and pathological fractures are common.
Ch. 78 Osteosarcoma, p 1671.

A 7.34. *The Typical Features of Osteosarcoma Are*

FALSE   A. Male:female = 2:1
Ch. 78 Osteosarcoma, p 1671.

TRUE   B. Other common sites are the proximal humerus and the proximal femur.
Ch. 78 Osteosarcoma, p 1671.

TRUE   C. Metastases are blood-borne to the lungs. Regional lymphadenopathy is usually late.
Ch. 78 Osteosarcoma, p 1671.

FALSE   D. Osteosarcoma cells always stain for alkaline phosphatase.
Ch. 78 Osteosarcoma, p 1671.

TRUE   E. This type of extension is well seen on cross-sectional imaging.
Ch. 78 Osteosarcoma, p 1671.

Q *7.35. The Radiological Features of Osteosarcoma Include*

    A. A laminated periosteal reaction

    B. A spiculated "sunburst" periosteal reaction

    C. A Codman's triangle

    D. The possible presence of a well-defined lytic lesion

    E. Features in an early osteosarcoma that may be impossible to distinguish from early myositis ossificans

Q *7.36. Concerning Malignant Osteoid Tumours of Bone*

    A. Most cases of parosteal osteosarcoma involve the proximal humerus, the distal femur and the proximal tibia

    B. Parosteal osteosarcoma exhibits a dense mass of new bone surrounding the bone

    C. Periosteal osteosarcomas are characterized by a low signal on T2-weighted MRI images

    D. Seventy to 90% of sarcomas secondary to Paget's disease are osteosarcomas

    E. Twenty to 30% of all patients with Paget's disease develop sarcomatous change

A *7.35. The Radiological Features of Osteosarcoma Include*

FALSE   A. This feature is more typical of a Ewing's sarcoma.
Ch. 78 Osteosarcoma, p 1671.

TRUE   B. This periosteal calcification follows the lines of Sharpey's fibres.
Ch. 78 Osteosarcoma, p 1671.

TRUE   C. This is ossified subperiosteal tissue. It is not unique to osteosarcoma and can be demonstrated in other diseases (e.g., osteomyelitis).

TRUE   D. This can make the lesion extremely difficult to distinguish from a benign lesion. MRI is necessary to assess the extra-osseous and medullary spread.
Ch. 78 Osteosarcoma, p 1671.

TRUE   E. As both lesions can present in the same way, the history may be unhelpful. A CT scan may be necessary to see if the extent of the soft-tissue involvement is greater than that of the calcification, followed by serial films at 2-weekly intervals. Biopsy at such an early stage is to be avoided.
Ch. 78 Osteosarcoma, p 1671.

A *7.36. Concerning Malignant Osteoid Tumours of Bone*

TRUE   A.
Ch. 78 Parosteal Osteosarcoma, p 1674.

TRUE   B. The radiology is often extremely helpful to the histopathologist when the diagnosis is difficult.
Ch. 78 Parosteal Osteosarcoma, p 1674.

FALSE   C. The lesion is of high signal, owing to the chondroid elements which are abundant in this variety of osteosarcoma.
Ch. 78 Parosteal Osteosarcoma, p 1674.

FALSE   D. The figure is in the region of 50%. Of the remainder, 25% are MFH (malignant fibrous histiocytoma) and fibrosarcoma, and the rest are of mixed cell types.
Ch. 78 Sarcoma in Paget's Disease, p 1676.

FALSE   E. A generally accepted figure is in the region of 1%.
Ch. 78 Sarcoma in Paget's Disease, p 1676.

Q *7.37. The Following Criteria Have to be Satisfied to Diagnose a Sarcoma in an Irradiated Bone as Having Arisen as a Result of the Radiation*

    A. A previous radiograph without any evidence of disease

    B. Evidence of radiation osteitis must be present

    C. A latent period of at least 10 years

    D. Histological evidence of a sarcoma

    E. A recorded minimum dose of 30 Gy

Q *7.38. Concerning Fibrous Tumours of Bone*

    A. MFH (malignant fibrous histiocytoma) occurs more frequently in the soft tissues than in bone

    B. MFH could easily be misdiagnosed as a metastasis

    C. Fibrosarcomas tend to exhibit extensive calcification on plain radiographs

    D. Periosteal reaction is a typical feature of fibrosarcoma

    E. There is a strong association between McCune-Albright syndrome and fibrosarcoma

A 7.37. *The Following Criteria Have to be Satisfied to Diagnose a Sarcoma in an Irradiated Bone as Having Arisen as a Result of the Radiation*

TRUE   A.
                  Ch. 78 Sarcoma Arising in Previously Irradiated Bone, p 1677.

FALSE   B. This may be helpful but is not necessary.
                  Ch. 78 Sarcoma Arising in Previously Irradiated Bone, p 1677.

FALSE   C. The minimum latent period is 4 years; it may be less in younger children.
                  Ch. 78. Sarcoma Arising in Previously Irradiated Bone, p 1677.

TRUE   D.
                  Ch. 78 Sarcoma Arising in Previously Irradiated Bone, p 1677.

FALSE   E. Most patients have received an excess of 30 Gy, but there is no known minimum dose.
                  Ch. 78 Sarcoma Arising in Previously Irradiated Bone, p 1677.

A 7.38. *Concerning Fibrous Tumours of Bone*

TRUE   A. This tumour was originally described as a soft-tissue tumour, although it is being diagnosed more frequently in bone. About 25% of these tumours are superimposed upon a pre-existing lesion.
                  Ch. 78 MFH, p 1677.

TRUE   B. Radiologically, this tumour may look like a metastasis or fibrosarcoma. Histologically, the tumour may have a large histocytic component that may mimic a pleomorphic carcinoma.
                  Ch. 78 MFH, p 1677.

FALSE   C. The pattern of bony destruction is that of a "moth eaten" appearance with no calcification.
                  Ch. 78 Fibrosarcoma, p 1678.

FALSE   D. Most fibrosarcomas do not demonstrate any periosteal reaction, although a soft-tissue component is usually demonstrated.
                  Ch. 78 Fibrosarcoma, p 1678.

FALSE   E. *Fibrous dysplasia* is associated with McCune-Albright syndrome (see "G and A," third edition); there is no increased risk of developing a bone tumour over and above that associated with the bone lesion per se.

Q *7.39. Regarding Ewing's Sarcoma*

    A. There is an associated chromosomal abnormality

    B. Most tumours occur between the ages of 5 and 15 years

    C. Asiatic races are more commonly affected than other racial groups

    D. The tumour readily metastasises to bone

    E. The tumour is usually medullary in origin

Q *7.40. The Radiological Features of Ewing's Sarcoma Include*

    A. Erosion of the outer cortex of the bone

    B. A Codman's triangle

    C. A soft-tissue mass that is disproportionately large in comparison with the bony involvement

    D. Matrix ossification as demonstrated on CT

    E. A frequent resemblance to other bone tumours

A 7.39. *Regarding Ewing's Sarcoma*

TRUE

A. There is a reciprocal chromosomal translocation between chromosomes 11 and 22.
Ch. 78 Ewing's Sarcoma, p 1680.

TRUE

B. Seventy-five percent below the age of 20 years.
Ch. 78 Ewing's Sarcoma, p 1680.

FALSE

C.
Ch. 78 Ewing's Sarcoma, p 1680.

TRUE

D.
Ch. 78 Ewing's Sarcoma, p 1680.

TRUE

E. Subperiosteal tumours may also occur.
Ch. 78 Ewing's Sarcoma, p 1680.

A 7.40. *The Radiological Features of Ewing's Sarcoma Include*

TRUE

A. The typical saucerization of bone.
Ch. 78 Ewing's Sarcoma, p 1680.

TRUE

B. This feature is not specific to osteosarcoma.
Ch. 78 Ewing's Sarcoma, p 1680.

TRUE

C. The soft-tissue mass may develop within weeks of presentation. The larger the mass, the poorer the prognosis.
Ch. 78 Ewing's Sarcoma, p 1680.

FALSE

D. This is not a feature of Ewing's sarcoma.
Ch. 78 Ewing's Sarcoma, p 1680.

FALSE

E. Although the lesion can occasionally resemble other bone tumours, the primary differential diagnosis is that of osteomyelitis.
Ch. 78 Ewing's Sarcoma, p 1680.

Q 7.41. *Concerning Primary Tumours of Bone*

A. Askin tumours occur in the pelvis in 50-60% of cases

B. Primary malignant lymphoma of bone is a form of non-Hodgkin's lymphoma

C. Chordomas can be demonstrated in the ribs on rare occasions

D. The third lumbar vertebra is the commonest site in the lumbar spine to be affected by chordoma

E. Chordomas at the base of the skull carry the worst prognosis

Q 7.42. *Concerning the Radiology of Sickle Cell Disease*

A. MRI or scintigraphy are the only methods by which early bone infarction can be demonstrated

B. A "bone within a bone" appearance can be demonstrated

C. Osteomyelitis tends to occur in necrotic bone

D. Bacteraemia due to salmonellae is due to the host's inability to mount an immune response to this species bacterium

E. All patients with sickle-cell trait demonstrate some degree of bony change

A 7.41. *Concerning Primary Tumours of Bone*

FALSE   A. Askin tumours occur in the *thoracic* region in children or young adults. Seventy percent of patients present with a pleural disorder.
Ch. 78 Askin Tumour, p 1682.

TRUE   B. To all intents and purposes, primary Hodgkin's lymphoma of bone does not exist.
Ch. 78 Primary malignant lymphoma of bone, p 1682.

FALSE   C. A chordoma arises from notochordal elements, none of which is found in the ribs.
Ch. 78 Chordoma, p 1684.

TRUE   D. Eighty-five to 90% of cases of chordoma affect the basi-sphenoid or the sacrum. The next most common site is the lumbar spine (L3).
Ch. 78 Chordoma, p 1684.

FALSE   E. Contrary to expectation, they carry the best prognosis, though 90% of all patients with chordoma are dead within 5-10 years.
Ch. 78 Chordoma, p 1684.

A 7.42. *Concerning the Radiology of Sickle Cell Disease*

TRUE   A. Many changes can be demonstrated on plain films, but these tend to reflect structural collapse or repair and are therefore generally regarded as late changes.
Ch. 79 Sickle Cell Disease, p 1693.

TRUE   B. This is due to infarction within the cortex producing cortical splitting.
Ch. 79 Sickle Cell Disease, p 1693.

TRUE   C. It is often difficult to detect infection when it is superimposed upon in-farcted bone.
Ch. 79 Sickle Cell Disease, p 1693.

FALSE   D. Gut infarcts are the reason why osteomyelitis is frequently caused by gut bacteria.
Ch. 79 Sickle Cell Disease, p 1693.

FALSE   E. Some patients do not demonstrate any bony changes.

Q *7.43. Concerning Bleeding Disorders and the Bones and Joints*

    A. Von Willebrand's disease is an autosomal dominant

    B. Small epiphyses may result when the corresponding joint is involved

    C. The weight-bearing hip is most commonly affected joint

    D. Avascular necrosis (AVN) is common in many joints

    E. The commonest reported site for a haemophilic pseudotumour is the pelvis

Q *7.44. Regarding Langerhans Cell Histiocytosis*

    A. Bone lesions predominate in Letterer-Siwe syndrome

    B. The triad of calvarial lesions, exomphalos and diabetes insipidus suggests the diagnosis of Hand-Schüller-Christian disease

    C. The typical bony sites for eosinophilic granuloma include the skull and proximal femur

    D. Vertebra plana is often associated with a soft-tissue mass

    E. Eosinophilic granuloma is a self-limiting disorder

A 7.43. *Concerning Bleeding Disorders and the Bones and Joints*

TRUE   A.
Ch. 79 p 1709.

FALSE   B. The epiphyses are usually *larger* than normal with altered modelling. Marginal erosions can be demonstrated that are similar to those produced by the pannus of rheumatoid arthritis.
Ch. 79 Haemophilia, p 1709.

FALSE   C. The joints that are affected in descending order of frequency are the knee, the ankle, the elbow, the wrist, the hip and the shoulder.
Ch. 79 Haemophilia, p 1709.

FALSE   D. The joint that is most susceptible to AVN is the hip joint in which the epiphysis is intracapsular. A tense effusion may interfere with the blood supply.
Ch. 79 Haemophilia, p 1709.

TRUE   E.
Ch. 79 Haemophilia, p 1709.

A 7.44. *Regarding Langerhans Cell Histiocytosis*

FALSE   A. This is predominantly a visceral disorder; bone lesions may never be identified in life.
Ch. 79 LCH, p 1705.

FALSE   B. Not exomphalos, but *exophthalmos*. The triad is found in only 10% of all patients with LCH.
Ch. 79 LCH, p 1705.

TRUE   C. Therefore, the SXR and pelvis are the best radiographs to obtain in these patients.
Ch. 79 LCH, p 1705.

TRUE   D. This probably represents haemorrhage associated with the compression fracture. Most affected vertebrae recover up to 2/3 of their predicted height.
Ch. 79 LCH, p 1705.

TRUE   E. Treatment is best avoided.
Ch. 79 LCH, p 1705.

Q 7.45. *The Following Features Suggest Myelomatosis Rather Than Metastases*

A. Destruction of the intervertebral discs

B. Lesions in the mandible

C. Very high levels of alkaline phosphatase

D. Destruction of the vertebral pedicles

E. A soft-tissue mass

Q 7.46. *Typical Features of Multiple Myeloma Include*

A. A 5 year survival rate in excess of 50%

B. Ten to 20% of cases demonstrate Bence-Jones proteinuria

C. Amyloidosis is reported in about 20% of patients

D. Complete absence of lesions on scintigraphic imaging

E. A periosteal reaction

A 7.45. *The Following Features Suggest Myelomatosis Rather Than Metastases*

TRUE   *A.*
                 Ch. 79 Myelomatosis, p 1703.

TRUE   *B.*
                 Ch. 79 Myelomatosis, p 1703.

FALSE   *C.* The alkaline phosphatase is usually normal.
                 Ch. 79 Myelomatosis, p 1703.

FALSE   *D.* This is more commonly seen with metastases.
                 Ch. 79 Myelomatosis, p 1703.

TRUE   *E.*
                 Ch. 79 Myelomatosis, p 1703.

A 7.46. *Typical Features of Multiple Myeloma Include*

FALSE   *A.* There is a varied survival rate; a generally accepted figure is 20% at 5 years.
                 Ch. 79 Myelomatosis, p 1703.

FALSE   *B.* Bence-Jones proteinuria is present in over half the patients.
                 Ch. 79 Myelomatosis, p 1703.

TRUE   *C.* The figure is probably higher in the light chain variety of myelomatosis.
                 Ch. 79 Myelomatosis, p 1703.

FALSE   *D.* Many lesions are "cold"; however, symptomatic lesions and rib lesions may be detected. Scintigraphy generally underestimates the extent of the disease.
                 Ch. 79 Myelomatosis, p 1703.

FALSE   *E.* Periosteal reactions are uncommon, even following infarction.
                 Ch. 79 Myelomatosis, p 1703.

Q *7.47. Concerning Myeloma and Plasma Cell Disorders*

A. Plasmacytoma commonly presents below the age of 40 years

B. Sixty to 70% of plasmacytomas rapidly progress to multiple myeloma

C. The radiological features of a solitary myeloma are often suggestive of a benign lesion

D. The vertebral pedicles are the preferred sites in the spine

E. Multiple myeloma is the commonest primary malignancy of bone

Q *7.48. Concerning Lymphoma*

A. Multiple bony involvement suggests stage IV disease

B. About 2% of patients with Hodgkin's disease have bony lesions discovered at presentation

C. Secondary malignancies complicate treated Hodgkin's disease in less than 1% of patients

D. One third of patients with Hodgkin's disease present with solitary bone lesions

E. Hodgkin's disease may produce an "ivory" vertebra

A 7.47. *Concerning Myeloma and Plasma Cell Disorders*

FALSE   A. Few cases occur below the age of 40.
Ch. 79 Solitary Myeloma, p 1702.

FALSE   B. A little over 30–35% will progress rapidly to multiple myeloma. High risk prognostic features of progression are immunoparesis and generalized osteopenia at presentation.
Ch. 79 Solitary Myeloma, p 1702.

TRUE   C. The margin is well defined; cortical thinning with expansion is usually present and apparent trabeculation or a "soap bubble" appearance is common.
Ch. 79 Solitary Myeloma, p 1702.

FALSE   D. The vertebral *body*.
Ch. 79 Solitary Myeloma, p 1702.

TRUE   E.
Ch. 79 Myelomatosis, p 1703.

A 7.48. *Concerning Lymphoma*

TRUE   A. Occasionally, a primary lymphoma of bone may be present, though this is extremely rare.
Ch. 79 Lymphoma, p 1700.

TRUE   B. The incidence of bony involvement at postmortem is in the region of 75%.
Ch. 79 Lymphoma, p 1700.

FALSE   C. Five to 10% of cases.
Ch. 79 Lymphoma, p 1700.

TRUE   D. Of these patients, the lesions may be mixed, lucent or sclerotic.
Ch. 79 Lymphoma, p 1700.

TRUE   E. Other causes include sclerotic metastases, Paget's disease and infection.
Ch. 79 Lymphoma, p 1700.

Q 7.49. *Concerning Leukaemia*

    A. Skeletal lesions in adults are uncommon

    B. The common sites for chloroma are the long bones

    C. Cortical destruction of the proximal medial aspect of the humerus is pathognomonic

    D. The marrow is more often involved in leukaemia than in lymphoma

    E. The absence of radiographic bone changes should suggest an alternative diagnosis in children

Q 7.50. *The Following are Typical Bone Changes Demonstrated in Children with Leukaemia*

    A. Epiphyseal lucencies

    B. Osteolytic lesions

    C. Osteoblastic lesions

    D. Soft-tissue mass with periosteal reaction

    E. Diffuse bony destruction

A 7.49. *Concerning Leukaemia*

TRUE

A. In children, they are common and reflect the widespread extent of the red marrow and active bone turnover.
Ch. 79 Leukaemia, p 1698.

FALSE

B. A chloroma (granulocytic sarcoma) is a collection of leukaemic cells that is commonly found in the skull, spine, ribs and sternum of leukaemic children.
Ch. 79 Leukaemia, p 1698.

FALSE

C. This can be demonstrated in many other malignancies, notably neuroblastoma.
Ch. 79 Leukaemia, p 1698.

TRUE

D. This is irrespective of radiological change.
Ch. 79 Leukaemia, p 1698.

FALSE

E.
Ch. 79 Leukaemia, p 1698.

A 7.50. *The Following are Typical Bone Changes Demonstrated in Children with Leukaemia*

FALSE

A. *Metaphyseal* lucencies.
Ch. 79 Leukaemia, p 1698.

TRUE

B.
Ch. 79 Leukaemia, p 1698.

TRUE

C.
Ch. 79 Leukaemia, p 1698.

FALSE

D. Most periosteal reactions are not associated with a soft-tissue mass.
Ch. 79 Leukaemia, p 1698.

TRUE

E.
Ch. 79 Leukaemia, p 1698.

Q *7.51. Concerning Myeloid Metaplasia*

    A. Polycythaemia is common

    B. Blurring of the cortico-medullary junction of bone can be demonstrated on plain radiography

    C. Periosteal new bone is formed in about 1/3 of cases

    D. Myelofibrosis is characterized by a high MRI signal intensity on T2W-images

    E. The natural history of myeloid metaplasia is that of rapid, fatal deterioration

Q *7.52. Concerning Sickle Cell Disease*

    A. The presence of the haematobium parasite within red blood cells causes them to sickle

    B. Cardiomegaly is only present in 20-30% of homozygotic sickle-cell subjects

    C. Most homozygotic subjects die before the age of 40 years

    D. Bone infarction tends to occur in the epiphyses and metaphyses of bones in adolescents and adults

    E. Stepped-end plate depression of the vertebrae is unique to sickle cell disease

A 7.51. *Concerning Myeloid Metaplasia*

TRUE   A. Polycythaemia is common in the early stages of the disease; most patients eventually develop a normochromic normocytic anaemia.
Ch. 79 Myeloid Metaplasia, p 1697.

TRUE   B.
Ch. 79 Myeloid Metaplasia, p 1697.

TRUE   C. This is most often demonstrated in the long bones of the legs.
Ch. 79 Myeloid Metaplasia, p 1697.

FALSE   D. The high signal of fat is replaced by a lower, homogeneous signal intensity.
Ch. 79 Myeloid Metaplasia, p 1697.

FALSE   E. The changes are usually slow and chronic, and may occur over a period exceeding 5 years.
Ch. 79 Myeloid Metaplasia, p 1697.

A 7.52. *Concerning Sickle Cell Disease*

FALSE   A. Schistosomiasis haematobium does not produce sickling. The merozoites of the malarial parasite do, and the ensuing disruption of the parasitic lifecycle affords some protection against malaria in endemic areas.
Ch. 79 Sickle Cell Disease, p 1693.

FALSE   B. Cardiomegaly is present in 80% of sickle-cell cases.
Ch. 79 Sickle Cell Disease, p 1693.

TRUE   C.
Ch. 79 Sickle Cell Disease, p 1693.

TRUE   D. Infarction may be massive or may be found incidentally.
Ch. 79 Sickle Cell Disease, p 1693.

FALSE   E. It is almost pathognomonic, but similar appearances can be demonstrated in Gaucher's disease and occasionally other haemoglobinopathies.
Ch. 79 Sickle Cell Disease, p 1693.

Q *7.53. Concerning Thalassaemia*

    A. In β-thalassaemia, the low level of HbA is partially replaced by HbF and HbA2

    B. The bony changes are usually most marked in the phalanges

    C. Erythropoiesis is rare outside the bone marrow, liver and spleen

    D. Ethmoidal hyperplasia is common in severe cases

    E. Radiological changes in the skeleton are rarely seen before 12 months of age

Q *7.54. The Following Disorders of Blood Cells are Correctly Associated with the Described Skeletal Changes on the Plain Radiograph*

    A. Aplastic anaemia and dense bones

    B. Thalassaemia major and the Erlenmeyer flask deformity

    C. Hb S-C disease and AVN of the femoral head

    D. Multiple bony changes in patients with hereditary spherocytosis

    E. Extramedullary haematopoiesis and myeloid metaplasia

A 7.53. *Concerning Thalassaemia*

TRUE
    A. None of these substitute haemoglobins is an effective oxygen carrier, hence the need for erythroid hyperplasia.
Ch. 79 Thalassaemia, p 1692.

TRUE
    B. The phalanges can become cylindrical and even biconvex.
Ch. 79 Thalassaemia, p 1692.

TRUE
    C. It is only seen in patients with severe childhood thalassaemia who survive to adulthood.
Ch. 79 Thalassaemia, p 1692.

FALSE
    D. The ethmoid air cells do not contain red marrow and are therefore unaffected by marrow hyperplasia.
Ch. 79 Thalassaemia, p 1692.

TRUE
    E.
Ch. 79 Thalassaemia, p 1692.

A 7.54. *The Following Disorders of Blood Cells are Correctly Associated with the Described Skeletal Changes on the Plain Radiograph*

FALSE
    A. Aplastic anaemia does not affect the skeletal radiograph.
Ch. 79 Red Cell Disorders, p 1691.

TRUE
    B. A similar radiological finding can be seen in other severe haemoglobinopathies, pyknodysostosis, Gaucher's disease and osteopetrosis.
Ch. 79 Red Cell Disorders, p 1691.

TRUE
    C. Hb S-C is five times more likely to affect the femoral head than HB SS (Hb SS is three times more common).
Ch. 79 Sickle Cell Disease, p 1693.

FALSE
    D. Bony changes are unusual in this disease.
Ch. 79 Hereditary Spherocytosis, p 1696.

TRUE
    E.
Ch. 79 Hereditary Spherocytosis, p 1696.

Q *7.55. Concerning Non-Hodgkin's Lymphoma of Bone*

    A. Bone lesions are more common than lesions in other organ systems in HIV related lymphoma

    B. Bone involvement is commoner in children than in adults

    C. The most common sites affected by Burkitt's lymphoma are the bones of the jaw and the abdominal viscera

    D. The treatment of Burkitt's lymphoma is primarily surgical

    E. Floating teeth are pathognomomic of Burkitt's lymphoma

Q *7.56. The Descriptions Attached to the Following Terms Are Accurate*

    A. Osteoporosis: a reduction in the bone quantity

    B. Halisteresis: demineralization

    C. Demineralization: osteomalacia

    D. Deossification: abnormal loss of bone

    E. Osteopenia: poverty of bone

A 7.55. *Concerning Non-Hodgkin's Lymphoma of Bone*

FALSE   A. The most commonly affected sites are the CNS and the GIT.
Ch. 79 NHL, p 1702.

TRUE   B. Bone involvement occurs in 15-25% of patients with NHL and is more common in children than in adults.
Ch. 79 NHL, p 1702.

TRUE   C. This tumour mainly affects African children. The jaw is the initial focus of the tumour in 50% of cases.
Ch. 79 NHL, p 1702.

FALSE   D. Treatment is primarily by cytotoxic drugs, which give a good cure rate and prognosis.
Ch. 79 NHL, p 1702.

FALSE   E. Floating teeth may be seen in Burkitt's lymphoma, but there are many other causes of this phenomenon.
Ch. 79 NHL, p 1702.

A 7.56. *The Descriptions Attached to the Following Terms Are Accurate*

TRUE   A. The quality of the bone is normal.
Ch. 80 Disease Conditions, p 1716.

TRUE   B. There is no loss of the normal organic component of bone.
Ch. 80 Disease Conditions, p 1716.

FALSE   C. Osteomalacia is an undermineralization of bone.
Ch. 80 Disease Conditions, p 1716.

TRUE   D. This is due to excessive bone resorption.
Ch. 80 Disease Conditions, p 1716.

TRUE   E. This is an acceptable nonspecific term for generalized or localized rarefaction of bone.
Ch. 80 Disease Conditions, p 1716.

Q *7.57. Disorders Associated with a Reduction in of Normal Bone Density Are*

    A. Osteogenesis imperfecta

    B. Hyperthroidism

    C. Hypothroidism

    D. Hypoparathyroidism

    E. Acromegaly

Q *7.58. Regarding Metabolic Bone Disease*

    A. Osteonecrosis of the femoral head is more commonly seen with endogenous than with exogenous Cushing's syndrome

    B. Neuropathic like joints are a feature of Cushing's syndrome

    C. The sesamoid indices increase in patients with hyperparathyroidism

    D. Posterior scalloping of the vertebral body is a feature of acromegaly

    E. Calvarial thickening occurs in hypoparathyroidism

A 7.57. *Disorders Associated with a Reduction in of Normal Bone Density Are*

TRUE   A.

Ch. 80 Table 80.1, p 1717.

TRUE   B.

Ch. 80 Table 80.1, p 1717.

TRUE   C.

Ch. 80 Table 80.1, p 1717.

FALSE   D.

Ch. 80 Table 80.1, p 1717.

TRUE   E.

Ch. 80 Table 80.1, p 1717.

A 7.58. *Regarding Metabolic Bone Disease*

FALSE   A. The other way around.
Ch. 80 Cushing's Disease, p 1719.

TRUE   B. Neuropathic like joints, tendon rupture, delayed skeletal maturation and decreased osteophyte formation are seen more frequently in exogenous Cushing's syndrome, more frequently than the exogenous type.
Ch. 80 Cushing's Disease, p 1719.

FALSE   C. The sesamoid index (the product of the length and diameter of the medial metacarpal is increased in acromegaly.
Ch. 80 Acromegaly, p 1729.

TRUE   D. This is often associated with ligamentous hypertrophy. The patient may develop spinal stenosis.
Ch. 80 Acromegaly, p 1729.

TRUE   E.

Ch. 80. Hypoparathyroidism, p 1743.

Q *7.59. The Following Disorders Produce Similar Radiological Appearances to Rickets and Have No Abnormality of Vitamin D or Phosphate Metabolism*

    A. Vitamin D dependent rickets

    B. Fanconi's anaemia

    C. Hypophosphatasia

    D. Metaphyseal chondrodysplasia (type Schmid)

    E. X-linked hyperphosphataemia

Q *7.60. The Following are Typical Features of Rickets*

    A. Bowing of the extremities

    B. Defective mineralization of the chondrocytes in the zone of provisional calcification produces irregular metaphyseal margins

    C. Pelkan's lines

    D. Widening of the physis

    E. Splaying and cupping of the metaphysis

A 7.59. *The Following Disorders Produce Similar Radiological Appearances to Rickets and Have No Abnormality of Vitamin D or Phosphate Metabolism*

TRUE   A. This is a deficiency of the enzyme that converts 15 (OH)D to 1,25 (OH)D.
              Ch. 80 Osteomalacia, p 1732.

FALSE   B. Fanconi's anaemia is a haematological disorder with skeletal manifesta-
              tions especially in the radial ray. Fanconi's syndrome is a disorder of renal
              tubular handling of phosphate.
              Ch. 80 Osteomalacia, p 1732.

TRUE   C. This is an autosomal recessive disorder in which patients have a low serum
              alkaline phosphatase.
              Ch. 80 Osteomalacia, p 1732.

TRUE   D.
              Ch. 80 Osteomalacia, p 1732.

FALSE   E. Hyperphosphataemia is associated with tumoral calcinosis and thus does
              not look like osteomalacia. It is not x-linked either.
              Ch. 80 Osteomalacia, p 1732.

A 7.60. *The Following are Typical Features of Rickets*

TRUE   A.
              Ch. 80 Rickets, p 1722.

TRUE   B.
              Ch. 80 Rickets, p 1722.

FALSE   C. These are found in scurvy.
              Ch. 80 Rickets, p 1722.

TRUE   D.
              Ch. 80 Rickets, p 1722.

TRUE   E.
              Ch. 80 Rickets, p 1722.

Q 7.61. The Following are Features of Renal Osteodystrophy

A. Brown tumours

B. Fractures of the lower ribs

C. Osteoporosis

D. Osteosclerosis

E. Looser's zones

A 7.61. *The Following are Features of Renal Osteodystrophy*

TRUE   A. Brown tumours are a feature of secondary hyperparathyroidism. Other features of secondary hyperparathyroidism include subperiosteal bone resorption and intracortical tunneling. Brown tumours were formally a well-described feature of patients with *primary* hyperparathyroidism; the earlier detection and treatment of these patients, however, and the increasing number of patients with chronic renal failure, now make brown tumours a common finding in secondary hyperparathyroidism.
Ch. 80 Renal Osteodystrophy, p 1723.

FALSE   B. Fractures of the *lower* ribs are not a feature of renal osteodystrophy. Fractures, particularly of the 2nd, 3rd and 4th ribs, are encountered with aluminium toxicity as a result of the use of aluminium phosphate binders and the decreased renal capacity to excrete aluminium.
Ch. 80 Renal Osteodystrophy, p 1723.

TRUE   C. This is due to the increased bone resorption resulting from the raised levels of PTH.
Ch. 80 Renal Osteodystrophy, p 1723.

TRUE   D. The reason for patients developing osteosclerosis is unclear; it is suggested that the presence of excessive osteoid may inhibit osteoclastic activity and simultaneously, the increased calcium and phosphate product may cause precipitation of mineral in the osteoid (i.e., "rugger-jersey-spine").
Ch. 80 Renal Osteodystrophy, p 1723.

TRUE   E.
Ch. 80 Renal Osteodystrophy, p 1723.

Q *7.62. The Radiological Appearances of Patients with Primary Hyperparathyroidism Include*

    A. Subperiosteal bone resorption in 50% of patients

    B. Cortical tunnelling in 10% of patients

    C. Diffuse osteosclerosis in some patients

    D. Brown tumours almost always involve multiple bones

    E. Renal stones and hypertension are the commonest clinical manifestations

A 7.62. *The Radiological Appearances of Patients with Primary Hyperparathyroidism Include*

FALSE

A. Subperiosteal bone resorption, which is very characteristic of hyperparathyroidism, is seen in only 10% of patients, most commonly along the radial aspect of the middle phalanges of the 2nd and 3rd digits.
Ch. 80 Primary Hyperparathyroidism, p 1726.

FALSE

B. Cortical tunnelling and intracortical tunnelling are due to osteolysis; these features are seen in more than 50% of patients with primary hyperparathyroidism.
Ch. 80 Primary Hyperparathyroidism, p 1726.

TRUE

C. Rarely, patients with primary hyperparathyroidism may have diffuse osteosclerosis. The reason for this is not clear, but it may be due to the fact that in addition to stimulating osteoclastic activity, PTH also stimulates osteoblastic activity.
Ch. 80 Primary Hyperparathyroidism, p 1726.

FALSE

D. They may be solitary or multifocal. Brown tumours contain collections of giant cells that are unusually responsive to PTH, thus the majority of these lesions heal after removal of the adenoma.
Ch. 80 Primary Hyperparathyroidism, p 1726.

TRUE

E. Other manifestations include peptic ulcers, pancreatitis, psychiatric disorders and bone pain.
Ch. 80 Primary Hyperparathyroidism, p 1726.

Q 7.63. *There is an Association Between the Following Bone Disorders and Radiological Features*

A. Scurvy: Wimberger's sign

B. Acromegaly: subligamentous bone deposition

C. Hyperthyroidism: cortical tunnelling

D. Osteogenesis imperfecta: wormian bones

E. Osteogenesis imperfecta: exuberant callus formation

A 7.63. *There is an Association Between the Following Bone Disorders and Radiological Features*

TRUE
A. Wimberger's sign is a ring of increased density surrounding the epiphysis in patients with scurvy.
Ch. 80 Scurvy, p 1727.

TRUE
B. Bone deposition produces prominent bony excrescenses at the sites of tendon insertions on the calcaneus and patella and the tuberosities of the trochanters.
Ch. 80 Acromegaly, p 1729.

TRUE
C. Cortical tunnelling occurs predominently in the long tubular bones of the hands and feet and is seen in up to 50% of patients.
Ch. 80 Hyperthyroidism, p 1730.

TRUE
D. There are many causes of wormian bones, which include types 1, 2 and 3 osteogenesis imperfecta.
Ch. 80 Osteogenesis Imperfecta, p 1732.

TRUE
E. Exuberant callus formation is a common feature secondary to a fracture in patients with osteogenesis imperfecta but is not specific and can be demonstrated in other conditions (e.g., patients receiving steroids).
Ch. 80 Osteogenesis Imperfecta, p 1732.

Q *7.64. The Following are Disorders That Demonstrate Generalised Osteopenia in Association with Delayed Skeletal Maturation*

    A. Hypothyroidism

    B. Addison's disease

    C. Turner's syndrome

    D. Klinefelter's syndrome

    E. Sickle cell disease

Q *7.65. Regarding Localized Loss of Bone Density*

    A. Patients with reflex sympathetic dystrophy and disuse osteoporosis cannot be differentiated clinically

    B. Reflex sympathetic dystrophy is associated with thinning of the soft tissues

    C. Gorham's disease demonstrates progressive involvement of contiguous bones

    D. Transient regional osteoporosis is characterised by high levels of alkaline phosphatase

    E. Bilateral transient osteoporosis of the hips tends to occur in the first trimester of pregnancy

A 7.64. *The Following are Disorders That Demonstrate Generalised Osteopenia in Association with Delayed Skeletal Maturation*

TRUE	A.
	Ch. 80 Table 80.2, p 1725.
TRUE	B.
	Ch. 80 Table 80.2, p 1725.

TRUE   C. In patients with Turner's syndrome, skeletal maturation is usually normal until about the middle of the second decade. At that time, delay in epiphyseal closure becomes evident, particularly in the apophyses of the iliac crests though it should be emphasized that over half the patients with this disorder exhibit no radiographic abnormalities.
Ch. 80 Hypogonadism, p 1730.

TRUE   D. Klinefelter's syndrome (karyotype XXY) is the most common primary developmental abnormality causing hypogonadism; there may be associated mental retardation.
Ch. 80 Klinefelter's Syndrome, p 1739.

FALSE   E. Sickle cell disease produces a normal or dense skeleton.

A 7.65. *Regarding Localized Loss of Bone Density*

FALSE   A. Patients with disuse osteoporosis rarely have symptoms from the osteoporosis alone. This aids in differentiating disuse osteoporosis from the closely related disorder *reflex sympathetic dystrophy* in which pain is a prominent clinical feature.
Ch. 80 Disuse Osteoporosis, p 1739.

FALSE   B. Soft-tissue swelling, pain, tenderness, diminished function and trophic skin changes are the clinical features of this disorder.
Ch. 80 Reflex Sympathetic Dystrophy Syndrome, p 1740.

TRUE   C. The pathophysiology of bone loss in this entity is unclear. The pathological findings are similar to those of skeletal haemangiomas. The disorder usually occurs before the age of 40 and frequently involves the pelvis or shoulder region.
Ch. 80 Massive Osteolysis of Gorham, p 1741.

FALSE   D. The laboratory findings in this disorder are normal.
Ch. 80 Transient Regional Osteoporosis, p 1742.

FALSE   E. The association between transient bilateral osteoporosis of the hips and pregnancy is well recognised. It commonly occurs in the third trimester.
Ch. 80 Transient Regional Osteoporosis, p 1742.

Q *7.66. Regarding Disorders Associated with Diffuse Osteosclerosis*

    A. Hypoparathyroidism is usually the result of inadvertent surgical removal of the parathyroid glands

    B. Pseudohyperparathyroidism is a disorder in which there is a lack of response of the end organs to PTH

    C. Pseudopseudohypoparathyroidism is not associated with premature closure of the epiphyses

    D. Pseudohypohyperparathyroidism can be differentiated from pseudohypoparathyroidism

    E. Hypoplastic dentition is a prominent feature of hypoparathyroidism

Q *7.67. The Following Disorders are Associated with Hyperostosis of Cortical Bone*

    A. Camurati-Engelman disease

    B. Van Buchem's disease

    C. Caffey's disease

    D. Multiple epiphyseal dysplasia

    E. Diabetes insipidus

A 7.66. Regarding Disorders Associated with Diffuse Osteosclerosis

TRUE   *A.*
     Ch. 80 Hypoparathyroidism, p 1743.

FALSE   *B.* This defect describes pseudo*hypo*parathyroidism.
     Ch. 80 Pseudohypoparathyroidism, p 1743.

FALSE   *C.* Hypoparathyroidism, pseudophypoparathyroidism and pseudopseudohy-poparathyroidism are all associated with variable changes in bone density, basal ganglia calcification, falx calcification, calvarial thickening, soft-tissue calcification and premature closure of the epiphyses.
     Ch. 80 Hypoparathyroidism, p 1743.

TRUE   *D.* In the former condition the skeletal (but not the renal) response to PTH is preserved and therefore the radiographic features of hyperparathyroid bone disease may be superimposed on those of hypoparathyroidism.
     Ch. 80 Hypoparathyroidism, p 1743.

TRUE   *E.*
     Ch. 80 Hypoparathyroidism, p 1743.

A 7.67. The Following Disorders are Associated with Hyperostosis of Cortical Bone

TRUE   *A.* This rare congenital dystrophy of bone results in progressive bilaterally symmetrical diametaphyseal sclerosis of the long bones.
     Ch. 80 Table 80.6, p 1747.

TRUE   *B.* This is a disorder of endosteal hyperostosis in which the skull and facial bones are affected, in addition to the long bones.
     Ch. 80 Table 80.6, p 1747.

TRUE   *C.* Infantile cortical hyperostosis (Caffey's disease) characteristically produces hyperostosis of the cortical bone.
     Ch. 80 Table 80.6, p 1747.

FALSE   *D.*

FALSE   *E.*

Q *7.68. The Following Conditions are Associated with Dense Metaphyseal Bands*

      A. Phosphorus poisoning

      B. Hyperthyroidism

      C. Untreated rickets

      D. Normal variant

      E. Park's lines

Q *7.69. Regarding Skeletal Dysplasias and Malformation Syndromes*

      A. One percent of live births have clinically apparent skeletal abnormalities

      B. Mesomelic shortening of the upper limb refers to a short forearm

      C. Only 1% of patients can be regarded as having unclassifiable abnormalities

      D. A prenatal ultrasound diagnosis is often specific with regard to the disorder

      E. All lethal neonatal skeletal dysplasias can be diagnosed at 14-18 weeks gestation by ultrasound

A 7.68. *The Following Conditions are Associated with Dense Metaphyseal Bands*

TRUE

    A. Phosphorus is a bone toxin similar to lead.
Ch. 80 Table 80.5, p 1747.

FALSE

    B. Dense metaphyseal bands are seen with hypothyroidism.
Ch. 80 Table 80.5, p 1747.

FALSE

    C. Untreated rickets does not produce dense metaphyseal bands; after treatment, however, the density of the metaphyses increases in comparison to the remainder of the bone as a result of osteoid.
Ch. 80 Table 80.5, p 1747.

TRUE

    D.
Ch. 80 Table 80.5, p 1747.

TRUE

    E. Park's lines (growth arrest lines) are usually incidental findings that indicate some past episode of stress when growth was temporarily halted. They are rarely more than a mm wide and their width is not related to the duration of the interruption in growth.
Ch. 80 Table 80.5, p 1747.

A 7.69. *Regarding Skeletal Dysplasias and Malformation Syndromes*

TRUE

    A. This figure does not take into account the large numbers of spontaneous abortions that occur or elective terminations; the features in many of these have significant skeletal abnormalities.
Ch. 81 Incidence, p 1752.

TRUE

    B.
Ch. 81 Table 81.1, p 1752.

FALSE

    C. A significant proportion of cases, approximately 30%, are unclassifiable because they do not conform to any recognisable condition.
Ch. 81 Diagnoses, p 1752.

FALSE

    D. Skeletal ultrasound findings are highly significant but are not highly specific and, in general, it is unwise to offer a precise diagnosis solely on the basis of the ultrasound findings.
Ch. 81 Prenatal Diagnosis, p 1752.

TRUE

    E.
Ch. 81 Prenatal Diagnosis, p 1752.

Q *7.70. Concerning Individual Osteochondrodysplasias*

    A. Thanatophoric dysplasia is the most common lethal neonatal skeletal dysplasia

    B. Achrondroplasia is an autosomal dominant condition

    C. Ellis-van Creveld syndrome is associated with cor triatriatum

    D. Kniest dysplasia is characterized by saggital clefts of the vertebral bodies in infancy

    E. There is an association between the Stickler syndrome and the Pierre-Robin abnormality

Q *7.71. Concerning Dyostosis Multiplex*

    A. Hurler's syndrome is an X-linked recessive condition

    B. Hunter's syndrome is associated with normal intelligence

    C. All patients are short in stature

    D. Individuals with Morquio's syndrome have coxa vara

    E. Spinal cord compression occurs more frequently in Morquio's syndrome than the other syndromes

A 7.70. *Concerning Individual Osteochondrodysplasias*

TRUE   A.

Ch. 81 Thanatophoric Dysplasia, p 1756.

TRUE   B.

Ch. 81 Achrondroplasia, p 1756.

FALSE   C. The congenital cardiac defects associated with Ellis-van Creveld syndrome are atrial septal defect and single atrium.
Ch. 81 Ellis-van Creveld Syndrome, p 1759.

FALSE   D. Typically, Kniest is associated with coronal clefts.

TRUE   E.

Ch. 81 Stickler Syndrome, p 1760.

A 7.71. *Concerning Dyostosis Multiplex*

FALSE   A. All patients with a mucopolysaccharidosis (MPS) are autosomally recessive except those with type II MPS (Hunter).
Ch. 81 Dysostosis Multiplex Group, p 1762.

FALSE   B. Only Morquio's disease (MPS IV) is associated with normal intelligence; mental retardation is a feature of the other syndromes.
Ch. 81 Dysostosis Multiplex Group, p 1762.

TRUE   C. The short stature is associated with a distinctive coarse facial appearance.
Ch. 81 Dysostosis Multiplex Group, p 1762.

TRUE   D. As do those affected by any of the other MPS
Ch. 81 Morquio's Syndrome, p 1762.

TRUE   E. Absent odontoid peg with cervical instability leading to spinal cord compression is most commonly associated with Morquio's syndrome although the other syndromes may demonstrate a degree of odontoid hypoplasia.
Ch. 81 Morquio's Syndrome, p 1762.

Q *7.72. Concerning Patients with Osteogenesis Imperfecta*

    A. There is an abnormality of type II collagen

    B. Patients with type I osteogenesis imperfecta are stillborn

    C. The sclerae of patients with type IV osteogenesis imperfecta patients are normal in colour

    D. Patients with type III osteogenesis imperfecta have normal dentition

    E. Type IV is the most common of these disorders

Q *7.73. Concerning Fibrous Dysplasia*

    A. McCune-Albright syndrome is associated with mono-ostotic bone lesions

    B. There is an association with osteomalacia or rickets

    C. The disorder is an autosomal dominant mode of inheritance

    D. There is an association with congenital cardiac disease

    E. Localised or asymmetrical bone overgrowth can be demonstrated in some patients

A 7.72. *Concerning Patients with Osteogenesis Imperfecta*

FALSE
    A. The abnormality is of *type I* collagen.
        Ch. 81 Osteogenesis Imperfecta, p 1768.

FALSE
    B. These patients have a normal life span.
        Ch. 81 Table 81.4a, p 1758.

TRUE
    C. In the other types the sclerae are blue. In type III the sclerae ultimately turns to grey.
        Ch. 81 Osteogenesis Imperfecta, p 1768.

TRUE
    D. Teeth are abnormal in all patients with type III osteogenesis imperfecta.
        Ch. 81 Osteogenesis Imperfecta, p 1768.

FALSE
    E. Types I and II are commoner by far.
        Ch. 81 Osteogenesis Imperfecta, p 1768.

A 7.73. *Concerning Fibrous Dysplasia*

FALSE
    A. McCune-Albright syndrome is the association of polyostotic fibrous dysplasia, patchy cafe au lait skin pigmentation and sexual precocity, usually in females.
        Ch. 81 Fibrous Dysplasia, p 1774.

TRUE
    B.
        Ch. 81 Fibrous Dysplasia, p 1774.

FALSE
    C.
        Ch. 81 Fibrous Dysplasia, p 1774.

FALSE
    D. No such association is known.
        Ch. 81 Fibrous Dysplasia, p 1774.

TRUE
    E.
        Ch. 81 Fibrous Dysplasia, p 1774.

Q 7.74. *Regarding the Radiology of Rheumatoid Arthritis*

A.   Acrosclerosis of the terminal phalanges is a recognised feature of rheumatoid arthritis

B.   Periosteal reaction occurs in about 15% of cases

C.   Rotator cuff atrophy and tearing is a common sequel of shoulder involvement

D.   Involvement of the acromioclavicular joint most commonly results in narrowing of the joint space

E.   Bony ankylosis of the carpus does not occur

Q 7.75. *Regarding Juvenile Chronic Polyarthritis*

A.   Most cases present as a systemic disease (Still's Disease)

B.   When the patient presents with systemic symptoms, these are usually preceded by radiological abnormalities

C.   Phalangeal epiphyseal enlargement is a radiological feature

D.   A florid periosteal reaction indicates the presence of infection

E.   Carpal ankylosis is common

A 7.74. *Regarding the Radiology of Rheumatoid Arthritis*

TRUE   *A.* Productive bone changes are uncommon in rheumatoid hands but acrosclerosis is a recognized finding.
Ch. 82 Rheumatoid Arthritis, p 1782.

FALSE   *B.* Periosteal reaction is very rare (in contrast to the situation in juvenile polyarthritis (Still's Disease)).
Ch. 82 Rheumatoid Arthritis, p 1782.

TRUE   *C.* This causes superior subluxation of the humeral head, which in turn erodes the undersurface of the acromion.
Ch. 82 Rheumatoid Arthritis, p 1782.

FALSE   *D.* Resorption of the distal clavicle often causes the joint space to *widen*.
Ch. 82 Rheumatoid Arthritis, p 1782.

FALSE   *E.* Bony ankylosis is uncommon in rheumatoid arthritis, but, when it does, the wrist is the most common joint to be affected.
Ch. 82 Rheumatoid Arthritis, p 1782.

A 7.75. *Regarding Juvenile Chronic Polyarthritis*

FALSE   *A.* Approximately 20% of affected individuals present with systemic manifestations such as fever, rash, carditis, hepatosplenomegaly and anaemia.
Ch. 82 Juvenile Chronic Polyarthritis, p 1784.

FALSE   *B.* Radiographic changes are usually absent when patients present with systemic symptoms.
Ch. 82 Juvenile Chronic Polyarthritis, p 1784.

TRUE   *C.* Individual carpal bones and metacarpal and phalangeal epiphyses may enlarge as a consequence of the chronic synovitis and hyperaemia.
Ch. 82 Juvenile Chronic Polyarthritis, p 1784.

FALSE   *D.* Periosteal reaction is a common feature of uncomplicated juvenile chronic arthritis.
Ch. 82 Juvenile Chronic Polyarthritis, p 1784.

TRUE   *E.* Unlike adult rheumatoid arthritis, carpal ankylosis often occurs in end-stage wrist involvement.
Ch. 82 Juvenile Chronic Polyarthritis, p 1786.

Q *7.76. Concerning Joint Involvement in Systemic Lupus Erythomatosus (SLE)*

    A. Juxta-articular osteopenia is a prominent feature in most cases

    B. The most common manifestation is an asymmetrical pauci-articular erosive arthropathy of small joints

    C. Joint subluxation and dislocation are common

    D. Chondrocalcinosis supports the diagnosis

    E. Avascular necrosis of the humeral head is a recognized feature

Q *7.77. Regarding the Radiology of Joint Disease*

    A. Jaccoud's arthropathy causes subluxation of the small joints in the hands and feet

    B. "Hook"-like erosions of the metacarpal heads are pathognomonic of systemic lupus erythematosus

    C. Multicentric reticulohistiocytosis causes arthritis mutilans

    D. "Squaring" of vertebral bodies is a feature of ankylosing spondylitis

    E. Subluxation at the atlanto-axial articulation becomes fixed in ankylosing spondylitis

A 7.76. *Concerning Joint Involvement in Systemic Lupus Erythomatosus (SLE)*

FALSE   A. This feature occurs unusually in SLE and only in the presence of a severe, acute exacerbation.
Ch. 82 Systemic Lupus Erythematosus, p 1788.

FALSE   B. Erosions occur very rarely in this disorder.
Ch. 82 Systemic Lupus Erythematosus, p 1788.

TRUE   C. This is especially frequent in the hand where soft-tissue laxity results in nondestructive malalignment of multiple joints.
Ch. 82 Systemic Lupus Erythematosus, p 1788.

FALSE   D. Chondrocalcinosis is not a feature of SLE. The main causes of chondrocalcinosis Wilson's disease, Haemochromatosis, Ochronosis, Oxalosis, Pseudogout, 1° (Primary) Hyperparathyroidism, Normal old age and Gout (WHOOPING).
Ch. 82 Systemic Lupus Erythematosus, p 1788.

TRUE   E. Many arthritides and arteritides cause avascular necrosis of the humeral head. These include rheumatoid arthritis, SLE, scleroderma, Wegener's granulomatosis, psoriatic arthropathy, polyarteritis nodosa, subacute bacterial endocarditis and osteoarthritis.
Ch. 82 Systemic Lupus Erythematosus, p 1788.

A 7.77. *Regarding the Radiology of Joint Disease*

TRUE   A. This is a severe, largely nondestructive, polyarthropathy that occurs after rheumatic fever.
Ch. 82 Jaccoud's Arthropathy, p 1789.

FALSE   B. These occur also in Jaccoud's arthropathy and in rheumatoid arthritis.
Ch. 82 Jaccoud's Arthropathy, p 1789.

TRUE   C. This causes a relentlessly progressive, widespread, symmetrical arthropathy, characterized by large, punched-out erosions without juxta-articular osteopenia.
Ch. 82 Multicentric Reticulohistiocytosis, p 1789.

TRUE   D. Mineralization of the anterior longitudinal ligament contributes to this effect by filling in the normal concavity of the anterior vertebral body.
Ch. 82 Ankylosing Spondylitis, p 1790.

TRUE   E. Ankylosis eventually occurs at C1-C2 leading to fixation of the subluxed joint.
Ch. 82 Ankylosing Spondylitis, p 1790.

Q 7.78. *Regarding Enteropathic Arthropathy*

    A. Peripheral joint involvement is commoner than in ankylosing spondylitis

    B. Erosions are rare

    C. In ulcerative colitis—associated disease, spondylitis resolves after colectomy

    D. Enthesopathy is a recognized feature

    E. Fingertip calcification is a recognized feature

Q 7.79. *Regarding Psoriatic Arthritis*

    A. It affects less than 10% of patients with skin lesions

    B. Ankylosis of the interphalangeal joints is a feature

    C. Periarticular osteopenia does not occur

    D. Periosteal reaction and proliferative new bone formation are regular features of the condition

    E. Paravertebral ossification occurs from midvertebral body to midvertebral body

A 7.78. *Regarding Enteropathic Arthropathy*

FALSE   A. Peripheral joint involvement is much less common in enteropathic arthropathy than in ankylosing spondylitis.
Ch. 82 Enteropathic Arthropathies, p 1791.

TRUE   B. Unlike ankylosing spondylitis, the acute mild synovitis of enteropathic arthropathy is rarely associated with erosive disease.
Ch. 82 Enteropathic Arthropathies, p 1791.

FALSE   C. "Reactive" *peripheral* arthritis parallels the activity of bowel disease and tends to resolve after colectomy. *Spinal* arthritis is independent of the activity of the colitis and may progress despite colectomy.
Ch. 82 Enteropathic Arthropathies, p 1791.

TRUE   D. Causes of enthesitis include ankylosing spondylitis, enteropathic arthritis, psoriatic arthropathy, Reiter's syndrome, diffuse idiopathic skeletal hyperostosis, acromegaly and, occasionally, rheumatoid arthritis.
Ch. 82 Enthesitis, p 1790.

FALSE   E. The main differential diagnosis of this finding is: scleroderma/CREST, Raynaud's disease, SLE, dermatomyositis and hyperparathyroidism.
Ch. 82 Enteropathic Arthropathies, p 1791.

A 7.79. *Regarding Psoriatic Arthritis*

TRUE   A. Only about 7% of affected individuals have joint disease.
Ch. 82 Psoriatic Arthropathy, p 1792.

TRUE   B. The joint space may be severely narrowed leading to bony ankylosis or it may be widened owing to the interposition of fibrous tissue as the adjacent articular cortex is destroyed.
Ch. 82 Psoriatic Arthropathy, p 1792.

FALSE   C. During an acute severe attack, periarticular osteopenia may be present.
Ch. 82 Psoriatic Arthropathy, p 1792.

TRUE   D. These are important clues to the diagnosis along with an erosive arthropathy in the presence (usually) of normal bone mineralization.
Ch. 82 Psoriatic Arthropathy, p 1792.

TRUE   E. Unlike the syndesmophytosis of ankylosing spondylitis, paravertebral ossification in psoriatic arthropathy is thick, extends from midvertebral body to midvertebral body and may be separated from the vertebra by a radiolucent cleft.
Ch. 82 Psoriatic Arthropathy, p 1793.

Q 7.80. *Concerning Reiter's Syndrome*

    A. Foot involvement is more common than hand involvement

    B. Paravertebral ossification similar to psoriatic arthropathy is seen

    C. Periosteal reaction and prominent new bone formation are features

    D. HLA B27 is associated with recurrent attacks and crippling disease

    E. It is successfully treated with tetracyclines

Q 7.81. *The Following Statements About Crystal Deposition Arthropathies are True*

    A. Gout is complicated by bone infarcts and avascular necrosis

    B. Calcium pyrophosphate dihydrate deposition disease (CPPD) simulates a neuropathic joint

    C. The arthropathy of haemochromatosis can be distinguished from that of CPDDD by the presence in the former of calcification in the triangular cartilage of the wrist

    D. Hyperphosphatasia causes chondrocalcinosis

    E. Ochronosis may cause severe destruction of shoulders, hips and knees

A 7.80. *Concerning Reiter's Syndrome*

TRUE   A. The feet, knees and ankles are the joints most commonly affected.
Ch. 82 Reiter's Syndrome, p 1794.

TRUE   B. An isolated osteophyte in the thoracolumbar area, separate from the vertebral body, may be found.
Ch. 82 Reiter's Syndrome, p 1794.

TRUE   C. The findings are similar to those seen in psoriatic arthropathy, with a predilection for the lower extremities.
Ch. 82 Reiter's Syndrome, p 1794.

TRUE   D.
Ch. 82 Reiter's Syndrome, p 1794.

FALSE   E. Reiter's syndrome causes a reactive, immune-mediated arthritis that does not respond to tetracyclines. Gonococcal arthritis is a septic arthritis responsive to antibiotics.
Ch. 82 Reiter's Syndrome, p 1794.

A 7.81. *The Following Statements About Crystal Deposition Arthropathies are True*

TRUE   A.
Ch. 82 Gout, p 1796.

TRUE   B. Gross destructive changes with bone cysts and fragmentation may cause a "pseudoneuropathic" joint.
Ch. 82 Calcium Pyrophosphate Dihydrate Deposition Disease, p 1798.

FALSE   C. The radiographic appearances of CPPD and haemochromatosis are very similar. The metacarpal heads are said to be more severely affected in the latter, but the distribution of the arthritis and the presence and extent of chondrocalcinosis may be identical.
Ch. 82 Haemochromatosis and Hypophosphatasia, p 1798.

FALSE   D. *Hyperphosphatasia* ("Juvenile Paget's disease") does not cause a crystal deposition arthropathy. It is a cause of dwarfism, osteopenia and pathological fractures. *Hypophosphatasia* is a spectrum of rachitic disease in which the mild adult form causes chondrocalcinosis and an arthropathy similar to CPPD and haemochromatosis.
Ch. 82 Haemochromatosis and Hypophosphatasia, p 1798.

TRUE   E. In this disorder, a polymer of homogentisic acid accumulates in articular cartilage, heart and kidney and causes disc calcification in the spine, as well as severe destruction in large joints. Cardiac and renal failure occur.
Ch. 82 Alkaptonuria, p 1798.

Q 7.82. *Regarding the Radiology of Osteoarthritis*

    A. Erosive osteoarthritis is limited to the hands

    B. Involvement of the trapezio-scaphoid joint is a feature

    C. Periosteal new bone formation is seen in the femoral neck

    D. Valgus deformity at the knee is commoner than varus deformity

    E. Patellofemoral joint involvement usually spares the medial side of the patella

Q 7.83. *Regarding the Radiology of Joint Conditions*

    A. Epiphyseal overgrowth may occur in haemophilic arthropathy

    B. Juxta-articular osteopenia is usually found in neuropathic arthropathy

    C. In idiopathic skeletal hyperostosis (DISH), the sacroiliac joints are not involved

    D. Synovial chondromatosis occurs within bursae

    E. Pigmented villonodular synovitis causes predominantly intra-articular low signal on all sequences on MRI

A 7.82. *Regarding the Radiology of Osteoarthritis*

TRUE   A. Central erosions occur in the articular surfaces of the proximal and distal interphalangeal joints of the hands, giving a "seagull" appearance. Large joints are not involved.
Ch. 82 Osteoarthritis, p 1799.

TRUE   B. Wrist involvement in primary osteoarthritis is usually limited to this joint and to the first carpometacarpal joint.
Ch. 82 Osteoarthritis, p 1800.

TRUE   C. This "buttressing" occurs on the medial side of the femoral neck as a response to lateral subluxation of the femoral head which may precede radiological evidence of joint-space narrowing.
Ch. 82 Osteoarthritis, p 1800.

FALSE   D. Preferential involvement of the medial compartment of the knee joint causes a varus deformity.
Ch. 82 Osteoarthritis, p 1800.

TRUE   E. The lateral facet of the patella and the lateral femoral condyle are usually affected with the medial side being spared.
Ch. 82 Primary Osteoarthritis, p 1800.

A 7.83. *Regarding the Radiology of Joint Conditions*

TRUE   A. It is not often symmetrical. Epiphyseal overgrowth is a feature that is stimulated by recurrent hyperaemia of joints affected by haemarthrosis.
Ch. 82 Haemophilia, p 1800.

FALSE   B. In the presence of gross destruction and deformity, regional mineral content is usually maintained.
Ch. 82 Neuropathic Arthropathy, p 1802.

TRUE   C. This helps the condition to be distinguished from ankylosing spondylitis.
Ch. 82 Idiopathic Skeletal Hyperostosis (DISH), p 1802.

TRUE   D. This is a chondrometaplasia of subsynovial connective tissue that occurs in joints, bursae and rarely tendon sheaths. Many cartilaginous calcified loose bodies often result.
Ch. 82 Synovial Chondromatosis, p 1803.

TRUE   E. This is owing to iron deposition from haemorrhagic effusions.
Ch. 82 Pigmented Villonodular Synovitis, p 1804.

Q *7.84. Non-Vascular Soft-Tissue Calcification and Hypercalcaemia Occur in the Following Conditions*

    A. Hypoparathyroidism

    B. Secondary hyperparathyroidism

    C. Sarcoidosis

    D. Calcium pyrophosphate deposition disease

    E. Pseudopseudohyperparathyroidism

Q *7.85. Calcification in the Intervertebral Discs is a Recognized Finding in*

    A. Calcium pyrophosphate deposition disease

    B. Ochronosis

    C. Dermatomyositis

    D. Calcium hydroxyapatite deposition disease

    E. Immobilization

A 7.84. Non-Vascular Soft-Tissue Calcification and Hypercalcaemia Occur in the Following Conditions

FALSE   A. Although soft-tissue calcification occurs, hypercalcaemia is not a feature of this condition. Instead, *hypocalcaemia* and *hyperphosphataemia* are present.
Ch. 83 Calcification, p 1814.

FALSE   B. Hypercalcaemia is not a feature of this condition. The stimulus to produce more parathyroid hormone is *low* serum calcium. Soft-tissue calcification is a feature.
Ch. 83 Calcification, p 1814.

TRUE   C. Hypercalcaemia is a feature of sarcoidosis and may result in soft-tissue calcification.
Ch. 83 Calcification, p 1814.

FALSE   D. Hypercalcaemia is not a feature of this condition in which soft-tissue calcification, particularly around joints and in cartilage, occurs.
Ch. 83 Calcification, p 1814.

FALSE   E. Hypercalcaemia is not a feature of this condition, affected individuals being biochemically normal. Short stature, generalized osteosclerosis and soft-tissue calcification are features of this disorder and are also seen in pseudo-hyperparathyroidism and primary hypoparathyroidism.
Ch. 83 Calcification, p 1814.

A 7.85. Calcification in the Intervertebral Discs is a Recognized Finding in

TRUE   A. Disc calcification in this condition is associated with pain and may mimic the syndesmophytes of anklosing spondylitis.
Ch. 83 Calcification, p 1815.

TRUE   B. Alkaptonuria is caused by the congenital absence of homogentisic acid oxidase. Pigmentation of many soft tissues precedes their degeneration. Marked disc-space calcification occurs in association with gross osteophytosis and spinal ankylosis.
Ch. 83 Calcification, p 1815.

FALSE   C. The most severe form of this condition occurs in childhood when extensive muscle fibrosis and soft-tissue calcification result in immobility. Disc calcification is not a feature.
Ch. 83 Calcification, p 1815.

FALSE   D. Periarticular calcification occurs in this condition. It is often monoarticular, affecting the shoulder where it is manifested as calcific tendinitis.
Ch. 83 Calcification, p 1815.

TRUE   E. Extensive ossification around joints—particularly the hips—is seen following spinal trauma and other causes of immobility. Intervertebral discs may be affected.
Ch. 83 Calcification, p 1815.

Q *7.86. Soft-Tissue Tumours Giving a High Signal on T1W and T2W Images Include*

    A. Aggressive fibromatosis (desmoids)

    B. Subacute haematoma

    C. Giant-cell tumour

    D. Melanoma

    E. Well-differentiated liposarcoma

Q *7.87. Regarding the Radiology of Soft-Tissue Tumours*

    A. Malignant fibrous histiocytoma is the most common malignant soft-tissue tumour in adults

    B. Myositis ossificans enhances intensely and diffusely with GdDTPA on MRI

    C. An encapsulated soft-tissue tumour with well-defined margins and homogeneous signal intensity on MRI is unlikely to be malignant

    D. A water-filled capsule taped to the skin over a suspected lesion is recommended to ensure that the correct area has been imaged on MRI

    E. Lymphocele has a very low and a very high signal on T1W and T2W images, respectively

A *7.86. Soft-Tissue Tumours Giving a High Signal on T1W and T2W Images Include*

FALSE   A. The prominent fibrotic element in these tumours exhibits a low signal on both T1W and T2W images.
Ch. 83 Soft-Tissue Tumours, p 1826.

TRUE   B. Extracellular methaemoglobin has a high T1W and T2W signal.
Ch. 83 Soft-Tissue Tumours, p 1827.

FALSE   C. This tumour often exhibits a low signal on both T1W and T2W sequences.
Ch. 83 Soft-Tissue Tumours, p 1826.

TRUE   D. The paramagnetic properties of melanin confer a high signal on T1W images. Associated oedema may generate a high signal on T2W images.
Ch. 83 Soft-Tissue Tumours, p 1826.

TRUE   E. The high fat content of this tumour yields a high signal on T1W and T2W images. It is worth reviewing a list of circumstances in which a high T1W signal occurs: fatty tissue, flow artefact, gadolinium enhancement, extracellular methaemoglobin, proteinaceous fluid, "milk of calcium," melanoma.
Ch. 83 Soft-Tissue Tumours, p 1827.

A *7.87. Regarding the Radiology of Soft-Tissue Tumours*

TRUE   A. It accounts for approximately 30% of all soft-tissue tumours and closely resembles a high-grade fibrosarcoma on histology.
Ch. 83 Soft-Tissue Tumours, p 1828.

TRUE   B. The lesions of this disorder are usually isointense with muscle on T1W images, and hyperintense on T2W images. It may be hyperintense to fat on T2W images. A rim of ossification, if present, exhibits decreased signal intensity on all MRI sequences.
Ch. 83 Soft-Tissue Tumours, p 1828.

FALSE   C. This pattern occurs with several soft-tissue tumours, most notably leiomyosarcoma and low-grade liposarcoma. In these cases, the capsule is a pseudocapsule that contains malignant cells.
Ch. 83 Soft-Tissue Tumours, p 1828.

FALSE   D. Cod liver oil is greatly preferred to water as it generates a high signal on both T1W and T2W images.
Ch. 83 Soft-Tissue Tumours, p 1827.

TRUE   E.
Ch. 83 Soft-Tissue Tumours, p 1826.

Q 7.88. *The Following Disorders Commonly Occur at the Specified Ages*

A. Perthe's disease between 6 and 8 years of age

B. Slipped upper femoral epiphyses 5 and 10 years of age

C. Hip infection before the age of one

D. Blount's disease between 5 and 8 years of age

E. Congenital dislocation of the hip after the age of 6 weeks

Q 7.89. *Nonaccidental Injury in Children Should be Suspected If*

A. Fractures are present in the shafts of long bones

B. Bucket handle fractures of the metaphases are present

C. Fractures of the outer end of the clavicle are present

D. Sternal fractures are present

E. Vertebral fractures are present

A *7.88. The Following Disorders Commonly Occur at the Specified Ages*

TRUE   A. Boys are five times more frequently affected than girls, and 10% of cases are bilateral.
Ch. 84 Perthe's Disease, p 1837.

FALSE   B. This condition occurs before the epiphyses fuse and presents between 10 and 16 years of age. Boys are more frequently affected than girls in the ratio of 3:1. The condition is usually bilateral in 20% of patients.
Ch. 84 Slipped Femoral Epiphyses, p 1838.

FALSE   C. Hip infections can occur at any time and should not be excluded on the basis of age.

FALSE   D. This condition occurs between 1 and 3 years and resembles extreme physiological bowing. The proximal medial tibial epiphyses are compressed, and beak shaped, and may fragment.
Ch. 84 Infantile Tibia Vara, p 1843.

FALSE   E. Most patients with congenital dislocation of the hips present before 6 weeks: at 6 weeks, most hips have stabilised and only 0.15% of patients have dislocatable hips. Those in the latter group need treatment.
Ch. 84 Congenital Dislocation in the Hip, p 1841.

A *7.89. Nonaccidental Injury in Children Should be Suspected If*

FALSE   A. Fractures of the shafts of long bones are common but not specific.
Ch. 84 Characteristics of Fractures in NAI, p 1845.

TRUE   B. These fractures are very suggestive, or even characteristic of nonaccidental injury in children.
Ch. 84 Characteristics of Fractures in NAI, p 1845.

TRUE   C.
Ch. 84 Characteristics of Fractures in NAI, p 1845.

TRUE   D.
Ch. 84 Non-Accidental Injury, p 1845.

TRUE   E.
Ch. 84 Characteristics of Fractures in NAI, p 1845.

Q *7.90. Concerning the Dating of Fractures in Children with Non-Accidental Injury*

    A. Early periosteal new bone appears between 4 and 21 days

    B. Soft callus at 6-8 weeks

    C. Loss of fracture-line definition occurs up to 1 week

    D. Hard callus may appear at 80 days

    E. Remodelling of bone can take up to 2 years

Q *7.91. Regarding Periosteal Reaction*

    A. Periosteal reaction of the newborn may present with several layers of thin new bone along the diaphysis of the humerus

    B. Hypervitaminosis A causes painful soft-tissue lumps and periosteal reactions

    C. Periosteal elevation caused by pus is usually seen within the first 5 days of symptomatic osteomyelitis

    D. Brodie's abscess has some associated periosteal reaction in more than 80% of cases

    E. Sclerosing osteitis of Garré is seen most commonly in the mandible

A 7.90. *Concerning the Dating of Fractures in Children with Non-Accidental Injury*

TRUE
    A.
      Ch. 84 Table 84.2, p 1837.

FALSE
    B. Soft callus appears between 10 and 21 days.
      Ch. 84 Table 84.2, p 1837.

FALSE
    C. Loss of fracture line definition occurs between 10 and 21 days.
      Ch. 84 Table 84.2, p 1837.

TRUE
    D. The appearance time for hard callus is between 14 and 90 days.
      Ch. 84 Table 84.2, p 1837.

TRUE
    E.
      Ch. 84 Table 84.2, p 1837.

A 7.91. *Regarding Periosteal Reaction*

FALSE
    A. This normal variant occurs as a single thin layer of new bone along the diaphysis of the humerus, femur and radius. It is bilateral and symmetrical and does not form double or multiple layers of periosteal bone.
      Ch. 85 Terminology, p 1854.

TRUE
    B. The differential diagnosis includes infection and metastatic leukaemia and neuroblastoma.
      Ch. 85 Terminology, p 1855.

FALSE
    C. It usually takes at least two weeks after the onset of symptoms for the periosteal reaction to be radiologically visible.
      Ch. 85 Acute Osteomyelitis, p 1855.

FALSE
    D. Only 40% of these lesions have an associated periosteal reaction. Prominent dense new bone deposition simulating osteoid osteoma may occur in cortical abscesses.
      Ch. 85 Brodie's Abscess, p 1857.

TRUE
    E. This rare condition provokes dense endosteal and periosteal new bone formation, causing marked sclerosis.
      Ch. 85 Sclerosing Osteitis of Garré, p 1857.

Q 7.92. *The Changes of (or Resembling Those of) Osteitis Pubis Regularly Occur in the Following Conditions*

    A. Long distance runners

    B. Psoriatic arthropathy

    C. Paget's disease

    D. Following prostatic resection

    E. Secondary hyperparathyroidism

Q 7.93. *Regarding the Radiology of Spinal Infection*

    A. Vertebral body sclerosis in a caucasian patient favours a pyogenic rather than a mycobacterial cause

    B. Calcification in a paravertebral mass is more likely to be due to tuberculosis than salmonellosis.

    C. The thoracic spine is more frequently affected by pyogenic organisms than by *M. Tuberculosis*.

    D. Degenerative disc disease is commonly associated with a high signal on T2W images which extends to involve half of the vertebral body

    E. Early extensive bone destruction is the hallmark of juvenile discitis

A 7.92. *The Changes of (or Resembling Those of) Osteitis Pubis Regularly Occur in the Following Conditions*

TRUE   A. Owing to chronic stress and/or tendon avulsion.
Ch. 85 Pubis, p 1858.

TRUE   B. Resorption of the corticated margins of the symphysis pubis with or without juxta-articular sclerosis occurs in this condition.
Ch. 85 Pubis, p 1858.

FALSE   C.
Ch. 85 Pubis, p 1858.

TRUE   D. A low-grade infection of the symphysis pubis is a recognized sequel of prostatectomy.
Ch. 85 Pubis, p 1858.

TRUE   E. Subperiosteal bone resorption and osteosclerosis may closely resemble osteitis pubis.
Ch. 85 Pubis, p 1858.

A 7.93. *Regarding the Radiology of Spinal Infection*

TRUE   A. The pattern of vertebral infection varies among ethnic groups. Black patients more frequently demonstrate reactive new bone with tuberculous infection than caucasian patients.
Ch. 85 Pyogenic Spinal Infection, p 1859.

TRUE   B. Calcified paravertebral soft-tissue masses do not normally occur in pyogenic infections.
Ch. 85 Pyogenic Spinal Infection, p 1859.

FALSE   C. The lower lumbar spine is the usual site of pyogenic infection. Thoracic vertebral infection favours TB.
Ch. 85 Pyogenic Spinal Infection, p 1859.

FALSE   D. One of the distinguishing features of noninfective degenerative discitis is the limitation of marrow oedema to the region of the adjacent end-plates.
Ch. 85 Pyogenic Spinal Infection, p 1860.

FALSE   E. In the first and second decades, discitis has a slow and self-limiting course. Loss of disc-space height is accompanied by marginal erosion and sclerosis of the adjacent vertebral surfaces with little bone destruction.
Ch. 85 Intervertebral Disc: Discitis, p 1860.

Q *7.94. The Following Statements Apply to Septic Arthritis*

A. Primary haematogenous joint infection is much less frequent than infection of the joint secondary to an adjacent osteomyelitis

B. Rapid cartilage destruction favours a pyogenic rather than a mycobacterial cause

C. Bony ankylosis is more likely to occur following pyogenic infection than mycobacterial infection

D. Widening of the joint space occurs as an early temporary manifestation of the condition

E. Metaphyseal bone destruction implicates osteomyelitis as the source of the septic arthritis

Q *7.95. Regarding Bone Infection*

A. Periosteal reaction is a less prominent feature in the neonate than in the older patient

B. Normal radiographic density in the epiphysis of an involved bone in a young patient is a favourable sign

C. Diaphyseal involvement by tuberculosis is rare

D. Calcific debris around a diseased joint is a reliable indicator of tuberculous, as opposed to pyogenic, arthritis

E. The growth plate in childhood provides a potent barrier to the spread of tuberculous infection

A 7.94. The Following Statements Apply to Septic Arthritis

TRUE A.

Ch. 85 Septic (Infective) Arthritis, p 1861.

TRUE B. Joint-space narrowing due to cartilage destruction occurs late in tuberculous infection.

Ch. 85 Septic (Infective) Arthritis, p 1861.

TRUE C. This reflects the greater degree of cartilage destruction that occurs with untreated pyogenic infection.

Ch. 85 Septic (Infective) Arthritis, p 1862.

TRUE D. It is imperative that needle aspiration followed by microscopy and culture of the aspirate be performed at this stage so that the appropriate antibiotic therapy can be instituted.

Ch. 85 Septic (Infective) Arthritis, p 1861.

TRUE E. The likelihood of metaphyseal infection spreading to involve the epiphysis and joint space is increased in young patients in whom primitive vascular channels between metaphysis and epiphysis are present. Septic arthritis is more likely if the metaphysis lies within the joint capsule (e.g., in the hip).

Ch. 85 Septic (Infective) Arthritis, p 1861.

A 7.95. Regarding Bone Infection

FALSE A. The loose attachment of periosteum in the neonate is associated with early and extensive subperiosteal new bone formation.

Ch. 85 Acute Osteomyelitis in the Neonate, p 1862.

FALSE B. In osteomyelitis, hyperaemia causes the metaphysis and epiphysis to become osteopenic. Avascular necrosis of the epiphysis is identified by the presence of "normal" epiphyseal density on a background of osteopenia. At this stage, ischaemia is often irreversible.

Ch. 85 Acute Osteomyelitis in the Neonate, p 1863.

TRUE C. Bone involvement in this disorder is usually at the end of a long bone or within a tuberosity (e.g., tuberosities of the humerus or greater trochanter of the femur). In the latter case, caseous material may track down deep to the fascia lata to present as a cold abscess in the region of the knee.

Ch. 85 Tuberculosis, p 1864.

TRUE D.

Ch. 85 Tuberculosis, p 1864.

FALSE E. The growth plate is breached early so that epiphyseal and metaphyseal involvement are commonly already established at the time of presentation.

Ch. 85 Tuberculosis, p 1864.

Q 7.96. *Features of Tuberculous Infection of Bones and Joints Include*

    A. End-stage ankylosis

    B. Peripheral erosions which mimic those seen in rheumatoid arthritis

    C. Epiphyseal overgrowth in children

    D. Periosteal reaction in a swollen finger

    E. Calcification of peripheral nerves adjacent to a tuberculous bony focus

Q 7.97. *The Following are Features of Fungal Infections of Bones and/or Joints*

    A. Prominent periosteal reaction

    B. The joint space is commonly involved

    C. Rapid destruction of a vertebral body with preservation of the disc space

    D. A sclerotic or osteolytic rib lesion with an adjacent sinus track discharging onto the chest wall suggests coccidioidomycosis

    E. Widespread ankylosis in the foot accompanied by bone destruction and sinus tracks suggests actinomycosis

A 7.96. *Features of Tuberculous Infection of Bones and Joints Include*

TRUE

A. The ankylosis in tuberculosis is commonly fibrous in contradistinction to the bony ankylosis of pyogenic arthritis.
Ch. 85 Tuberculous Arthritis, p 1866.

TRUE

B. The absence of joint-space narrowing in the presence of juxta-articular osteopenia and marginal erosions should raise the suspicion of tuberculous arthritis.
Ch. 85 Tuberculous Arthritis, p 1866.

TRUE

C. Any chronic inflammatory arthritis in children may result in overgrowth of an epiphysis (e.g., coxa magna) and premature epiphyseal fusion due to hyperemia.
Ch. 85 Tuberculous Arthritis, p 1868.

TRUE

D. Subperiosteal new bone occurs in tuberculous dactylitis but when particularly prominent, it is more suggestive of syphilis or yaws dactylitis.
Ch. 85 Tuberculous Arthritis, p 1865.

FALSE

E. This is a rare but diagnostic sign of leprosy.
Ch. 85 Tuberculous Arthritis, p 1871.

A 7.97. *The Following are Features of Fungal Infections of Bones and/or Joints*

FALSE

A. Periosteal reaction occurs more commonly in children than in adults but is not usually a prominent feature.
Ch. 85 Mycotic (Fungal) Infections, p 1871.

FALSE

B. Articular cartilage is a potent barrier to fungal infection making fungal arthritis a rarity.
Ch. 85 Mycotic (Fungal) Infections, p 1871.

TRUE

C. Fungal infection may be difficult to differentiate from malignant destruction of a vertebral body.
Ch. 85 Mycotic (Fungal) Infections, p 1871.

FALSE

D. This is a typical presentation of *actinomycosis*. Coccidioidomycosis affects bone as a complication of disseminated pulmonary infection and has a predilection for long bones and bony prominences.
Ch. 85 Mycotic (Fungal) Infections, p 1871.

FALSE

E. This is a typical presentation of *maduromycosis*. "Madura foot"—a tropical fungal infection that occurs among people who do not wear shoes. *Actinomycosis* classically affects the mandible, maxilla and thorax.
Ch. 85 Mycotic (Fungal) Infections, p 1872.

Q 7.98. *The Following Statements Regarding Bone Conditions Apply*

A. In a diabetic foot, the presence of gas produced by bacteria in the soft tissues implies that gangrene is present

B. [67]Gallium scanning allows an infected loose prosthesis to be distinguished reliably from a non-infected loose prosthesis

C. Hand radiographs may be of diagnostic value in sarcoidosis in the absence of any other evidence of the disease on clinical examination

D. In Infantile Cortical Hyperostosis (Caffey's disease), the skull is characteristically not involved

E. Ainhum (fibrosis occuring in the fifth toe) is frequently complicated by infection and osteomyelitis

Q 7.99. *The Following Have a Low Signal Intensity on T1 and T2-Weighted Images*

A. Gas

B. Hyaline cartilage

C. Fibrocartilage

D. Red marrow

E. Cortical bone

A *7.98. The Following Statements Regarding Bone Conditions Apply*

FALSE
A. Gas may be Clostridial in origin or produced by certain strains of *E. coli*. Gas does not necessarily mean that gangrene is present as tissue viability may still be present.
Ch. 85 Diabetic Osteopathy, p 1874.

FALSE
B. The appearances are often indistinguishable, particularly if the infection is low-grade—as is usually the case. The best scintigraphic discrimination between these two conditions is probably achieved by sequential nuclear medicine studies with a ^{99m}Tc bone scan and an ^{111}In-labelled leucocyte scan.
Ch. 85 Infected Prostheses, p 1874.

FALSE
C. Skeletal involvement is closely associated with skin involvement by sarcoidosis. If there are no cutaneous manifestations, hand radiographs have no diagnostic value.
Ch. 85 Sarcoidosis, p 1875.

FALSE
D. In order of frequency, the mandible, clavicle, tubular bone diaphyses and ribs are most commonly affected. Involvement of the latter gives a plain chest radiograph appearance of "double exposure." The skull, but not vertebrae, may also be involved.
Ch. 85 Infantile Cortical Hyperostosis, p 1876.

TRUE
E. It is of unknown origin, occuring in bare-footed persons in the tropics.
Ch. 85 Ainhum, p 1877.

A *7.99. The Following Have a Low Signal Intensity on T1 and T2-Weighted Images*

TRUE
A.
Ch. 87 Table 87.1, p 1894.

FALSE
B. The signals are intermediate in both cases.
Ch. 87 Table 87.1, p 1894.

TRUE
C.
Ch. 87 Table 87.1, p 1894.

FALSE
D. The signals are intermediate in both cases.
Ch. 87 Table 87.1, p 1894.

TRUE
E.

Q *7.100. Concerning Bone Marrow Imaging*

    A. Yellow marrow contains 40% fat

    B. Red marrow contains 40% water

    C. Yellow marrow appears black on STIR sequences

    D. MRI can in most cases reliably distinguish benign marrow replacement from malignant infiltration

    E. MRI is much more sensitive than radiography in the detection of nondisplaced fractures

Q *7.101. Concerning MRI Imaging of the Joints*

    A. An injury or partial tear of any of the knee ligaments is detected by an increased signal within the ligament on most pulse sequences

    B. The anterior cruciate ligament inserts more anteriorly on the femur than the posterior cruciate ligament

    C. CT is superior to MRI in the assessment of the anterior ligaments of the shoulder joint

    D. The intra-articular disc of the temporomandibular joint is similar in composition to the menisci of the knee and hence produces a low signal on MR sequences

    E. MR is reliable in demonstrating communicating defects in the intrinsic ligaments of the wrist

A 7.100. *Concerning Bone Marrow Imaging*

FALSE   A. Yellow marrow contains 15% water, 80% fat and 5% protein.
Ch. 87 Red and Yellow Marrow, p 1898.

TRUE   B. Red marrow contains a further 40% of fat and 20% of protein.
Ch. 87. Red and Yellow Marrow, p 1898.

TRUE   C.
Ch. 87 Imaging Characteristics of Bone Marrow, p 1898.

FALSE   D. Unfortunately, this is not the case.
Ch. 87 Neoplastic Infiltration, p 1899.

TRUE   E. MRI will usually beat diagnostic radiography immediately after injury.
Ch. 87 Trauma, p 1901.

A 7.101. *Concerning MRI Imaging of the Joints*

TRUE   A.
Ch. 87 The Knee Joint, p 1907.

FALSE   B. This is of considerable importance when planning surgery.
Ch. 87 The Knee Joint, p 1907.

FALSE   C.
Ch. 87 The Shoulder Joint, p 1908.

TRUE   D.
Ch. 87 The TMJ, p 1910.

FALSE   E. Unfortunately, this has not so far proved to be the case though smaller coils may be helpful in the future.
Ch. 87 Other Joints, Ligaments and Tendons, p 1910.

Q *7.102. Concerning Radionuclide Bone Scanning*

    A. Following injection of ^{99m}Tc labelled MDP, 10% is deposited within bone within one hour

    B. The gallium ion shares certain physiological properties with the ferrous ion

    C. Gallium localises to normal bone by binding to phosphate

    D. Giant cell tumours of bone demonstrate intense uptake of ^{99m}Tc MDP

    E. In patients with bone trauma, a negative bone scan effectively excludes significant bony injury

A *7.102. Concerning Radionuclide Bone Scanning*

FALSE   A. Fifty percent is deposited within bone within one hour.
              Ch. 88 Technetium^{99m} Labelled Bone Seekers, p 1916.

FALSE   B. The ferric ion.
              Ch. 88 Gallium^{67} Citrate, p 1917.

TRUE   C. Gallium localises to a mild degree in normal bone by binding to phosphate
              to produce insoluable complexes.
              Ch. 88 Gallium^{67} Citrate, p 1917.

TRUE   D. Giant cell tumours and osteomas are unusual examples of benign tumours
              demonstrating increased bone tracer uptake.
              Ch. 88. Benign Giant Cell Tumours and Osteoid Osteomas, p 1921.

TRUE   E. A negative bone scan which effectively excludes significant bony injury does
              not exclude damage to soft tissue or cartilage. A positive bone scan, how-
              ever, is objective evidence of significant trauma and is useful in cases of
              litigation.

8

The Female Reproductive System

Q 8.1. Concerning the Diagnosis of Pregnancy and Assessment of Gestational Age

A. Using transvaginal sonography, a gestational sac can be seen only when the Beta Human Chorionic Gonadotrophin (BHCG) level is greater than 1500 mIu. ml^{-1}

B. Transabdominal scanning can detect a gestational sac within the choriodecidual mass at 4-5 weeks amenorrhoea

C. Between 8 and 10 weeks transvaginal assessment of crown rump length is the preferred method of determining gestational age

D. Fetal abdominal circumference is a reliable measurement of the assessment of gestational age after 12 weeks

E. A crescentic hyporeflective area beneath the choriodecidua is a normal finding

Q 8.2. Features Consistent with Ectopic Pregnancy on Transvaginal Ultrasound Include

A. Uterine decidual thickening

B. Uterine intraluminal fluid

C. An echogenic adnexal ring on the side of the pain

D. A corpus luteal cyst in the ovary contralateral to the side of the pain

E. Absence of fluid in pouch of Douglas

A 8.1. *Concerning the Diagnosis of Pregnancy and Assessment of Gestational Age*

FALSE A. This level applies to *transabdominal* scanning. For *transvaginal* sonography, a sac can be seen when the BHCG is between 500 and 1500 mIu. ml^{-1}.
Ch. 89 Confirm Intrauterine Pregnancy/Exclude Extrauterine Pregnancy, p 1934.

FALSE B. This is true of *transvaginal* scanning.
Ch. 89 Establish Gestational Age, p 1934.

FALSE C. Crown rump length is measured *transabdominally* by ultrasound.
Ch. 89 Establish Gestational Age, p 1934.

FALSE D. It allows an assessment of head/body proportionality and an approximate evaluation of fetal weight.
Ch. 89 Establish Gestational Age, p 1934.

FALSE E. This indicates retrochorionic haemorrhage. If greater in size than the gestational sac, a poor outcome is likely.
Ch. 89 Evaluate Fetal Viability, p 1937.

A 8.2. *Features Consistent with Ectopic Pregnancy on Transvaginal Ultrasound Include*

TRUE A.
Ch. 89 Fig. 89.3, p 1936.

TRUE B.
Ch. 89 Fig. 89.3, p 1936.

TRUE C.
Ch. 89 Fig. 89.3, p 1936.

TRUE D.
Ch. 89 Fig. 89.3, p 1936.

TRUE E.
Ch. 89 Fig. 89.3, p 1936.

Q 8.3. Regarding Sonography in Pregnancy

A. Scanning with the bladder maximally distended is the most accurate method of assessing placenta praevia

B. Chorionic villus sampling is best performed in the second trimester

C. High impedance in uteroplacental arteries is a sign of intra-uterine growth retardation (IUGR)

D. Transperineal sonography is used to evaluate cervical incompetence

E. Umbilical cord torsion is associated with fetal hydrops

Q 8.4. Pelvic Neoplasm is Suspected When

A. Ascites accompanies an ovarian cyst

B. There is low impedance, high-velocity flow in an ovarian cystic mass

C. The endometrial thickness is greater than 5 mm in a post-menopausal woman

D. There are papillary excrescences related to the ovary

E. Thick irregular septae are present within an ovarian cystic mass

A 8.3. *Regarding Sonography in Pregnancy*

FALSE   A. Scans with the bladder both full and empty are required to avoid errors resulting from compression of the lower uterine segment, which can simulate placenta praevia.
Ch. 89 Placental Disorders, p 1939.

FALSE   B. The optimal time for this is between 8 and 11 weeks to allow the early detection of anomalies.
Ch. 89 Guidance for Obstetric Intervention, p 1939.

TRUE   C. Increased vascular resistance occurs in IUGR.
Ch. 89 Placental Disorders, p 1939.

TRUE   D. Dilation of the cervical canal is readily shown by this method.
Ch. 89 Other Applications, p 1939.

TRUE   E. A twisted cord also occurs with cord tumours such as angiomyxoma.
Ch. 89 Fetal Anomalies (Table 84.5), p 1939.

A 8.4. *Pelvic Neoplasm is Suspected When*

TRUE   A.
Ch. 89 Pelvic Mass evaluation, p 1942.

TRUE   B. Tumour neo-vascularity characteristically produces abnormal shunts, which lead to a decrease in the resistance of the neo-vascular bed and an increase in the velocity of its arterial supply.
Ch. 89 Ovarian Cancer: Early Detection, p 1944.

TRUE   C. Normal secretory-phase endometrium is regularly 15 mm thick in the pre-menopausal woman. The normal post-menopausal endometrium is less than 5 mm thick. Hyperplasia and carcinoma are the main differential diagnoses of a thicker endometrium (above 5 mm) in a post-menopausal patient.
Ch. 89 Endometrial Disorders, p 1944.

TRUE   D. Best seen on transvaginal scanning.
Ch. 89 Ovarian Cancer: Early Detection, p 1944.

TRUE   E. More complex cysts have a higher chance of being malignant.
Ch. 89 Ovarian Cancer: Early Detection, p 1944.

Q 8.5. *Regarding Obstetric Radiology*

A. Transurethral US-guided aspiration of follicles is useful for ovaries located in the cul-de-sac

B. As ovulation approaches, the endometrium becomes less reflective on transabdominal ultrasound

C. The most important single measurement in pelvimetry is the AP diameter of the outlet

D. The average AP outlet diameter is 7.5 cm

E. An AP diameter of pelvic inlet of less than 11.5 cm is likely to result in a difficult vaginal delivery of a full term fetus in vertex presentation

Q 8.6. *Concerning Hysterosalpingography*

A. The optimal time to perform the examination is in the second half of the cycle

B. All water-soluble contrast medium disappears normally within an hour

C. A large globular atonic uterine cavity with a "shaggy" outline and a rounded filling defect is likely to represent endometrial polyposis

D. Venous intravasation of water-soluble contrast medium is a significant cause of morbidity

E. The cervix is seen as a shorter structure after childbirth

A 8.5. *Regarding Obstetric Radiology*

FALSE   A. This technique is used when the ovaries are located near the dome of the bladder.
Ch. 89 Guided Follicular Aspiration, p 1949.

FALSE   B. More reflective, owing to the distended, fluid-filled, tortuous gland architecture of the endometrium.
Ch. 89 Endometrial Assessment, p 1949.

FALSE   C. The AP diameter of the **inlet** is the most important single measurement. It has an average value of 12.5 cm.
Ch. 89 Pelvimetry, p 1952.

TRUE   D.
Ch. 89 Pelvimetry, p 1952.

FALSE   E. Delivery with an AP inlet diameter exceeding 10.5 cm is likely to proceed without difficulty.
Ch. 89 Pelvimetry, p 1952.

A 8.6. *Concerning Hysterosalpingography*

FALSE   A. At the end of the first week.
Ch. 90 Hysterosalpingography, p 1956.

TRUE   B. In hydrosalpinx, opacification of the occluded tubes may persist for several hours.
Ch. 90 Hysterosalpingography, p 1956.

FALSE   C. Globular uterine enlargement occurs in *early pregnancy* when endometrial thickening causes an irregular outline. A *trophoblast* appears as a rounded filling defect.
Ch. 90 Hysterosalpingography, p 1956.

FALSE   D. This complication is largely avoided by performing the examination when endometrium is neither too thin nor too thick; at the end of the first week is optimal. Its importance is obscuration of detail, not morbidity.
Ch. 90 Hysterosalpingography, p 1957.

TRUE   E.
Ch. 90 Radiological Anatomy, p 1957.

Q 8.7. *Normal Findings on Ultrasound of the Female Pelvis Include*

A. Pre-menopausal uterine dimensions of $9 \times 7 \times 5$ cm

B. A prepubertal uterine length of 5 cm with a vestigial cervix

C. A hyporeflective lumen in the extra-isthmic Fallopian tube

D. Ovaries not longer than 3 cm in any two planes or 5 cm in any one plane

E. Free fluid in the pouch of Douglas during ultrasound hystero-salpingography

Q 8.8. *Regarding Gynaecological Imaging*

A. Pelvic kidney is an association of bicornuate uterus

B. Tubo-ovarian abscess is a common sequel of primary gono-coccal infection

C. Fitz-Hugh Curtis syndrome (Gonococcal perihepatitis) results from rupture of a gonococcal adnexal abscess

D. Most tubo-ovarian abscesses cause ureteric obstruction at or just below the pelvic brim

E. Crohn's disease causes acute salpingitis

A 8.7. *Normal Findings on Ultrasound of the Female Pelvis Include*

TRUE   *A.*
             Ch. 90 Ultrasound, p 1958.

FALSE   *B.* The normal prepubertal uterus is 2-3 cm long and the cervical portion accounts for most of this length.
             Ch. 90 Anatomy (Ultrasonic), p 1959.

FALSE   *C.* The Fallopian tubes are not normally seen on ultrasound beyond the isthmus.
             Ch. 90 Anatomy (Ultrasonic), p 1959.

TRUE   *D.* The volume of the ovary can be calculated by multiplying length by width by breadth and dividing by two. The normal volume is less than 9 cm^3.
             Ch. 90 Anatomy (Ultrasonic), p 1959.

TRUE   *E.* This technique involves the injection of saline or US contrast medium into the uterine cavity. The identification of free fluid in the pouch of Douglas implies that at least one Fallopian tube is patent.
             Ch. 90 Hysterosalpingography, p 1957.

A 8.8. *Regarding Gynaecological Imaging*

TRUE   *A.* Renal ectopia and agenesis are also associations of bicornuate uterus.
             Ch. 90 Congenital Anomalies of the Female Genital Tract, p 1960.

FALSE   *B.* It occurs with recurrent gonococcal infection, or secondary bacterial invasion by other organisms. It is a rare complication of primary gonococcal infection.
             Ch. 90 Inflammatory Disease of the Female Genital Tract, p 1961.

TRUE   *C.* A generalized peritonitis or more rarely perihepatitis may occur.
             Ch. 90 Inflammatory Disease of the Female Genital Tract, p 1961.

TRUE   *D.* This is reported to occur in 80% of tubo-ovarian abscesses.
             Ch. 90 Inflammatory Disease of the Female Genital Tract, p 1961.

TRUE   *E.* Crohn's disease may present as acute salpingitis when adjacent terminal ileal or rectosigmoid disease is present.
             Ch. 90 Pelvic Inflammatory Disease of Extragenital Origin, p 1962.

Q 8.9. *Regarding the Following Gynaecological Conditions*

A. In salpingitis isthmica nodosa, the Fallopian tubes are often blocked bilaterally

B. Emphysematous vaginitis is commonly caused by clostridia

C. Fibroids are rarely single

D. Clinical staging is more accurate than ultrasound and CT in the staging of stage 1 and stage 2a carcinoma of cervix

E. Malignant degeneration within a fibroid is readily diagnosed on MRI

Q 8.10. *Concerning Pelvic Tuberculous Infection*

A. Tubal calcification may be seen on the plain film

B. Bilateral ampullary occlusion is often seen during hysterosalpingography

C. "Pipe-stem" fallopian tubes are found

D. Polypoid lesions occur in the uterine cavity

E. Small gas bubbles are seen above and behind the symphysis pubis on plain abdominal radiography

A 8.9. *Regarding the Following Gynaecological Conditions*

TRUE	A.	It is not clear whether infection is the sole cause of this condition—it may be a secondary phenomenon. The consistently nodular and uniform appearance of the diverticula differentiates the disorder from tuberculosis. *Ch. 90 Pelvic Inflammatory Disease of Extragenital Origin, p 1962.*
FALSE	B.	Emphysematous vaginitis is a benign and self-limiting infection caused by Trichomonas vaginalis. Gas gangrene of the uterus is usually due to clostridial infection following septic abortion. *Ch. 90 Uterine Infections, p 1963.*
TRUE	C.	They are almost always multiple. (Small fibroids are easy to miss on ultrasound.) *Ch. 90 Uterine Tumours, p 1963.*
TRUE	D.	Stage 1 is carcinoma confined to the cervix. Stage 2a extends beyond the cervix without reaching the pelvic wall or the lower third of the vagina. Parametrial invasion advances the staging to 2b and requires CT for its early detection. *Ch. 90 Carcinoma of the Cervix, p 1964.*
FALSE	E.	High or low signal occurs in benign fibroids owing to necrosis and haemorrhage. The appearances of malignant change are nonspecific and nondiagnostic on MRI. *Ch. 90 Uterine Tumours, p 1964.*

A 8.10. *Concerning Pelvic Tuberculous Infection*

TRUE	A.	*Ch. 90 Tuberculosis, p 1963*
TRUE	B.	This may be ampullary or isthmic and is nonspecific. *Ch. 90 Tuberculosis, p 1963.*
TRUE	C.	Multiple strictures, however, with or without sinus tracts and cavities, are more common. *Ch. 90 Tuberculosis, p 1963.*
TRUE	D.	*Ch. 90 Tuberculosis, p 1963.*
FALSE	E.	Gas-fluid levels in the adnexae due to fistulae into adjacent bowel do occur in pelvic TB. The appearance described above, however, is a feature of *emphysematous vaginitis*. *Ch. 90 Tuberculosis, p 1963.*

Q *8.11. The Following CT Features are Indicative of Extension of Carcinoma of the Cervix*

     A. Fluid in pouch of Douglas

     B. Low-density rim around the urethra

     C. Parametrial strands of soft-tissue density

     D. Hydronephrosis

     E. An eccentric soft-tissue mass

Q *8.12. The Following Statements Apply to Carcinoma of Cervix*

     A. Ureteric obstruction is most commonly caused by radio-therapy

     B. Vesicovaginal fistula is usually due to direct tumour spread

     C. Cavitation in lung metastases suggests the presence of a second, different primary tumour

     D. The presence of lymphangitis carcinomatosa of lung suggests a separate pathological process

     E. Direct involvement of the rectum is a common finding

A *8.11. The Following CT Features are Indicative of Extension of Carcinoma of the Cervix*

FALSE A. This is a nonspecific finding which of itself does not indicate extension of cervical carcinoma.
Ch. 90 Carcinoma of the Cervix, p 1964.

FALSE B. Obliteration of the normal peri-urethral fat plane is a sign of invasion.
Ch. 90 Carcinoma of the Cervix, p 1964.

TRUE C. These extend towards the obturator internus and/or pyriformis. Involvement of the pelvic wall advances the staging to 3b.
Ch. 90 Carcinoma of the Cervix, p 1964.

TRUE D. This is also a sign of 3b spread, which may be due to direct ureteric involvement, uterine enlargement or para-aortic or iliac lymph node disease.
Ch. 90 Carcinoma of the Cervix, p 1965.

TRUE E.
Ch. 90 Carcinoma of the Cervix, p 1964.

A *8.12. The Following Statements Apply to Carcinoma of Cervix*

FALSE A. It is almost always due to recurrent tumour and has a grave prognosis—less than half of patients with this complication survive a year.
Ch. 90 Carcinoma of the Cervix, p 1965.

FALSE B. This is usually due to radiotherapy or a complication of hysterectomy.
Ch. 90 Carcinoma of the Cervix, p 1965.

FALSE C. Cavitating lung metastases are a recognized occurrence in this disorder. The differential diagnosis includes squamous-cell carcinoma, colonic carcinoma, melanoma, transitional-cell carcinoma, sarcoma and response to chemotherapy.
Ch. 90 Carcinoma of the Cervix, p 1965.

FALSE D. This is also a well-recognized feature of cancer of the cervix. The differential diagnosis includes cancers of the lung, breast, stomach, colon, pancreas, thyroid and larynx.
Ch. 90 Carcinoma of the Cervix, p 1965.

FALSE E. The pouch of Douglas acts as a barrier to spread and direct rectal involvement is uncommon.
Ch. 90 Carcinoma of the Cervix, p 1964.

Q 8.13. *Choriocarcinoma Produces the Following*

A. Multiple luteal cysts

B. Subarachnoid haemorrhage

C. Pseudomyxoma peritonei

D. Highly attenuating cerebral masses on MRI that enhance following IV contrast medium

E. Calcified lung metastases after chemotherapy

Q 8.14. *Multiple Ovarian Cysts are Features of*

A. Infantile polycystic kidney disease

B. Oldfield's syndrome

C. Stein-Leventhal syndrome

D. Gardner's syndrome

E. Metropathia Haemorrhagia

A 8.13. Choriocarcinoma Produces the Following

TRUE
    A. These occur in nearly 50% of patients owing to excess gonadotrophin production.
Ch. 90 Choriocarcinoma, p 1966.

TRUE
    B. Brain metastases may bleed into the subarachnoid space.
Ch. 90 Choriocarcinoma, p 1966.

FALSE
    C. This is caused by rupture of a mucinous cystadenocarcinoma, usually of appendiceal or ovarian origin.
Ch. 90 Choriocarcinoma, p 1966.

TRUE
    D. The increased density is caused by haemorrhage.
Ch. 90 Choriocarcinoma, p 1966.

TRUE
    E. Calcification of lung metastases unrelated to treatment occurs with breast, thyroid and gonadal primaries, as well as mucinous adenocarcinoma and osteosarcoma.
Ch. 90 Choriocarcinoma, p 1966.

A 8.14. Multiple Ovarian Cysts are Features of

TRUE
    A. This causes cyst development in kidneys with fibrotic changes in liver and pancreas, and lung hypoplasia.
Ch. 90 Non-neoplastic Cysts of the Ovaries, p 1966.

FALSE
    B. This is a colonic multiple polyposis syndrome that is associated with sebaceous cysts.
Ch. 90 Non-neoplastic Cysts of the Ovaries, p 1966.

TRUE
    C. This is caused by deficient androgen conversion to oestrogen resulting in the accumulation of atretic ovarian follicles which fail to mature into Graafian follicles. More than 5 small subcapsular cysts suggests the diagnosis. It is associated with obesity, hirsutism and, less commonly, breast hypoplasia.
Ch. 90 Non-neoplastic Cysts of the Ovaries, p 1966.

FALSE
    D. Ovarian cysts are not a feature of this condition.
Ch. 90 Non-neoplastic Cysts of the Ovaries, p 1966.

TRUE
    E. This is characterized by cystic hyperplasia of the endometrium due to unopposed oestrogen stimulation.
Ch. 90 Non-neoplastic Cysts of the Ovaries, p 1966.

Q *8.15. Regarding MRI of the Female Pelvis*

A. The normal uterus has a central low-intensity stripe on T2W images that represents endometrium

B. On T_1W images the normal uterine body has a homogeneously low signal intensity

C. During staging of cervical carcinoma, on T2W images the presence of a complete ring of low signal around a tumour mass is an accurate indication of stage 1b

D. Calculated relaxation times allow reliable discrimination between lymph nodes infiltrated by malignancy, nonspecific lymphadenopathy and granulomatous disease

E. Brenner tumours of the ovary have a low signal on T1W and T2W images

Q *8.16 Regarding MR Imaging in Obstetrics*

A. Current NRPB guidelines exclude women in the first trimester of pregnancy from having MRI

B. MR pelvimetry is more useful in breech presentations than in cephalic presentations

C. MRI is accurate at determining the relationship between the lower edge of the placenta and the cervical os

D. Intra-uterine growth retardation may be better assessed by MRI than ultrasound

E. Fetal lung has high signal on T2W images

A *8.15. Regarding MRI of the Female Pelvis*

FALSE   A. The normal endometrium has high signal intensity on T2W images. The surrounding low signal area is a junctional layer of inner *myometrium*. The outermost layer has intermediate signal and represents fibrous stroma.
Ch. 91 Normal Anatomy, p 1978.

TRUE   B.
Ch. 91 Normal Anatomy, p 1978.

TRUE   C. Stage 1b is invasive tumour confined to the cervix.
Ch. 91 Cervical Carcinoma, p 1980.

FALSE   D. MRI, like CT, has to rely on size criteria to assess malignant involvement. An axial measurement of 1 cm is currently deemed to discriminate between benign and malignant lymph nodes.
Ch. 91 Cervical Carcinoma, p 1981.

TRUE   E. This characteristic is shared with fibrothecoma, and Sertoli-Leydig cell tumours. *Malignant* tumours tend to exhibit hyperintensity on T2W imaging.
Ch. 91 Ovarian Neoplasms, p 1986.

A *8.16 Regarding MR Imaging in Obstetrics*

TRUE   A. There are no known adverse chromosal effects of MR in vitro or in vivo. No mutagenic or lethal effects have been observed in bacterial culture. Despite this, extra caution is exercised during the period of organogenesis.
Ch. 91 MR Imaging in Obstetrics, p 1988.

TRUE   B. Most clinicians consider pelvic measurements to have little value in cephalic presentations as soft tissue dystocia is the most significant factor in difficult childbirths; however, there is a definite role for MR pelvimetry in breech presentations as a guide to the need for caesarian section, as it demonstrates all relevant bony landmarks.
Ch. 91 Pelvimetry, p 1988.

TRUE   C. The cervix has a distinctive trilaminar appearance on T2W images that can be distinguished accurately from the high signal of the placenta.
Ch. 91 Placental Localization, p 1988.

TRUE   D. Reliable estimates of fetal fat are possible using MRI.
Ch. 91 Fetal Anatomy, p 1989.

TRUE   E. The fetal lung has a distinctive appearance on MRI with a high signal intensity on T2W images.
Ch. 91 Fetal Anatomy, p 1989.

Q 8.17 *Concerning Mammography Technique, Equipment and Quality Control*

A. A single film-screen system is used because it allows a lower dose than that obtained by film alone without screen

B. A mediolateral oblique (MLO) view images more of the posterior breast and axillary tail than a 90° lateral view

C. The pectoralis major muscle should be visualized down to the level of the nipple

D. Breast compression reduces geometric unsharpness, motion unsharpness and radiation dose at the expense of reduced tissue contrast

E. At higher kVp settings, the dose is lower because of greater tissue penetration but contrast is reduced

Q 8.18. *Regarding the Radiology of Benign Breast Conditions*

A. Adenosis causes an increase in the expected density of the breast

B. Foci of calcification in adenosis have irregular borders and vary in size and shape

C. Fibroadenomas rarely develop or grow after menopause

D. The rapid growth of a mass prior to menstruation is strongly suggestive of a benign cyst

E. On ultrasound, a well-circumscribed smooth round lesion with a bright posterior wall, absent internal echoes and through transmission is definitely benign

A 8.17 *Concerning Mammography Technique, Equipment and Quality Control*

TRUE A. A double-screen system would allow a further reduction in dose but at the expense of resolution.
Ch. 92A Technical Requirements for Mammography, p 1995.

TRUE B. In the MLO view, the pectoralis major muscle is parallel to the plane of compression, allowing the breast to be pulled away from the chest and onto the film. Compression for the 90° view does not allow this to occur equally well.
Ch. 92A Positioning, p 1996.

TRUE C. This ensures inclusion of the posterior breast.
Ch. 92A Positioning, p 1996.

FALSE D. Contrast is ***improved*** by compression as scatter is reduced and a lower kVp can be used to penetrate the reduced thickness of breast.
Ch. 92A Breast Compression, p 1996.

TRUE E. There is a reduction in photo-electric absorption at higher kVp. This causes a reduction in contrast.
Ch. 92A Technical Factors, p 1997.

A 8.18. *Regarding the Radiology of Benign Breast Conditions*

TRUE A. Adenosis represents an increase in the number of breast lobules and acini within each lobule. The breasts, therefore, appear denser than would be expected for the patient's age and parity.
Ch. 92A Adenosis, p 2003.

TRUE B. The areas of calcification in this condition are usually bilateral, symmetrical and punctate. Variation in size and shape is seen. The borders may be smooth or irregular.
Ch. 92A Adenosis, p 2003.

TRUE C. They generally arise in younger women and regress after menopause.
Ch. 92A Fibroadenoma, p 2003.

TRUE D. A feature which distinguishes cysts is their tendency to grow rapidly, often prior to menstration and diminish in size equally rapidly.
Ch. 92A Cysts, p 2005.

TRUE E. These are strict ultrasonographic criteria which, if all are met, define a benign simple cyst.
Ch. 92A Cysts, p 2005.

Q *8.19. Regarding the Assessment of Breast Lumps*

    A. The demonstration of fatty density in a circumscribed mass excludes the possibility of malignancy

    B. Lack of change in a lesion for over 12 months excludes malignancy

    C. A rapidly enlarging breast mass occurs in cystosarcoma phylloides

    D. Traumatic fat necrosis always has at least some central fat density

    E. Ultrasound can detect less than 10% of cancers seen only as areas of microcalcifications on mammography

A *8.19. Regarding the Assessment of Breast Lumps*

TRUE   *A.*
                    Ch. 92A Circumscribed Carcinoma, p 2008.

FALSE   *B.* It is well documented that some malignant lesions may remain circum-
                    scribed and "dormant" for months or even years.
                    Ch. 92A Circumscribed Carcinoma, p 2009.

TRUE   *C.* This tumour is best thought of as a giant fibroadenoma that has a low
                    malignant potential and goes through periods of rapid growth.
                    Ch. 92A Fibroadenoma, p 2003.

FALSE   *D.* Many cases of fat necrosis are indistinguishable from carcinoma on mam-
                    mography and contain no fat density.
                    Ch. 92A Differential Diagnosis, p 2007.

TRUE   *E.* The quoted figure is 6%.
                    Ch. 92A Limitations of Ultrasound, p 2020.

9

The Central Nervous System

Q *9.1. Regarding Imaging Techniques of the Skull and Brain*

    A. The antero posterior projection is generally preferable to the postero anterior in frontal skull radiography

    B. Contrast-enhanced MRI is more sensitive than contrast-enhanced CT for detecting breakdown in the blood-brain barrier

    C. Cochlear implants are an absolute contraindication to MRI

    D. A 15 ml bolus of intravenous GdDTPA is adequate for MR angiography

    E. In the investigation of clinically typical Bell's palsy, MRI of the petrous temporal bone has replaced CT

Q *9.2. Regarding Cranial Anatomy*

    A. The foramen ovale and foramen spinosum extend from the middle cranial fossa to the pterygopalatine fossa

    B. The temporal lobes occupy the whole of the temporal fossae

    C. The internal carotid artery enters the subarachnoid space at the level of the anterior clinoid process

    D. The artery of Heubner arises from the middle cerebral artery

    E. Symmetry of the temporal fossae is the best method of assessing rotation on an occipitofrontal radiograph

A   9.1. *Regarding Imaging Techniques of the Skull and Brain*

FALSE
A. Improved definition of the more important anterior structures is obtained with an occipito frontal radiograph.
Ch. 93 Plain Radiography, p 2040.

TRUE
B.
Ch. 93 Other Imaging Techniques, p 2045.

TRUE
C.
Ch. 93 Magnetic Resonance Imaging, p 2049.

FALSE
D. Intravenous contrast medium is not required for this technique.
Ch. 93 Angiography, p 2049.

FALSE
E. Bell's palsy does not require imaging of the petrous bone.
Ch. 93 Acute Presentations, p 2063.

A   9.2. *Regarding Cranial Anatomy*

FALSE
A. They act as conduits for the passage of the mandibular division of trigeminal nerve and the middle meningeal artery respectively to the infratemporal fossa.
Ch. 93 The Cranial Foramina and Canals, p 2044.

FALSE
B. The temporal fossae are extracranial (facial) spaces deep to the zygomatic arches.
Ch. 93 Plain Radiography, p 2042.

TRUE
C.
Ch. 93 Anatomy of the Cerebral Arteries and Veins, p 2055.

FALSE
D. It is the major branch of the first segment of the anterior cerebral artery. It arcs to join the lenticulostriate branches of the middle cerebral artery.
Ch. 93 Anatomy of the Cerebral Arteries and Veins, p 2056.

FALSE
E. The temporal fossae are often asymmetrical. Rotation is best assessed by noting if the odontoid process (posterior) is in the same sagittal plane as the nasal septum.
Ch. 93 Plain Radiography, p 2040.

Q 9.3. *Regarding CNS Mass Lesions*

A. In children, continuously raised intracranial pressure is associated with thickening of the skull vault

B. Most brain tumours in children are primary CNS tumours

C. Most astrocytomas are cortically based

D. T2W images allow tumour to be differentiated from oedema

E. Oligodendrogliomas enhance with GdDTPA in under 10% of cases

Q 9.4. *Concerning Supratentorial Tumours*

A. Colloid cysts of the third ventricle are associated with slit-like third ventricles

B. Colloid cyst has a short T1 and long T2

C. Choroid plexus papillomas are dense on non-contrast-enhanced CT

D. Pineal germinomas are hyperdense on CT but are virtually never calcified

E. Germinomas may present as an enhancing suprasellar mass

A 9.3. *Regarding CNS Mass Lesions*

FALSE A. If the increase in pressure is intermittent, the vault may be thick and laminated.
Ch. 94 The Skull in Raised Intracranial Pressure, p 2068.

TRUE B. In children, three-quarters are primary, half of which are gliomas. In adults, metastases are more frequent than primary CNS tumours.
Ch. 94 Cerebral Tumours, p 2069.

FALSE C. They are more frequently located in deep white matter.
Ch. 94 Cerebral Tumours, p 2069.

FALSE D. Both are high-signal lesions. Their differentiation requires contrast medium (Gadolinium) administration, although areas in which the blood-brain barrier is apparently undisturbed may also contain many tumour cells. This is particularly true of low-grade astrocytomas.
Ch. 94 Cerebral Tumours, p 2070.

FALSE E. About 50% show some enhancement.
Ch. 94 Cerebral Tumours, p 2070.

A 9.4. *Concerning Supratentorial Tumours*

TRUE A. Unilateral or more commonly bilateral enlargement of the lateral ventricles also occurs.
Ch. 94 Colloid Cyst, p 2071.

TRUE B. This gives a characteristally high signal on T1W images and a high signal on T2W images. No contrast enhancement occurs.
Ch. 94 Colloid Cyst, p 2071.

TRUE C. These are usually well-defined, rounded tumours situated near the trigone or at the outlet foramina of the 4th ventricle. Marked contrast enhancement is seen.
Ch. 94 Choroid Plexus Papilloma, p 2072.

TRUE D. Uniform hyperdensity is a feature. They have long T1 and T2 on MRI.
Ch. 94 Pineal Region Tumours, p 2073.

TRUE E. Pineal tumours can appear in this location owing to subependymal spread along the third ventricle. Primary suprasellar germinomas also occur.
Ch. 94 Pineal Region Tumours, p 2073.

Q *9.5. Regarding Infratentorial Tumours*

    A. Cyst formation, calcification and haemorrhage are the hall-marks of brain stem gliomas

    B. Brain stem gliomas frequently occlude the basilar artery

    C. Cerebellar astrocytomas are seen as cystic tumours with enhancing mural nodules

    D. Medulloblastoma is the most common intracranial tumour in childhood

    E. A high signal on T1W images is present in 70% of medulloblastomas

Q *9.6. Concerning Tumour Spread in the Brain*

    A. Post-resection cranial CT with contrast enhancement is sufficient for medulloblastoma surveillance

    B. Subependymal nodules may be rendered invisible by periventricular oedema on T2W images of pineal germinomas

    C. In a child, a calcified tumour filling the fourth ventricle extending into cerebellar hemisphere and pons is likely to be a medulloblastoma

    D. Over 90% of all metastases to the brain from distant primary sites enhance with contrast medium

    E. Metastasis is the most common cerebellar tumour in the adult

A 9.5. Regarding Infratentorial Tumours

FALSE   A. These features are rare.
         Ch. 94 Brain Stem Gliomas, p 2073.

FALSE   B. However, they may grow around and "engulf" the artery.
         Ch. 94 Brain Stem Gliomas, p 2073.

TRUE   C. Ring enhancement is more frequent. The differential diagnosis of this appearance includes haemangioblastoma and, in adults, cystic metastases.
         Ch. 94 Cerebellar Tumours, p 2073.

TRUE   D.
         Ch. 94 Cerebellar Tumours, p 2073.

FALSE   E. A low T1W signal is the most common appearance and is nonspecific. A strikingly low T1W signal intensity may be present, however, and suggests the diagnosis.
         Ch. 94 Cerebellar Tumours, p 2074.

A 9.6. Concerning Tumour Spread in the Brain

FALSE   A. GdDTPA-enhanced MRI of the brain is required to detect subarachnoid seeding into the cisterns and sulci. The spinal canal should be checked for "drop" metastases.
         Ch. 94 Cerebellar Tumours, p 2074.

TRUE   B. Subependymal spread along lateral and third ventricles regularly occurs. Nodules may be masked by oedema and are best shown on GdDTPA-enhanced T1W images.
         Ch. 94 Pineal Region Tumours, p 2072.

FALSE   C. Calcification makes an ependymoma the likelier diagnosis.
         Ch. 94 Ependymoma, p 2075.

TRUE   D. Absence of contrast enhancement puts the diagnosis of metastasis in doubt.
         Ch. 94 Metastases to the Brain, p 2076.

TRUE   E. Even in specialist neurological centres, this is the case.
         Ch. 94 Metastases to the Brain, p 2077.

Q 9.7. *Concerning Pituitary Tumours*

A. Gd-DTPA administration allows more than 90% of microadenomas to be identified as small, high-signal areas on T1W images

B. Macroadenomas usually fail to enhance

C. Most craniopharyngiomas appear as cystic, calcified, peripherally contrast-enhancing suprasellar masses

D. MRI is the most useful technique for diagnosing craniopharyngioma

E. Undercutting of the planum sphenoidale characteristically occurs with optic nerve sheath meningioma.

Q 9.8. *Features Firmly Supporting Diagnosis of Meningioma Include*

A. White matter oedema

B. An intraventricular location in the right lateral ventricle

C. A lucent or fatty non-enhancing centre on CT

D. A broad base abutting the posterior surface of the petrous bone giving rise to a mass which reaches the midline

E. Widening of the internal auditory meatus

A 9.7. *Concerning Pituitary Tumours*

FALSE   A. Precontrast T1W images show microadenomas as low-signal areas against intermediate-signal normal pituitary tissue. After contrast medium administration, microadenomas are identified as areas of relative nonenhancement.
Ch. 94 Pituitary Tumours, p 2080.

FALSE   B. They generally exhibit homogeneous enhancement unless cystic or haemorrhagic areas are present.
Ch. 94 Pituitary Tumours, p 2080.

TRUE   C. Two thirds of these tumours show all these features.
Ch. 94 Pituitary Tumours, p 2082.

FALSE   D. The failure of MRI to appreciate calcification is a major weakness in the diagnosis of craniopharyngioma. CT is much better in this regard.
Ch. 94 Other Tumours in the Sellar Region, p 2083.

FALSE   E. This feature occurs when an optic chiasm *glioma* enlarges and erodes the anterior half of the sella turcica to give an omega-shaped sella.
Ch. 94 Optic Chiasm Glioma, p 2083.

A 9.8. *Features Firmly Supporting Diagnosis of Meningioma Include*

TRUE   A. This is detectable in the majority but is often minimal. It may be extensive and out of proportion to the size of the tumour bulk.
Ch. 94 Meningiomas, p 2084.

FALSE   B. Intraventricular meningiomas are almost always situated in the trigone of the *left* lateral ventricle.
Ch. 94 Meningiomas, p 2084.

FALSE   C. This is a recognized appearance that may cause diagnostic difficulty, but it is uncommon and not firmly supportive of the diagnosis.
Ch. 94 Meningiomas, p 2084.

TRUE   D. Acoustic neuroma tends to have no such base and only uncommonly reaches the midline.
Ch. 94 Meningiomas, p 2085.

FALSE   E. This is a feature which favours the diagnosis of acoustic neuroma but may occasionally occur in meningioma.
Ch. 94 Meningiomas, p 2085.

Q 9.9. *Enlargement of the Internal Auditory Meatus May Be Caused by*

    A. Meningioma

    B. Brain stem glioma

    C. Vertebrobasilar arterial ectasia

    D. Raised intracranial pressure

    E. Cholesteatoma

Q 9.10. *Concerning Intracranial Tumours*

    A. Contrast enhancement of cerebello-pontine angle epidermoids is an expected finding

    B. Virtually all imaging manifestations of chordomas can be mimicked by chondromas and chondroblastomas

    C. A glomus jugulare tumour is associated with a high signal within the ipsilateral internal jugular vein on T1W images

    D. Markedly homogeneous contrast enhancement is characteristic of a glomus jugulare tumour after GdDTPA administration

    E. Extracranial epidermoids tend to occur at the medial canthus of the eye in over 70% of cases

A 9.9. *Enlargement of the Internal Auditory Meatus May Be Caused by*

TRUE   A. Rarely.
Ch. 94 Acoustic Neuromas, p 2087.

TRUE   B.
Ch. 94 Acoustic Neuromas, p 2087.

TRUE   C. It is classically associated with pulsatile tinnitus.
Ch. 94 Acoustic Neuromas, p 2087.

TRUE   D. Raised intracranial pressure may cause bilateral enlargement.
Ch. 94 Acoustic Neuromas, p 2087.

TRUE   E. In the context of massive bony destruction in adults, or in congenital cholesteatoma (epidermoid tumour), erosion of the porus acousticus by a cerebello-pontine angle tumour may occur.
Ch. 94 Acoustic Neuromas, p 2087.

A 9.10. *Concerning Intracranial Tumours*

FALSE   A. They enhance poorly; dermoids behave similarly.
Ch. 94 Pearly Tumours, p 2089.

TRUE   B. Chordomas classically appear as dense, partly calcified masses with associated bone destruction arising in the midline at the clivus. None of these features is specific, and even histological differentiation from chondroid tumours may be difficult.
Ch. 94 Chordoma, p 2089.

TRUE   C. Ipsilateral jugular venous thrombosis, which causes high signal on T1W images, often occurs.
Ch. 94 Glomus Tumours, p 2089.

FALSE   D. Large vessels within the mass persist as flow voids even after enhancement.
Ch. 94 Glomus Tumours, p 2089.

FALSE   E. The lateral canthus is the more common site.
Ch. 94 Pearly Tumours, p 2088.

Q *9.11. Concerning the Neuroradiology of HIV Infection*

    A. Most asymptomatic HIV positive individuals have some abnormality on cranial MRI

    B. CNS tuberculosis indicates probable intravenous drug abuse

    C. Multiple high T2W signal white matter lesions combined with positive papova virus serology is diagnostic of progressive multifocal leukoencephalopathy (PML)

    D. Necrotizing ventriculitis is usually caused by cytomegalovirus

    E. Kaposi's sarcoma commonly metastasizes to the brain

Q *9.12. Regarding the Diagnosis of CNS Disease in HIV Positive Patients*

    A. Large, poorly-defined symmetrical white matter lesions that are isointense on T1W and hyperintense on T2W images are more likely to be due to HIV encephalopathy than to Progressive Multifocal Leukoencephalopathy (PML)

    B. Rim enhancement of a mass failing to regress on anti-toxoplasma therapy puts the diagnosis of toxoplasmosis in doubt

    C. Lymphoma presents as multifocal haemorrhagic lesions which often contain calcium

    D. A ring-enhancing lesion exhibiting subependymal spread is almost certainly lymphoma

    E. Cryptococcal meningitis causes prominent but non-specific meningeal enhancement

A 9.11. Concerning the Neuroradiology of HIV Infection

FALSE   A. Abnormalities in the asymptomatic patient are rarely encountered.
Ch. 95B Introduction, p 2119.

TRUE   B. Nearly all CNS TB and nocardia occurs in IV drug abusers.
Ch. 95B Introduction, p 2119.

FALSE   C. This is a demyelinating disease caused by reactivation of a latent viral infection of oligodendrocytes. The virus responsible is usually the JC papovavirus, but as half of the UK population has positive JC virus serology, this test is useless in diagnosing this condition.
Ch. 95B Progressive Multifocal Leukoencephalopathy, p 2124.

TRUE   D. Less commonly caused by herpes simplex.
Ch. 95B Herpes, p 2125.

FALSE   E. Metastatic CNS involvement by Kaposi's sarcoma is very rare.
Ch. 95B Kaposi's sarcoma, p 2126.

A 9.12. Regarding the Diagnosis of CNS Disease in HIV Positive Patients

TRUE   A. Large PML lesions are usually hypointense on T1W images. They are generally less symmetrically orientated.
Ch. 95B HIV Encephalopathy, p 2120.

FALSE   B. One third of confirmed toxoplasma abscesses show no imaging response on treatment.
Ch. 95B Cerebral Toxoplasmosis, p 2122.

FALSE   C. Although commonly multifocal, haemorrhage is unusual, and calcification does not occur.
Ch. 95B Primary Cerebral Lymphoma, p 2123.

TRUE   D. Ring enhancement is common in AIDS-related lymphoma and subependymal spread is not a feature of toxoplasmosis.
Ch. 95B Primary Cerebral Lymphoma, p 2123.

FALSE   E. There is little or no meningeal enhancement.
Ch. 95B Cryptococcosis, p 2123.

Q 9.13. *Regarding Plain Radiology of the Spine*

    A. During radiography of the cervical spine 30° caudal angulation of the beam is used to demonstrate the lateral masses

    B. The cervical foramina shown *en face* are contralateral to the side to which the head is rotated

    C. In the "swimmer's" view, the arm adjacent to the film remains down by the side

    D. In the presence of a thoracic scoliosis, a lateral thoracic spine radiograph should be taken with the concavity of the scoliosis adjacent to the film

    E. More than 70° of obliquity best demonstrates the lumbar neural exit foramina of the side towards which the body is rotated

Q 9.14. *Concerning MR Imaging of the Spine*

    A. A band of high signal in the centre of spinal cord on midsagittal images is caused by truncation artefact

    B. The FLAIR sequence is heavily T2 weighted and CSF appears as a signal void

    C. Dura mater is separated by fat from the bony walls of the spinal canal

    D. Dorsal root ganglia enhance strongly with IV gadolinium, unlike normal intradural roots

    E. The commonest conjoined roots are L5/S1

A 9.13. Regarding Plain Radiology of the Spine

TRUE A.
Ch. 97 Plain Radiography, p 2149.

TRUE B. The opposite is true of the lumbar spine.
Ch. 97 Plain Radiography, p 2149.

FALSE C. The arm adjacent to the film is elevated and stretched towards the head. The other arm is dropped to the patient's side.
Ch. 97 Thoracocervical Spine, p 2150.

FALSE D. If the convexity should be positioned adjacent to the film, the divergent beam is more parallel to the disc spaces. This also holds true for cervical or lumbar scoliosis.
Ch. 97 Thoracic Spine, p 2150.

FALSE E. Thirty to 40° of obliquity is required to achieve this.
Ch. 97 Lumbar Spine, p 2150.

A 9.14. Concerning MR Imaging of the Spine

TRUE A. Truncation artefact is responsible for high or low signal central bands projected over the middle of the cord in the sagittal plane.
Ch. 97 Motion Artefacts, p 2151.

TRUE B. All CSF signal is suppressed. All cysts and cystic lesions in the spinal cord are similarly suppressed. There is paradoxical null CSF signal despite the heavy T2 weighting.
Ch. 97 Advanced MRI of the spine, p 2153.

TRUE C. Especially in the thoracic region where the fat layer may be 5 mm thick posteriorly. It should not be confused with epidural lipomatosis.
Ch. 97 Ligaments and epidural soft tissues, p 2157.

TRUE D.
Ch. 97 Spinal Nerves, p 2157.

TRUE E. Conjoined roots simulate an elongated epidural mass at the site of the "missing" root level because the thecal sac shows a long smooth cavity. Careful analysis of the conjoined root and its upper and lower neighbour is essential.
Ch. 97 Normal Myelographic Anatomy, p 2159.

THE CENTRAL NERVOUS SYSTEM

Q *9.15. Regarding MRI of the Spine*

    A. Fast spin-echo (FSE) techniques improve contrast resolution

    B. The spinal cord oscillates anteroposteriorly with cardiac systole

    C. Truncation artefact causes high or low signal near the centre of the cord on mid-sagittal images

    D. Titanium causes a severe metallic artefact, particularly during gradient echo imaging

    E. Fluid attenuation inversion recovery (FLAIR) removes motion artefact from CSF

A *9.15. Regarding MRI of the Spine*

FALSE   A. FSE reduces data acquisition time and improves resolution by using several phase-encoding steps per excitation rather than just one. The disadvantages are an increased susceptibility to motion artefact and a slight reduction in contrast.

Ch. 97 Magnetic Resonance Imaging, p 2151.

TRUE   B. This is caused by expansion of the brain during systole, which causes downward descent of the brain stem and cord accompanied by anteroposterior oscillation. This motion causes a linear artefact that may mimic intramedullary pathology.

Ch. 97 Motion Artefacts, p 2151.

TRUE   C. Truncation artefact is generated at CSF-cord boundaries by image processing. It may cause difficulties in trying accurately to define the true CSF-cord boundary.

Ch. 97 Motion Artefacts, p 2152.

FALSE   D. Titanium is non-ferromagnetic and causes little interference to the MRI image. Gradient echo imaging greatly magnifies the metallic artefact from ferromagnetic materials.

Ch. 97 Motion Artefacts, p 2153.

TRUE   E. This sequence removes all signal from CSF on heavily T2W images. The disadvantages at present are the prolonged duration of data acquisition, low resolution and null signal from cysts and cystic lesions.

Ch. 97 Advanced MRI of the spine, p 2153.

Q 9.16. *Concerning Imaging of the Normal Spine*

    A. The spinal canal is widest at C7/T1

    B. The normal intervertebral foramen contains only nerve roots and fat

    C. Perineural cysts are most common and largest at S2

    D. Dorsal root ganglion on CT, MR or both, enhancement is an indirect sign of nerve root impingement

    E. Conjoined nerve roots occur most commonly at L5/S1

Q 9.17. *Regarding Myelography*

    A. A laminectomy defect provides an optimal portal for administering intrathecal contrast

    B. Congenital absence or defect in the posterior neural arches is a contraindication to lumbar myelographic puncture at that level

    C. Lateral cervical punctures at C1-C2 should be avoided in patients with spina bifida

    D. Epilepsy is a contraindication to myelography with water soluble media

    E. Adhesive arachnoiditis has not been observed using modern non-ionic water-soluble contrast media

A 9.16. Concerning Imaging of the Normal Spine

FALSE   A. Widest at C1.
Ch. 97 Normal Anatomy, p 2155.

FALSE   B. The foramina normally contain nerve roots, dorsal root ganglia, epidural fat and fascia, and radicular arteries and veins.
Ch. 97 The Intervertebral Foramina, p 2156.

TRUE   C. Perineural (Tarlov) cysts are common at all levels, but particularly so at S2.
Ch. 97 Spinal Nerves, p 2157.

FALSE   D. The normal dorsal root ganglion enhances avidly with contrast. Normal intradural roots barely enhance.
Ch. 97 Spinal Nerves, p 2157.

TRUE   E. Less commonly at L4/5 and rarely at other levels.
Ch. 97 Normal Myelographic Anatomy, p 2159.

A 9.17. Regarding Myelography

FALSE   A. It is best to avoid laminectomy sites, if at all possible. If feasible, puncture two disc spaces away—even if this is L1/2. The reasoning is that postoperative infection at a laminectomy site can be chronic and occult. Furthermore, postoperative adhesions can render a puncture excruciatingly painful and more difficult.
Ch. 97 Special Situations, p 2160.

TRUE   B. The spinal cord may be low or tethered posteriorly where such defects exist.
Ch. 97 Special Situations, p 2160.

TRUE   C. Owing to the frequently associated Chiari type 2 malformation.
Ch. 97 Special Situations, p 2160.

FALSE   D. Seizures previously presented problems when the older water-soluble contrast media were used. Modern water-soluble media are thought to be safe to use in patients with epilepsy.
Ch. 97 Complications of Myelography, p 2161.

TRUE   E.
Ch. 97 Complications of Myelography, p 2161.

Q *9.18. The Following Statements Apply to Chiari Malformations*

      A. All the features of a Chiari type 1 malformation may develop after birth

      B. Kinking of the medulla oblongata occurs in over 90% of cases of Chiari 1 malformation

      C. In Chiari type 2 malformation, a cervical myelomeningocele occurs in over 90-98% of cases

      D. Chiari type 2 malformation is associated with basilar invagination

      E. Imaging in the sagittal plane is the optimal MRI method of showing the extent of tonsillar descent

Q *9.19. Dural Ectasia is an Association of*

      A. Neurofibromatosis

      B. Marfan's syndrome

      C. Ankylosing spondylitis

      D. Gaucher's disease

      E. Ehlers-Danlos syndrome

A *9.18. The Following Statements Apply to Chiari Malformations*

TRUE A. The mechanism of this acquired deformity appears to be that the posterior fossa grows at a slower rate than the hindbrain.
Ch. 98 Chiari Malformations, p 2169.

FALSE B. This feature occurs in only 15% when elongation is so marked that a posterior kink occurs.
Ch. 98 Chiari Malformations, p 2169.

FALSE C. A meningomyelocoele is almost invariable in this condition. Its location, however, is in the *lumbar spine*.
Ch. 98 Chiari Malformations, p 2169.

FALSE D. There is no such association. Chiari type 1 (acquired cerebellar ectopia) may occur as a result of basilar invagination, Klippel-Feil deformity, occipitalization of the atlas and craniosynostosis.
Ch. 98 Chiari Malformations, p 2170.

FALSE E. The coronal plane is preferable because partial volume effects from the laterally placed biventral lobules may lead to overdiagnosis of tonsillar descent in the sagittal plane.
Ch. 98 Chiari Malformations, p 2170.

A *9.19. Dural Ectasia is an Association of*

TRUE A.
Ch. 98 Meningoceles, p 2170.

TRUE B. This causes posterior vertebral scalloping and widening of the interpedicular distance. Focal ectasia may be seen as presacral and lateral sacral meningoceles.
Ch. 98 Meningoceles, p 2170.

TRUE C. Pocket-like, CSF-filled spaces invaginate the posterior elements of the lumbar spine in this condition. The vertebral bodies may also be affected. Cauda equina syndrome is a potential complication.
Ch. 98 Meningoceles, p 2170.

FALSE D. Multiple vertebral compression fractures and end-plate infractions occur in this condition. Dural ectasia is not a feature.
Ch. 98 Meningoceles, p 2170.

TRUE E.
Ch. 98 Meningoceles, p 2170.

Q *9.20. Regarding the Radiology of Syringomyelia*

A. At least 90% of cases are associated with cerebellar ectopia

B. Focal accumulation of contrast medium within the spinal cord after intra-thecal injection is a pathognomonic finding

C. A flow void is demonstrated on T2W images

D. The size of the syrinx bears a close relationship to the clinical severity of the condition

E. The cervical spinal cord is of normal size or small in more than 60% of patients

Q *9.21. Concerning Degenerative Disease of the Spine*

A. Most acute disc herniations extend or herniate through the posterior longitudinal ligament

B. An increased vertebral signal on T1W and isointensity on T2W images indicates fatty replacement of red marrow

C. An increased MR signal in an intervertebral disc on T1W images may be seen in degenerative disease

D. In postoperative MRI, recurrent or residual disc material is distinguished reliably from epidural fibrosis by the lack of gadolinium enhancement in the former

E. A mid-sagittal cervical canal diameter of less than 20 mm on the plain film indicates that cord compression is probably present

A 9.20. *Regarding the Radiology of Syringomyelia*

FALSE   A. At most 70%. In these cases, the cerebellar tonsils lie at the C1 or C2 level. It is postulated that they cause intermittent obstruction of the outlet foramina of the fourth ventricle. The increased CSF pressure is then transmitted downwards through a communication between the fourth ventricle and the central canal. This is referred to as primary syringohydromyelia.
Ch. 98 Syringomyelia, p 2173.

FALSE   B. Late filling of spinal cord cavities occurs due to diffusion and is seen in a variety of other conditions (e.g., post-myelitic cord necrosis).
Ch. 98 Syringomyelia, p 2174.

TRUE   C. When the syrinx is pulsatile, this is the case.
Ch. 98 Syringomyelia, p 2173.

FALSE   D. Clinical symptoms are loss of pain and temperature sensation. Muscular weakness and pyramidal tract involvement do not parallel the size of the cavity, the distention of the cord or the amount of cord thinning. Furthermore, clinical outcome and further extension of the cavity are not related to successful operative decompression/collapse of the existing cavity.
Ch. 98 Syringomyelia, p 2173.

FALSE   E. This is the case in 20% of patients
Ch. 98 Syringomyelia, p 2173.

A 9.21. *Concerning Degenerative Disease of the Spine*

FALSE   A. Only 10% extend through this ligament or its lateral membrane. This is because the posterior longitudinal ligament is tightly adherent to the posterior margins of the disc.
Ch. 98 Degenerative Spinal Disease, p 2175.

TRUE   B.
Ch. 98 Degenerative Spinal Disease, p 2175.

TRUE   C. This paradoxical feature is occasionally seen and may represent calcium precipitation. Usually, however, the signal from degenerate discs is lower than from healthy discs.
Ch. 98 MRI, p 2179.

TRUE   D. Such enhancement generally persists to a greater or lesser degree for years.
Ch. 98 The Postoperative Spine, p 2181.

FALSE   E. A cervical sagittal diameter of less than 10 mm indicates the likelihood of cord compression.
Ch. 98 Plain Radiographs, p 2179.

Q 9.22. *Concerning the Extradural Space*

A. The most common extradural tumour of the spine is a metastasis

B. Fifty to 60% of the bone mass of a vertebral body needs to be destroyed before it becomes visible on plain radiography

C. Displacement of the spinal cord substance away from the margin of the thecal sac is the characteristic appearance of an extradural obstruction

D. A densely calcified mass within the spinal canal is likely to be extradural

E. Spinal meningiomas seldom cause conspicuous hyperostosis of adjacent bone

Q 9.23. *Concerning Meningioma Within the Spinal Canal*

A. An associated extradural component occurs more commonly with meningiomas than with neurinomas

B. Calcification within an intraspinal tumour is diagnostic of meningioma

C. The thecal sac is expanded and the cord is displaced away from the tumour

D. A conspicuously increased signal on T2W images favours neurinoma over meningioma

E. Diffuse enlargement of spinal nerve roots occurs in neurofibromatosis

A *9.22. Concerning the Extradural Space*

TRUE   A. Vertebral body and neural arch involvement are usually associated.
Ch. 98 Extradural Tumours, p 2182.

TRUE   B. In particular, the sacrum is a site where extensive lysis is necessary before abnormal lucency of bone can be detected reliably on plain radiography.
Ch. 98 Extradural Tumours, p 2183.

FALSE   C. Extradural obstruction displaces the *dura* away from the bony walls of the spinal canal.
Ch. 98 Extradural Tumours, p 2184.

TRUE   D. Heavy calcification is rare in neurofibromas and meningiomas and usually represents calcified extruded disc material.
Ch. 98 Intradural Extramedullary Tumours, p 2185.

TRUE   E.
Ch. 98 Intradural Extramedullary Tumours, p 2185.

A *9.23. Concerning Meningioma Within the Spinal Canal*

FALSE   A. A significant extradural component is more common with neurinomas (30%) than with meningiomas (7%).
Ch. 98 Intradural Extramedullary Tumours, p 2185.

FALSE   B. Eighty percent of spinal meningiomas are thoracic and occur in women over 40 years of age. These tumours may calcify but not as often as their intracranial counterparts. Neurinomas also exhibit tumoral calcification, and calcification is therefore not a good discriminating feature.
Ch. 98 Intradural Extramedullary Tumours, p 2185.

TRUE   C. These are the hallmarks of an intradural extramedullary tumour on MRI, myelography and CT myelography.
Ch. 98 Intradural Extramedullary Tumours, p 2186.

TRUE   D. Both are often isointense compared to spinal cord substance on T1W images.
Ch. 98 MRI Intradural Extramedullary Tumours, p 2185.

TRUE   E. This occurs also in hereditary sensorimotor neuropathies.
Ch. 98 Intradural Extramedullary Tumours, p 2185.

Q 9.24. *Regarding Intramedullary Pathology*

A. Gliomas are commonly associated with syrinx (spinal cord cavity) formation

B. Expansion of the spinal canal on a plain film is most likely to be detected in the lumbosacral spine

C. Astrocytoma and ependymoma can be reliably distinguished on MRI

D. The great majority of spinal cord gliomas enhance at least partially on MRI following IV contrast medium, unlike similar tumours in the brain

E. Enlarged vessels visible on the surface of the spinal cord are pathognomonic and are seen only in haemangioblastoma

Q 9.25. *Regarding the Imaging of Spinal Pathology*

A. Atlanto-axial subluxation in patients with rheumatoid arthritis causes a clinical compressive myelopathy in about 70% of cases

B. Intraspinal extension from disco-vertebral osteomyelitis occurs more commonly in TB than in infections due to *Salmonella* or *Staph. aureus*

C. Arachnoiditis caused by myelography with Myodil (iophendylate oil) is always most severe at the lower end of the spinal canal

D. 70% of patients with spinal plaques of demyelination have no intracranial involvement

E. CT contrast enhancement of a focus of myelitis persisting for many months suggests that multiple sclerosis is not the cause

A 9.24. *Regarding Intramedullary Pathology*

TRUE

A. Syringomyelia occurs in association with almost 50% of spinal cord tumours including metastases.
Ch. 98 Intramedullary Tumours, p 2186.

TRUE

B. The most frequent cause of spinal canal expansion by tumour is the giant myxopapillary ependymoma of the cauda equina, which occurs in childhood.
Ch. 98 Intramedullary Tumours, p 2187.

FALSE

C. Not only are these two tumours difficult to distinguish, but other processes (including inflammatory) may cause diagnostic confusion.
Ch. 98 Intramedullary Tumours, p 2187.

TRUE

D. MRI contrast enhancement allows for greater discrimination of tumour extent and is particularly valuable in the diagnosis of haemangioblastomas and metastases.
Ch. 98 Intramedullary Tumours, p 2187.

FALSE

E. This feature occurs in 80% of haemangioblastomas but also in 10% of ependymomas and in many arterio-venous malformations of the cord.
Ch. 98 Intramedullary Tumours, p 2187.

A 9.25. *Regarding the Imaging of Spinal Pathology*

FALSE

A. A clinical myelopathy develops in only 2-6% of patients with atlantoaxial subluxation. The subluxation is often vertical or subaxial and in 30% of cases is not reducible.
Ch. 98 Inflammatory Diseases, p 2189.

TRUE

B. Intraspinal extension occurs in less than 1% of pyogenic disco-vertebral infections. It occurs in up to 40% of infections with non-pyogenic organisms, the commonest of which is TB.
Ch. 98 Vertebral Osteomyelitis, p 2190.

TRUE

C.
Ch. 98 Spinal Meningitis (Arachnoiditis), p 2191.

FALSE

D. Seventy percent of patients *do* have coexisting brain involvement.
Ch. 98 Myelitis, p 2191.

TRUE

E. Enhancement of individual lesions in Multiple Sclerosis does not persist for long. An alternative diagnosis (e.g., sarcoidosis) should be considered.
Ch. 98 Myelitis, p 2192.

Q *9.26. Consider the Following Statements Regarding Spinal Disorders*

A. Pagetic involvement of a vertebra causes it to be enlarged in over 80% of cases

B. Pseudogout affects the spine more commonly than gout

C. Spinal arteriovenous malformations are often simple fistulae which shunt into a single draining vein

D. Spinal arteriovenous malformations are usually high-flow lesions

E. The MRI findings in Acute Disseminated Encephalomyelitis affecting the cord often resolve completely

Q *9.27. Regarding Ultrasound of the Infant Brain*

A. Transcranial scanning through the temporal bone detects contralateral subdural haematoma

B. The internal carotid bifurcation is regularly seen on coronal section through the anterior fontanelle

C. An isolated hyperreflective focus anterior to the caudothalamic groove at 31 weeks is an indicator of severe intracranial haemorrhage and poor prognosis

D. Decreased reflectivity in periventricular white matter is suggestive of early leukomalacia

E. A wedge-shaped area of hyperreflective cortex indicates recent infarction

A 9.26. *Consider the Following Statements Regarding Spinal Disorders*

FALSE   A. The vertebral body is enlarged in only about 20% of cases.
Ch. 98 Paget's Disease, p 2194.

TRUE   B. The lumbar intervertebral discs are particularly likely to be involved by calcium pyrophosphate dihydrate crystal deposition. Gout rarely affects the spine.
Ch. 98 Crystal Deposition Disease, p 2194.

TRUE   C.
Ch. 98 Spinal Arteriovenous Malformations, p 2192.

FALSE   D. Symptomatic lesions have very slow anomalous venous drainage. Venous stagnation is a very important part of the clinical myelopathy, which may result in venous infarction of the cord.
Ch. 98 Spinal Arteriovenous Malformations, p 2192.

TRUE   E. A characteristic finding in this autoimmune postencephalitic state is that existing lesions tend to regress and no new lesions appear over time, unlike Multiple Sclerosis.
Ch. 98 Myelitis, p 2192.

A 9.27. *Regarding Ultrasound of the Infant Brain*

TRUE   A. A low frequency (3.5 MHz) transducer provides good definition of the opposite hemisphere and brain surface.
Ch. 100 Technique, p 2212.

TRUE   B.
Ch. 100 Normal Anatomy, p 2213.

FALSE   C. This is the description of a grade 1 germinal matrix haemorrhage that is associated with little or no longterm morbidity.
Ch. 100 Intracranial Haemorrhage, p 2216.

FALSE   D. Leukomalacia initially appears as heterogeneous periventricular white matter hyperreflectivity. This may subsequently break down into hyporeflective cystic cavities which coalesce with the adjacent ventricle.
Ch. 100 Hypoxic Ischaemic Encephalopathy, p 2217.

TRUE   E. Arterial infarction typically has this appearance early on, conforming to a vascular territory, most commonly the middle cerebral artery in the term infant.
Ch. 100 Hypoxic Ischaemic Encephalopathy, p 2217.

Q 9.28. *In Non-Accidental Injury of the Infant Brain (NAI)*

    A. Subdural haematomas are most often bilateral

    B. Ultrasound is very sensitive at detecting shear injuries

    C. CT scanning is mandatory in suspected acute brain injury

    D. Hydranencephaly is a potential sequal of NAI

    E. Thalamic infarction is characteristic of NAI

Q 9.29. *Ultrasound Features Suspicious of Congenital Brain Anomalies Include*

    A. Radiating sulci above the third ventricle

    B. Nonvisualization of the cingulate gyri

          hyporeflective midline structure between the ventri-

               the post-trigonal white matter

                 choroid plexus in the lateral

A 9.28. *In Non-Accidental Injury of the Infant Brain (NAI)*

TRUE   *A.* Subdural haematomas are bilateral in 75% of cases. Typical locations are the posterior interhemispheric and parieto-occipital areas. Only 10% are infratentorial.
Ch. 100 Trauma, p 2219.

TRUE   *B.* These devastating injuries appear at the cortico-medullary junction as slit-like cavities parallel or perpendicular to brain surface. They also occur within the corpus callosum and brain stem.
Ch. 100 Trauma, p 2219.

TRUE   *C.* CT is more sensitive than US or MRI in acute haemorrhage.
Ch. 100 Trauma, p 2220.

FALSE   *D.* This occurs owing to bilateral internal carotid artery occlusion *early in gestation*, causing loss of the cerebral mantle with preservation of posterior fossa structures.
Ch. 100 Hypoxic Ischaemic Encephalopathy, p 2217.

FALSE   *E.* This is the classical consequence of *birth hypoxia*. The infarcted thalami appear hyperreflective on US.
Ch. 100 Hypoxic Ischaemic Encephalopathy, p 2217.

A 9.29. *Ultrasound Features Suspicious of Congenital Brain Anomalies Include*

TRUE   *A.* This is a feature of callosal dysgenesis, which in turn may be accompanied by other features of the Chiari II malformation.
Ch. 100 Pathology, Congenital, p 2220.

TRUE   *B.* These parallel gyri are normally visible. They are absent in the Chiari II malformation.
Ch. 100 Pathology, Congenital, p 2220.

TRUE   *C.* This describes an interhemispheric cyst. Cavum septum pellucidum and cavum septum vergae (normal variants) also appear as fluid-filled structures between the lateral ventricles, but their shape is angular.
Ch. 100 Pathology, Congenital, p 2220.

FALSE   *D.* This is a normal appearance of the corona radiata in this location.
Ch. 100 Normal Anatomy, p 2212.

FALSE   *E.* This is a normal finding.
Ch. 100 Normal Anatomy, p 2213

Q *9.30. Structures Hyperreflective on Transcranial Ultrasound of the Infant Brain*

    A. Corpus callosum

    B. Choroid plexus

    C. Brain surface

    D. Third ventricle

    E. Cerebellar hemispheres

Q *9.31. Regarding Intracranial Infection*

    A. Most brain abscesses are streptococcal

    B. Cerebral abscesses are more likely to contain central high density before contrast enhancement than brain tumours

    C. Intracranial empyema occurs more commonly in the subdural space than in the extradural space

    D. Tuberculous meningitis causes basal ganglial infarction in children

    E. Calcification in a cerebral cyst suggests a diagnosis of hydatid disease

A 9.30. *Structures Hyperreflective on Transcranial Ultrasound of the Infant Brain*

FALSE   *A.* The corpus callosum is normally echo-poor.
Ch 100. Normal Anatomy, p 2213.

TRUE   *B.*
Ch. 100 Normal Anatomy, p 2212.

TRUE   *C.*
Ch. 100 Normal Anatomy, p 2212.

TRUE   *D.* This often appears as a hyperreflective slit.
Ch. 100 Normal Anatomy, p 2213.

FALSE   *E.* The vermis is hyperreflective whereas the hemispheres are normally echo-poor.
Ch. 100 Normal Anatomy, p 2213.

A 9.31. *Regarding Intracranial Infection*

TRUE   *A.* They are the result of local disease (e.g., direct extension from paranasal sinus or mastoid disease) in about half of cases. In the remainder, haematogenous spread is the mode of entry.
Ch. 95A Brain Abscess, p 2095.

FALSE   *B.* The reverse is the case: central high density pre-contrast enhancement makes tumour more likely.
Ch. 95A Brain Abscess, p 2095.

TRUE   *C.* Empyema is more often subdural, appearing as a crescentic collection over a cerebral hemisphere, widening of the interhemispheric fissure or in relation to the tentorium.
Ch. 95A Intracranial Empyema, p 2097.

TRUE   *D.* This occurs because a chronic granulomatous reaction in the basal cisterns tracks along the major arteries with a consequent arteritis.
Ch. 95A Tuberculosis, p 2097.

FALSE   *E.* Hydatid cysts appear as round water density lesions, usually without oedema or contrast enhancement. They virtually never calcify.
Ch 95A Parasite Infestations, p. 2099

Q *9.32. Regarding Degenerative Disorders of the Central Nervous System*

A. Huntington's chorea causes focal atrophy predominantly affecting the corpus callosum

B. High density lesions seen on CT in the brain stem and basal ganglia suggest a diagnosis of Wilson's disease

C. Cerebellar atrophy is a recognized finding in patients with chronic epilepsy

D. Generalized cerebral atrophy is a manifestation of HIV infection

E. In progressive supranuclear palsy, the midbrain and superior colliculi are shrunken

Q *9.33. Regarding Demyelinating Disorders*

A. Ovoid plaques perpendicular to the lateral ventricular surfaces are suggestive of multiple sclerosis

B. Congenital leukodystrophies cause reduced water content of the cerebral white matter leading to areas of increased density on CT

C. Marked mass effect is not seen in relation to the plaques of multiple sclerosis

D. Almost complete failure of myelination is a feature of Pelizaeus-Merzbacher's disease

E. Diffuse white matter hyperintensity on T2W images is seen in the mucopolysaccharidoses

A 9.32. *Regarding Degenerative Disorders of the Central Nervous System*

FALSE
A. Atrophy mainly affects the heads of the caudate nuclei, causing the frontal horns of the lateral ventricles to have a "rounded-off" appearance.
Ch. 95A Degenerative Disorders, p 2100.

FALSE
B. Wilson's disease (hepaticolenticular degeneration) does not cause hyperdense basal ganglia—the white matter degeneration is seen as low density lesions on CT.
Ch. 95A Degenerative Disorders, p. 2100.

TRUE
C. Along with calvarial thickening, it is a recognized side effect of chronic phenytoin ingestion.
Ch. 95A Degenerative Disorders, p. 2100.

TRUE
D. Normal appearances and generalized atrophy are more common than focal lesions in symptomatic patients.
Ch. 95A Acquired Immune Deficiency Syndrome, p. 2099.

TRUE
E.
Ch. 95A Degenerative Disorders, p. 2100.

A 9.33. *Regarding Demyelinating Disorders*

TRUE
A. These are known as Dawson's fingers, which together with involvement of the septal surface of the corpus callosum and lesions of the cerebellum and brain stem strongly suggest this diagnosis.
Ch. 95A Multiple Sclerosis, p. 2102.

FALSE
B. Demyelination causes an increase in water content that is seen as reduced density on CT and increased signal on T2W images with MRI.
Ch. 95A Demyelinating Disorders, p. 2101.

FALSE
C. Occasionally marked mass effect is seen along with contrast enhancement. This can simulate intracerebral neoplasia.
Ch. 95A Multiple Sclerosis, p. 2101.

TRUE
D. This is an X-linked recessive disorder that causes early psychomotor developmental arrest in children. Residual white matter hyperintensity is prominent on T2W MR images.
Ch. 95A Demyelinating Disorders, p. 2101.

TRUE
E. Many metabolic diseases produce changes of demyelination. These include the mucopolysaccharidoses, gangliosidoses, and leukodystrophies.
Ch. 95A Demyelinating Disorders, p. 2101.

Q 9.34. *Concerning Subarachnoid Haemorrhage*

    A. The prognosis is better when no underlying cause can be found

    B. MRI, where available, is the diagnostic test of choice for acute subarachnoid haemorrhage

    C. High signal in the subarachnoid space is seen on MRI after blood is no longer detectable as increased density on CT

    D. Ischaemic infarction occurs as a result of subarachnoid haemorrhage

    E. A concentric "onion-skin" appearance of high and low signal on MRI is virtually pathognomonic of an aneurysm.

A 9.34. *Concerning Subarachnoid Haemorrhage*

TRUE A. About 75% are caused by berry aneurysms at the circle of Willis. Most of the remainder are caused by arteriovenous malformations. In 10–15% of cases no cause is found; in these, the long-term prognosis is generally better.
Ch. 95A Subarachnoid Haemorrhage, p. 2102.

FALSE B. Currently, CT is the radiological investigation of choice. Recently the FLAIR (fast low-angle inversion recovery) sequence has been reported as having a 100% sensitivity for the detection of acute subarachnoid blood. This is because the protein content of blood shortens its T1 value, rendering it bright on this sequence.
Ch. 95A Subarachnoid Haemorrhage, p. 2102.

TRUE C. On T1W images, high signal, due to the presence of methemoglobin, may persist even when the blood is no longer visible on CT.
Ch. 95A Subarachnoid Haemorrhage, p. 2103.

TRUE D. This is due to intense vasospasm and is responsible for much of the morbidity of sub-arachnoid haemorrhage. Reversible ischemia may appear as an area of low density on CT or of increased signal on T2W images, often with mild mass effect. Subsequently, this can resolve completely.
Ch. 95A Subarachnoid Haemorrhage, p. 2103.

TRUE E. Central flow void appears as an area of low intensity. This is surrounded by the high signal of methemoglobin. An outer layer of dark signal is caused by hemosiderin.
Ch. 95A Subarachnoid Haemorrhage, p. 2104.

Q *9.35. Concerning Cerebral Angiography*

    A. Angiography is the diagnostic study of choice in traumatic aneurysms

    B. Multiple intracerebral aneurysms are demonstrated on angiography in about 20% of cases

    C. Aneurysms arising from the internal carotid artery within the cavernous sinus usually present as massive subarachnoid haemorrhage

    D. The combination of subdural and intra-axial haemorrhage is suggestive of an intra-axial arteriovenous fistula or malformation

    E. An ulcerated plaque is a more accurate predictor of stroke than a high-grade stenosis

A 9.35. *Concerning Cerebral Angiography*

TRUE A. This is because they are usually overlooked on CT—obscured by concomitant haemorrhage. A signal void may be seen on MRI, but angiography is the diagnostic study of choice.
Ch. 95A Subarachnoid Haemorrhage, p. 2104.

TRUE B. The largest or most irregular aneurysm is usually found to be responsible for the haemorrhage. A focal haematoma or localized arterial spasm also points to the offending lesion.
Ch. 95A Subarachnoid Haemorrhage, p. 2104.

FALSE C. They do not cause subarachnoid haemorrhage. Enlargement causes compression of the 3rd and 6th cranial nerves within the cavernous sinus. Percutaneous transcatheter embolization with balloons and coils is often successful treatment.
Ch. 95A The Angiography of Subarachnoid Haemorrhage and Intracranial Aneurysms, p. 2105.

FALSE D. This combination suggests the presence of an extra-axial dural arteriovenous fistula or malformation. These are often caused by a pathological connection between meningeal artery and vein near the lateral, superior sagittal or cavernous sinuses. They may cause subarachnoid haemorrhage.
Ch. 95A Angiography, p 2106.

FALSE E. Multicentre trials have shown that the surface morphology of a plaque is not associated with an increased risk of stroke.
Ch. 95A Imaging of the Cerebral Vessels, p. 2113.

Q *9.36. Regarding Cerebral Malformation and Abnormal Development*

A. If only part of the corpus callosum is missing, it is usually the posterior part

B. The commonest cause of obstructive hydrocephalus in young children is aqueduct stenosis

C. The fundamental anomaly in Dandy-Walker syndrome is hypoplasia of the cerebellar vermis and hemispheres

D. Premature fusion of the sutures occurs most commonly as a result of an underlying metabolic defect or bone dysplasia

E. Basilar invagination is usually developmental rather than caused by a bone softening condition

Q *9.37. Concerning Trauma to the Brain and Skull*

A. Skull fractures do not branch

B. "Growing fractures" (leptomeningeal cysts) usually present with headache

C. A biconvex collection of CSF density may indicate a chronic subdural collection

D. In traumatic CSF fistulae, identification of the point of external leakage is the best guide to the site of the fistula

E. Following head injury, a low density rim surrounding an acute intracerebral haematoma indicates clot retraction

A 9.36. *Regarding Cerebral Malformation and Abnormal Development*

TRUE

A. This is associated with enlargement of the posterior horns of the lateral ventricles.
Ch. 96 Corpus Callosum Defects, p. 2128.

TRUE

B. This condition may present in adulthood. Enlargement of the lateral and third ventricles in the presence of a normal fourth ventricle suggests the diagnosis.
Ch. 96 Aqueduct Stenosis, p. 2130.

TRUE

C. This is associated with enormous dilation of the fourth ventricle because of atresia of the outlet foramina.
Ch. 96 The Dandy-Walker Syndrome, p. 2130.

FALSE

D. The commonest cause is idiopathic (i.e., no underlying pathological process).
Ch. 96 Abnormalities of the Cranial Sutures, p. 2132.

TRUE

E. In this condition the margins of the foramen magnum are inverted. It may complicate rickets or Paget's disease but is usually developmental.
Ch. 96 Abnormalities of the Skull Base and Foramen Magnum, p. 2132.

A 9.37. *Concerning Trauma to the Brain and Skull*

FALSE

A. They are characteristically linear but sometimes branch and must be differentiated from vascular markings. Fractures are more radiolucent than vascular markings, are usually straighter and do not have corticated margins.
Ch. 96 Fractures of the Skull, p. 2135.

FALSE

B. The enlarging poorly defined bone defect occurs as a result of exposure of bone to CSF pulsation owing to a traumatic dural tear. It usually presents as a large extracranial soft tissue mass which contains herniated brain.
Ch 96 Fractures of the Skull, p. 2136.

TRUE

C. A biconvex shape does not, therefore, necessarily imply an extradural collection.
Ch 96 Extradural and Subdural Haematomas, p. 2138.

FALSE

D. CSF may fistulate into the ear and track via the eustachian tube so that it exits from the nose.
Ch 96 The Late Effects of Head Injury: Fistulae, p. 2140.

TRUE

E.
Ch 96 Other Findings in Acute Trauma, p. 2140, Fig. 96.24.

Q *9.38. Regarding Pathology of the Cranial Vault*

    A. The sclerotic form of fibrous dysplasia is commoner than the cystic type

    B. In Paget's disease, the inner table is most affected

    C. Loss of the outer table and diploe occurs in thinning of the parietal bones

    D. Patients in whom incidental basal ganglial calcification is discovered require biochemical investigation

    E. Haemangioma of the skull vault presents as a palpable lump or area of tenderness

Q *9.39. The Following Features Favour a Diagnosis of Communicating Hydrocephalus Over Atrophy*

    A. Enlarged cerebral sulci

    B. A callosal angle of less than 120 degrees

    C. Diffuse periventricular low attenuation on CT

    D. Plateau waves on intracranial pressure monitoring

    E. Commensurate enlargement of temporal horns with the remainder of the lateral ventricles

A 9.38. *Regarding Pathology of the Cranial Vault*

TRUE   A. Dense expanded dysplasia is the commonest appearance. This most often involves the skull base and/or facial bones. The less common cystic type usually produces a small "blistered" lesion of the skull vault.
Ch. 96 Fibrous Dysplasia, p. 2142.

FALSE   B. The outer and middle tables are most affected by sclerosis and expansion.
Ch. 96 Paget's Disease, p. 2143.

TRUE   C. Sharply demarcated marked thinning of the outer table and diploe occurs in this uncommon condition of unknown aetiology.
Ch. 96 Thinning of the Parietal Bones, p. 2144.

FALSE   D. Calcification of the basal ganglia is a frequent finding in normal older people. Disturbances of calcium metabolism are so rarely causative that biochemical testing is performed only if there is another indication.
Ch. 96 Calcification of the Basal Ganglia, p. 2145.

TRUE   E. There may be prominent vascularity seen on external carotid angiography adjacent to this benign tumour. It is indolent and treatment is not usually required.
Ch. 96 Tumours of the Skull, p. 2143.

A 9.39. *The Following Features Favour a Diagnosis of Communicating Hydrocephalus Over Atrophy*

FALSE   A. Enlarged sulci are features of atrophy. The sulci are often less prominent than normal in communicating hydrocephalus.
Ch. 96 Table 96.1, p. 2147.

TRUE   B. This may be accompanied by rounding of the frontal horns of the lateral ventricles.
Ch. 96 Table 96.1, p. 2147.

TRUE   C. This occurs owing to transependymal flow of CSF.
Ch. 96 Table 96.1, p. 2147.

TRUE   D. These do not occur in cerebral atrophy.
Ch. 96 Table 96.1, p. 2147.

TRUE   E. This is one of the more reliable discriminating signs.
Ch. 96 Table 96.1, p. 2147.

Q 9.40. Concerning Functional Imaging of the Brain

A. PET (positron emission tomography) results in better image quality for much less radiation exposure than SPECT (single photon emission computed tomography)

B. During cerebral activity, there is a regional increase in blood flow with a decrease in local oxygen concentration

C. Glucose and oxygen consumption in the brain is normal in Parkinson's disease

D. In Friedreich's ataxia, ambulant patients have a generalized increase in glucose metabolism as shown by PET

E. Using 18-fluorodeoxyglucose PET scanning, increased metabolism of glucose is demonstrated in oligodendrogliomas

A *9.40. Concerning Functional Imaging of the Brain*

TRUE   A. This is because a pair of gamma photons is released in opposite directions when a positron is annihilated. This allows for precise calibration of activity, and precise electronic delineation of the field of view. SPECT observes only a single gamma ray and requires heavy collimation to get sufficient spatial resolution. This results in decreased sensitivity.
Ch. 99 PET and SPECT, p. 2197.

FALSE   B. Local blood flow increases but there is no decrease in oxygen concentration. In fact, the reverse is true—there is an increase in local venous oxygen concentration. This increase causes an increase in signal of activated areas of the brain on T2W images.
Ch. 99 Blood Oxygenation Level Dependent (BOLD) Contrast, p. 2197.

TRUE   C. Idiopathic Parkinson's disease has been investigated with (^{18}F)DOPA. In Parkinson's disease uptake of this compound is reduced in the basal ganglia with relative sparing of the caudate nucleus.
Ch. 99 Parkinson's Disease, p. 2202.

TRUE   D. This increase is evident throughout the cortex, basal ganglia, and cerebellum. In chairbound patients, activity decreases to normal levels in all areas apart from the caudate and lentiform nuclei.
Ch. 99 Friedreich's Ataxia and Other Cerebellar Degenerative Syndromes, p. 2203.

FALSE   E. This tumour, and other low-grade cerebral tumours, show hypometabolism. Conversely, high-grade tumours show large increases in glucose metabolism.
Ch. 99 Staging, p. 2206.

10

The Orbit: Ear, Nose & Throat, Face, Teeth

Q *10.1. Concerning the Anatomy of the Orbit*

    A. The lateral wall is the strongest of the orbital walls

    B. The 2nd cranial nerve and ophthalmic artery pass through the superior orbital fissure

    C. The four rectus muscles are inserted into the greater wing of sphenoid

    D. On coronal CT, or MRI, the superior rectus muscle is demonstrated as muscle mass immediately inferior to the levator palpebrae superioris

    E. The largest orbital muscle is the inferior rectus

Q *10.2. Regarding Ultrasound of the Orbit*

    A. The scan is performed through the closed lid

    B. The optimal frequency for examination of the orbit is 7.5-8 MHz.

    C. Ultrasound is the imaging method of choice for demonstrating the degree of retinal detachment

    D. "Blow-out" fractures are readily detected

    E. Muscles enlarged by Graves' Disease are hyperreflective

A *10.1. Concerning the Anatomy of the Orbit*

TRUE   A. The medial wall is papyraceous and the floor of the orbit is also thin and prone to fracture. The lateral wall, formed by the greater wing of sphenoid and the malar bone, is the most resistant to fracture.
Ch. 101 Anatomy, p 2227.

FALSE   B. These structures pass through the *optic canal*, which lies between the two roots of the lesser wing of sphenoid. The superior orbital fissure transmits the 3rd, 4th and 6th nerves and an arterial connection between the middle meningeal and ophthalmic arteries.
Ch. 101 Anatomy, p 2227.

FALSE   C. They arise from the inferior root of the lesser wing of the sphenoid.
Ch. 101 The Orbital Contents, p 2228.

TRUE   D.
Ch. 101 The Orbital Contents, p 2228.

TRUE   E. This can be seen to be the case on coronal imaging of the orbit.
Ch. 101 Fig. 101.1, p 2228.

A *10.2. Regarding Ultrasound of the Orbit*

TRUE   A. Local anaesthetic drops are applied to the eye prior to the examination, which may proceed with the probe directly on the conjunctiva or coupled to the closed eyelid with methyl cellulose gel.
Ch. 101 Ultrasound, p 2229.

TRUE   B. This frequency allows structures at the back of the orbit to be interrogated. The globe itself is best imaged with a 10 MHz probe.
Ch. 101 Ultrasound, p 2229.

TRUE   C. The sensitivity of ultrasound in this regard exceeds CT or MRI.
Ch. 101 Retinal Lesions, p 2232.

FALSE   D. The role of ultrasound in suspected blow-out fracture is to assess associated globe lesions, in particular lens subluxation, intraocular haemorrhage and retinal detachment.
Ch. 101 Fractures of the Orbit, p 2235.

TRUE   E. The early deposition of protein and polysaccharides is followed by collagen deposition and ultimately fibrosis.
Ch. 101 Graves' Orbitopathy, p 2237.

Q 10.3. Regarding Retinoblastoma

A. Involvement of the choroid precipitates metastases to bones, lung, liver and brain

B. Calcification in a cystic orbital mass makes hydatid disease the likely diagnosis

C. Eighty-five percent of cases occur before three years of age

D. Retinal detachment after subretinal spread occurs in more than 80% of cases

E. Optic nerve enlargement is not a feature

A 10.3. *Regarding Retinoblastoma*

TRUE   A. The highly vascular choroid allows for the rapid dissemination of tumour and prominent choroidal involvement signals a poor prognosis.
Ch. 101 Ocular Tumours, p 2232.

FALSE   B. Calcification occurs in the majority of retinoblastoma cases. The differential diagnosis of retinoblastoma includes retrolental fibroplasia, Coats' disease and persistent hyperplastic primary vitreous, but calcification is not a feature of the two latter disorders. Hydatid disease may calcify but is usually retrobulbar.
Ch. 101 Ocular Tumours, p 2232.

TRUE   C. The mean age of presentation is 18 months and almost all occur by 5 years of age.
Ch. 101 Ocular Tumours, p 2232.

FALSE   D. The posterolateral wall of the globe is the aspect most frequently affected by retinoblastoma and a retrolental mass is the most common appearance. Subretinal spread and retinal detachment occur only in 25% of cases.
Ch. 101 Ocular Tumours, p 2232.

FALSE   E. Retinoblastoma spreads by direct extension into the optic nerve and orbit.
Ch. 101 Ocular Tumours, p 2232.

Q 10.4. The Following are Associated

A. Microphthalmia and congenital rubella

B. Absence of the iris and nephroblastoma

C. Congenital cataract and Down's syndrome

D. Congenital glaucoma and neurofibromatosis

E. Von Hippel–Lindau disease and retinal angiomas

A 10.4. The Following are Associated

TRUE   A. Growth retardation, cataract, deafness and microphthalmia occur in congenital rubella infection. The absence of intracerebral calcification helps to distinguish the imaging findings of Rubella from those of Cytomegalovirus infection.
Ch. 101 Orbital Malformations, p 2234.

TRUE   B. Wilms' tumour has an associated sporadic aniridia in about 10% of cases.
Ch. 101 Orbital Malformations, p 2234.

TRUE   C. Many congenital syndromes are associated with cataract formation. These include chondrodysplasia punctata, congenital rubella infection, Lowe's syndrome and Down's syndrome.
Ch. 101 Orbital Malformations, p 2234.

TRUE   D. Abnormal tissue accumulates in the vicinity of the canal of Schlemm causing obstruction and buphthalmos. Congenital glaucoma also occurs in Lowe's syndrome and Sturge-Weber syndrome.
Ch. 101 Orbital Malformations, p 2235.

TRUE   E. Retinal angiomatosis causes retinal haemorrhage and inflammation leading to detachment. A thick, calcified retinal haematoma is a further complication.
Ch. 101 Orbital Malformations, p 2235.

Q *10.5. Regarding Graves' Disease*

A. The severity of Graves' ophthalmopathy parallels the degree of thyroid dysfunction

B. In Graves' disease, glycoprotein deposition in the anterior tendinous parts of the muscles occurs in the majority of cases

C. The MRI signal characteristics allow differentiation of Graves' disease from orbital pseudotumour in over 50% of cases

D. Painful proptosis is commoner with orbital pseudotumour than with Graves' disease

E. Dermoid cyst is the commonest benign tumour of the orbit in adulthood

Q *10.6. Regarding Orbital Imaging*

A. Calcification in an orbital mass in a young child favours a benign lesion

B. A focally thickened posterior wall of the globe with an increased signal on T1W on MRI is typical of a glioma

C. Marked contrast enhancement on CT of a thickened calcified optic nerve suggests meningioma

D. Orbital metastasis is usually suspected because of known disseminated malignant disease

E. A young child presenting with a blind white "cat's eye" is a frequent presentation of retinoblastoma.

A 10.5. Regarding Graves' Disease

FALSE   A. There is *no* correlation between the two. Thyroid function is normal in 10-20% of patients with eye involvement by Graves' disease.
Ch. 101 Graves' Orbitopathy, p 2237.

FALSE   B. In almost every case, only the *extraocular muscle bellies* are thickened. This helps in differentiating the condition from pseudotumour (idiopathic orbital inflammation), which usually involves the anterior tendinous insertion into the globe.
Ch. 101 Graves' Orbitopathy, p 2237.

FALSE   C. The signal characteristics are indistinguishable—enlarged and isointense to normal muscle on T1W images and a high T2W signal during active inflammation in Graves' disease.
Ch. 101 Graves' Orbitopathy, p 2237.

TRUE   D. The combination of unilateral painful proptosis, lacrimal gland involvement, tendinous muscle swelling and marked scleral and optic nerve enhancement is very suggestive of orbital pseudotumour.
Ch. 101 Idiopathic Orbital Inflammation (IOI), p 2238.

FALSE   E. Dermoid cyst contains fat, hair and dermal appendages; occurs up to the age of 10 years. It is characterized by fat density on CT and high signal intensity on T1W and T2W MR images.
Ch. 101 Tumours with Intra- and Extra-orbital Components, p 2244.

A 10.6. Regarding Orbital Imaging

FALSE   A. Retinoblastoma classically has punctate areas of calcifications best identified on orbital CT and readily visible on orbital ultrasound.
Ch. 101 Ocular Tumours, p 2232.

FALSE   B. A high T1 signal is characteristic of melanin as in melanoma. Gliomas cause optic nerve thickening which is distinguishable from the choroidal thickening of melanoma.
Ch. 101 Optic Nerve Glioma, p 2239 & p 2240.

TRUE   C. Gliomas enhance much more variably and rarely calcify.
Ch. 101 Meningioma of the Optic Nerve Sheaths, p 2240.

FALSE   D. Orbital metastasis often occurs before the primary tumour has been identified.
Ch. 101 Lyphoma, Metastasis, Myeloma, p 2243.

TRUE   E. This is the most frequent presentation.
Ch. 101 Ocular Tumours, p 2232.

Q 10.7. Regarding ENT Radiology

A. Choanal atresia is usually bilateral

B. Choanal atresia is more commonly caused by bony obstruction than membranous obstruction

C. If present, a thick bony septum is usually identified on plain radiography on the frontal projection

D. Uncertainty regarding sinus mucosal thickening is resolved by comparison with the other side

E. A sinus air-fluid level is not a good discriminating feature between infective and allergic sinusitis

Q 10.8. Concerning Imaging of the Ear, Nose and Throat

A. An antral signal void on T1 and T2 sequences rules out significant sinusitis

B. Amorphous calcification in a maxillary antral mass is compatible with a diagnosis of aspergillus infection

C. In contrast-enhanced CT, identification of the carotid artery within the cavernous sinus is a sign of cavernous sinus thrombosis

D. Mucoceles occur most commonly in the maxillary antrum

E. Frontal mucoceles present as increased sinus lucency owing to bony erosion

A 10.7. Regarding ENT Radiology

TRUE   A.
            Ch. 102 Choanal Atresia, p 2250.

TRUE   B.
            Ch. 102 Choanal Atresia, p 2250.

FALSE   C. Even thick septa may not be visible, because they are viewed *en face* on a frontal radiograph.
            Ch. 102 Choanal Atresia, p 2251.

FALSE   D. Bilateral disease is very common and often asymmetric and renders comparison between the sides unreliable.
            Ch. 102 Infection and Allergy, p 2251.

FALSE   E. An air-fluid level implies infection for all practical purposes.
            Ch. 102 Acute Sinusitis, p 2252.

A 10.8. Concerning Imaging of the Ear, Nose and Throat

FALSE   A. Highly proteinaceous, inspissated and dehydrated mucus has a low T1 and T2 signal that may be confused with air.
            Ch. 102 Acute Sinusitis, p 2252.

TRUE   B. This feature is seen more commonly on CT but is occasionally present on plain films.
            Ch. 102 Granulomatous and Fungal Infection, p 2253.

TRUE   C. The thrombosed sinus fails to opacify, whereas contrast in the arterial lumen allows it to stand out within the sinus.
            Ch. 102 Granulomatous and Fungal Infection, p 2254.

FALSE   D. Frontal and ethmoidal sinuses are the commonest locations.
            Ch. 102 Mucoceles, p 2255.

TRUE   E. Despite the fluid content of these lesions, a paradoxical increase in lucency may be seen.
            Ch. 102 Mucoceles, p 2255.

Q   *10.9. Regarding the Imaging of Paranasal and Nasal Masses*

    A. A high signal, soft-tissue sinus mass on both T1 and T2W images indicates a likely diagnosis of cholesterol granuloma

    B. A sinus soft-tissue mass which has a high signal on T2W images and which enhances brightly with gadolinium-DTPA is likely to be neoplastic

    C. A calcified tumour mass arising from the nasal septum which has a high T2W signal and peripheral Gd-DTPA enhancement is likely to be a chondrosarcoma

    D. Most extramedullary plasmacytomas arise in the paranasal sinuses or the nasopharynx

    E. Adenoid cystic carcinoma extends into the orbit, middle cranial fossa and along nerves

Q   *10.10. Concerning Cholesteatoma*

    A. The tympanic membrane is usually intact

    B. The soft-tissue component is hyperintense on T1W images

    C. MR enhancement with GdDTPA is usually present

    D. Ossicle erosion is readily detectable on MRI

    E. Erosion of the tegmen tympani renders the patient liable to temporal lobe abscess

A 10.9. Regarding the Imaging of Paranasal and Nasal Masses

TRUE   A. Owing to the presence of cholesterol and methaemoglobin.
Ch. 102 Cholesterol Granuloma, p 2257.

FALSE   B. These features describe inflamed mucosa. Tumours generally have an intermediate T2 signal and moderate enhancement.
Ch. 102 Malignant Tumours of the Nasal Cavity and Paranasal Sinuses, p 2261.

TRUE   C.
Ch. 102 Chondrosarcoma, p 2264.

TRUE   D.
Ch. 102 Plasmacytoma, p 2263.

TRUE   E. It typically spreads perineurally along the mandibular division of trigeminal nerve through the foramen ovale.
Ch. 102 Adenoid Cystic Carcinoma, p 2262.

A 10.10. Concerning Cholesteatoma

FALSE   A. Most cases of acquired cholesteatoma have a history of chronic suppurative otitis media and the tympanic membrane is usually perforated.
Ch. 102 Cholesteatoma, p 2267.

FALSE   B. The soft-tissue component is usually isointense on T1 and hyperintense on T2 imaging. A high T1W signal suggests a cholesterol granuloma. Both cholesterol granuloma and cholesteatoma have a high T2W signal.
Ch. 102 Cholesteatoma, p 2269.

FALSE   C. Cholesteatoma, unlike granulation tissue, does not enhance.
Ch. 102 Cholesteatoma, p 2268.

FALSE   D. Erosion of the ossicles is poorly seen on MRI and certainly much less reliably than on CT, owing to the low MRI signal of these calcified structures.
Ch. 102 Cholesteatoma, p 2268.

TRUE   E. This heralds invasion of the middle cranial fossa.
Ch. 102 Cholesteatoma, p 2268.

Q 10.11. The Following Lesions Can Erode the Petrous Apex

A. Cholesteatoma

B. Cholesterol granuloma

C. Rasmussen aneurysm

D. Nasopharyngeal angiofibroma

E. Arachnoid cyst

Q 10.12. Regarding the Investigation of Acoustic Neuroma

A. Loss of the corneal reflex is an unexpected finding

B. If the 7th and 8th nerves can be seen clearly on T1W images from the cerebello-pontine angle to the outer end of internal auditory canal, an acoustic neuroma can be excluded

C. An acoustic neuroma exhibits an intermediate signal intensity in contrast to the high-signal CSF on T2W images

D. An intracanalicular high-signal lesion demonstrated on contrast-enhanced T1W images is diagnostic of acoustic neuroma

E. An intracanalicular neuroma found incidentally on imaging is likely to remain clinically silent

A 10.11. *The Following Lesions Can Erode the Petrous Apex*

TRUE   A.

   Ch. 102 Tumours and Other Destructive Lesions of the Petrous Apex, p 2274.

TRUE   B.

   Ch. 102 Tumours and Other Destructive Lesions of the Petrous Apex, p 2274.

FALSE   C. This is a pseudoaneurysm which occurs in the lung secondary to inflammation caused by a tuberculous focus.
   Ch. 16 Post-primary Tuberculosis, p 316.

TRUE   D.

   Ch. 102 Tumours and Other Destructive Lesions of the Petrous Apex, p 2274.

TRUE   E.

   Ch. 102 Tumours and Other Destructive Lesions of the Petrous Apex, p 2274.

A 10.12. *Regarding the Investigation of Acoustic Neuroma*

FALSE   A. Tumour pressure on the trigeminal nerve often causes an absent corneal reflex.
   Ch. 102 Acoustic Neuroma, p 2275.

TRUE   B.

   Ch. 102 Acoustic Neuroma, p 2276.

TRUE   C.

   Ch. 102 Acoustic Neuroma, p 2277.

FALSE   D. Intracanalicular lipoma simulates acoustic neuroma on T1W contrast-enhanced images. Pre-enhancement T1W images reveal the fatty nature of a lipoma.
   Ch. 102 Acoustic Neuroma, p 2277.

TRUE   E.

   Ch. 102 Acoustic Neuroma, p 2278.

Q *10.13. Concerning Juvenile Angiofibroma*

A. It occurs most commonly in females over the age of seven

B. It arises in the region of the sphenopalatine foramen adjacent to the superior part of the medial pterygoid plate

C. The diagnosis is best established on biopsy

D. On the plain lateral film it appears as a sessile, rounded mass anterior to the adenoids

E. Erosion of the lateral pterygoid plate on CT is characteristic

Q *10.14. Regarding Tumours of the Head and Neck*

A. Neural tumours usually displace the carotid artery anteriorly while tumours of salivary gland origin displace it posteriorly

B. Occult primary tumours of head and neck demonstrate uptake of 18 FDG on PET scanning

C. Low density in the centre of a lymph node on CT scanning suggests its involvement by malignancy

D. Mixed high and low signal on T1W and T2W images in a para-pharyngeal mass which exhibits ring enhancement is diagnostic of a glomus tumour

E. In left-sided vocal palsy, in the presence of a normal chest X-ray, CT from skull base to aortic arch is required

A 10.13. *Concerning Juvenile Angiofibroma*

FALSE   A. Almost all are boys from 7–29 years of age.
Ch. 102 Juvenile Angiofibroma, p 2285.

TRUE   B.
Ch. 102 Juvenile Angiofibroma, p 2285.

FALSE   C. Biopsy is hazardous owing to severe bleeding and is generally not required for diagnosis.
Ch. 102 Juvenile Angiofibroma, p 2285.

TRUE   D. This causes anterior bowing of the posterior wall of the maxillary antrum.
Ch. 102 Juvenile Angiofibroma, p 2285.

FALSE   E. The *medial* pterygoid plate is characteristically eroded—a feature that is useful in distinguishing angiofibroma from other nasopharyngeal masses.
Ch. 102 Juvenile Angiofibroma, p 2285.

A 10.14. *Regarding Tumours of the Head and Neck*

TRUE   A.
Ch. 102 Neurofibromas, p 2292.

TRUE   B. This is a promising test for the investigation of a solitary enlarged metastatic cervical lymph node.
Ch. 102 Malignant Tumours, p 2287.

TRUE   C.
Ch. 102 Malignant Tumours, p 2288.

FALSE   D. Renal and thyroid metastases, and haemangiomas can all cause this appearance and mimic glomus tumours.
Ch. 102 Benign Tumours, p 2292.

TRUE   E. This is required to diagnose a lesion affecting the left recurrent laryngeal nerve.
Ch. 102 Vocal Cord Palsy, p 2297.

Q *10.15. Concerning Facial Fractures*

    A. In a Le Fort 1 fracture the tooth-bearing part of the maxilla becomes separated from the rest of the maxilla

    B. Both zygomatic arches are fractured in a Le Fort 111 fracture

    C. When fractured as a result of direct trauma, the zygomatic arch is usually fractured in two places

    D. In a "blow-out" fracture the orbital rim remains intact

    E. A fracture of the body of mandible, which runs inferiorly and anteriorly, is more stable than a fracture which runs inferiorly and posteriorly

A *10.15. Concerning Facial Fractures*

TRUE

A. This is a consequence of a fracture through both the medial and lateral walls of the maxillary antra as well as a fracture through the lower part of the nasal septum.
Ch. 103 Fractures of the Maxilla, p 2303.

TRUE

B. In "craniofacial dysjunction," the combination of fractures through the nasal bones, medial and lateral walls of the orbits and zygomatic arches separates the face from the remainder of the skull.
Ch. 103 Fractures of the Maxilla, p 2303.

FALSE

C. There are usually three fracture lines.
Ch. 103 Fractures of the Zygoma, p 2304.

TRUE

D. The increase in intra-orbital pressure causes the thin orbital floor to fracture. The rim remains intact.
Ch. 103 Blow-out Fractures of the Orbital Floor, p 2305.

TRUE

E. The former type of fracture is described as "horizontally favourable," as muscle groups tend to pull the fragments together. In the latter type, the opposite is true.
Ch. 103 Fractures of the Mandible, p 2307.

Q *10.16. Regarding Lesions of the Mandible*

    A. The commonest radiolucent lesion of the mandible is a dentigerous cyst

    B. Multiple odontogenic keratocysts are a feature of Gardner's syndrome

    C. Unicameral bone cysts are invariably asymptomatic and never become infected

    D. A giant-cell tumour of the mandible tends to recur after surgical excision

    E. Caffey's disease tends to spare the mandible

A *10.16. Regarding Lesions of the Mandible*

FALSE

A. An apical *dental* cyst is the commonest cyst of the jaw. It occurs at the apex of a non-vital permanent tooth and is the result of necrosis within a granuloma. A *dentigerous* cyst develops from the enamel-forming tissue of a developing permanent tooth.
Ch. 103 Dental Cyst, p 2309.

FALSE

B. They are a feature of *Gorlin's* syndrome. This is basal cell naevus syndrome characterized by multiple cutaneous basal cell carcinomas, odontogenic keratocysts, ectopic calcification and skeletal anomalies. Multiple osteomas occur in *Gardner's* syndrome.
Ch. 103 Odontogenic Keratocyst, p 2310.

TRUE

C. These are rare, noncorticated cysts which usually cause no expansion and are incidental findings. They may resolve spontaneously.
Ch. 103 Nonepithelial Bone Cyst, p 2310.

TRUE

D. Many benign jaw tumours and cysts tend to recur after excision. Among these are giant-cell tumours, chondromas, odontogenic keratocysts, amelo-blastomas and ossifying fibromas.
Ch. 103 Tumours of Bone and Cartilage, p 2311.

FALSE

E. Infantile cortical hyperostosis usually affects the mandible as well as the ribs, clavicle, radius and ulna. It presents in the first five months of life and appears as florid periosteal reaction in affected areas.
Ch. 103 Caffey's Disease, p 2317.

Q *10.17. Regarding Imaging of the Salivary Glands*

    A. The sublingual glands are situated deep to the mylohyoid muscle

    B. The facial nerve divides the parotid gland into a larger deep lobe and a much smaller superficial lobe

    C. Pertechnetate scanning identifies Warthin's tumour as an area of reduced uptake

    D. Benign pleomorphic adenoma has a higher attenuation value than normal parotid gland on unenhanced CT scans

    E. Sjögren's syndrome is associated with sialectasis

A 10.17. *Regarding Imaging of the Salivary Glands*

FALSE

A. They are situated in the floor of the mouth *above* the mylohyoid muscles. The submandibular glands are situated below the mylohyoid muscle.
Ch. 103 General Considerations, p 2322.

FALSE

B. The superficial lobe is the larger entity. Superficial tumours are therefore removed with less risk of facial nerve damage.
Ch. 103 General Considerations, p 2322.

FALSE

C. This rare adenoma ("adenolymphoma") is exceptional in that, unlike other adenomas, it appears as a "hotspot."
Ch. 103 General Considerations, p 2322.

TRUE

D. This is the commonest salivary gland tumour. The presence of myxoid elements gives a characteristically high signal on T2-weighted MR images.
Ch. 103 Tumours, p 2323.

TRUE

E. Multiple punctate "cavities" occur in the salivary glands in this condition. There may be associated main duct dilatation. Sialectasis is seen in a wide variety of other connective tissue disorders such as rheumatoid disease, SLE, ankylosing spondylitis, Reiter's disease, polyarteritis nodosa and scleroderma.
Ch. 103 Sialectasis, p 2325.

11

Angiography, Interventional Radiology & Other Techniques

Q *11.1. Regarding Vascular Imaging*

   A. During intravenous digital subtraction angiography (IVDSA) undiluted contrast medium is routinely used

   B. Closure of a haemodynamically significant arteriovenous fistula results in an immediate and dramatic bradycardia

   C. Saccular aneurysms are more likely to rupture than fusiform aneurysms

   D. MRA is as effective as contrast angiography at distinguishing high-grade stenosis from occlusion of the carotid arteries

   E. MRA detects the response to treatment of tumour neovascularity

A *11.1. Regarding Vascular Imaging*

TRUE   A. An important aspect of IVDSA is its dependence on a good contrast medium bolus. 40 ml of undiluted contrast medium (350 mg iodine per ml) is injected at 20 ml/sec into the right atrium or one of the great veins.
Ch. 105 Intravenous Digital Subtraction Angiography, p 2375.

TRUE   B. This is called *Branham's sign.*
Ch. 105 Arteriovenous Fistula, p 2375.

TRUE   C.
Ch. 105 Degenerative Aneurysms, p 2371.

FALSE   D. Because slow flow is often present in the recirculation zone of the carotid bulb, saturation of the imaged volume can occur leading to a reduced signal. Slow flow can thus be confused with no flow. Contrast angiography remains the most sensitive method of detecting the remaining lumen in barely patent vessels.
Ch. 105 Clinical Applications, p 2414.

TRUE   E. It is particularly useful in this regard when assessing treatment response in osteogenic sarcoma.
Ch. 105 Pelvis and Lower Extremity, p 2418.

Q *11.2. Concerning Arteriography*

    A. A 7 French catheter would be appropriate for trans-radial arteriography

    B. The maximum dose of 1% lignocaine in an average adult is 20 ml

    C. Intravascular contrast agents (e.g., IV or IA) are necessary to provide good quality arteriograms

    D. Excessive bleeding from a puncture site is usually the result of poor puncture technique

    E. If the principal feeding artery to an organ is obstructed, this becomes clinically manifest in most cases

Q *11.3. The Following Entities Are Usually Associated*

    A. Arteritis: specific arteriographic changes

    B. AIDS vasculitis: predominantly cerebral vascular changes

    C. Necrotizing angiitis: Churg-Strauss syndrome

    D. Takayasu's syndrome: pulmonary vasculitis

    E. Behçet's disease: venous and arterial involvement

A 11.2. Concerning Arteriography

FALSE

A. Modern catheters for trans-brachial and trans-radial arteriography are usually 3–4 French.
Ch. 105 Arteriography, p 2341.

TRUE

B. The recommended maximum dose is 200 mg for a 70 kg man. A 1% solution contains 1 g/100 ml = 1000 mg/100 ml = 100 mg/10 mls. Hence 20 ml will contain 200 mg. See BNF.
Ch. 105 Arteriography, p 2351.

FALSE

C. MRA is now an extremely important tool in the investigation of vascular disease of the neck vessels and the cerebral circulation.
Ch. 105 Arteriography, p 2364.

TRUE

D. Other contributory factors include hypertension, anti-coagulation and the use of large diameter catheters.
Ch. 105 Arteriography, p 2365.

FALSE

E. With some notable exceptions (e.g., brain, kidney) most organs continue to receive blood via a collateral circulation following principal artery obstruction.
Ch. 105 Arteriography, p 2367.

A 11.3. The Following Entities Are Usually Associated

FALSE

A. The changes of arteritis include narrowing, dilatation ectasia and aneurysm formation. Similar changes can, however, be seen in other disorders.
Ch. 105 Arteritis, p 2381.

TRUE

B.
Ch. 105 Arteritis, p 2383.

TRUE

C. Many of the vascular changes are microscopic, however, and cannot be demonstrated angiographically.
Ch. 105 Arteritis, p 2383.

TRUE

D.
Ch. 105 Arteritis, p 2383.

TRUE

E.
Ch. 105 Arteritis, p 2384.

Q *11.4. The Following Entities Are Usually Associated*

A. Syphilis: saccular aneurysm of the proximal aorta

B. Mycotic aneurysms: fungal infections

C. Dissecting aneurysms: haemorrhage into the tunica albuginea

D. DeBakey type III dissections: Marfan's syndrome

E. Cirsoid aneurysm: Behçet's syndrome

Q *11.5. Regarding the Central Veins of the Chest*

A. 90% of patients who present with the superior vena caval syndrome have mediastinal neoplasia

B. Histiocytosis is a common cause of mediastinal fibrosis producing the superior vena caval syndrome

C. An aneurysm of the left subclavian artery may produce the superior vena caval syndrome

D. A double superior vena cava is commoner than an isolated left-sided superior vena cava

E. Superior vena caval stenting is contraindicated in patients with complete occlusion of the vessel

A 11.4. The Following Entities Are Usually Associated

FALSE   A. The aneurysm is fusiform in nature.
Ch. 105 Aneurysms, p 2376.

FALSE   B. Most mycotic aneurysms are produced by bacterial infections
Ch. 105 Aneurysms, p 2376.

FALSE   C. The tunica albuginea covers the testis! Vascular mural bleeding normally occurs into the tunica media.
Ch. 105 Aneurysms, p 2377.

FALSE   D. Marfan's syndrome is typically associated with type II dissection of the aorta (localized to the ascending aorta).
Ch. 105 Aneurysms, p 2377.

FALSE   E. Behçet's syndrome is an arteritis of unknown aetiology that may cause vascular thrombosis and aneurysm formation that can rupture. A cirsoid aneurysm is a dated surgical term for a type of arteriovenous communication.
Ch. 105 Aneurysms, p 2380.

A 11.5. Regarding the Central Veins of the Chest

TRUE   A. This syndrome is characterized by cyanosis, swelling of the face, neck and arms, orbital oedema, proptosis and distension of the veins of the neck and trunk.
Ch. 106 S.V.C. Syndrome, p 2428.

FALSE   B. *Histoplasmosis*, T.B. Sarcoidosis, actinomycosis and cryptococcosis are common benign causes of mediastinal fibrosis.
Ch. 106 S.V.C. Syndrome, p 2428.

FALSE   C. The *right* subclavian artery.
Ch. 106 S.V.C. Syndrome, Table 106.1, p 2429.

TRUE   D. The left superior vena cava usually drains into the coronary sinus.
Ch. 106 Persistent Left S.V.C., p 2430.

FALSE   E. In a symptomatic patient, complete occlusion is an excellent indication for the procedure.
Ch. 106 S.V.C. Stenting, p 2430.

Q *11.6. Concerning Venous Angiography and Intervention*

A. The right gonadal vein is usually difficult to catheterize

B. Communications may exist between the left testicular vein and the inferior mesenteric vein and portal vein

C. In Klippel-Trenaunay syndrome, the deep veins are usually hypoplastic or absent

D. Inferior petrosal vein sampling is used to differentiate Cushing's syndrome from ectopic ACTH syndrome

E. The commonest indication for cavernosography is arteriogenic impotence

Q *11.7. Regarding Vascular Disorders*

A. The anomalous artery that supplies a sequestered pulmonary segment is usually demonstrated arising from the thoraco-abdominal aorta on the right

B. The arc of Bühler is a congenital communication between the coeliac axis and the superior mesenteric artery

C. A "strawberry naevus" is unlikely to resolve spontaneously

D. Angiodysplasia is a vascular disorder that predominantly affects the small bowel

E. Branham's sign is bradycardia engendered by the temporary occlusion of a haemodynamically significant arteriovenous fistula

A *11.6. Concerning Venous Angiography and Intervention*

TRUE   A. This relates to the anatomy of the gonadal veins.
              Ch. 106 Gonadal Venography, p 2441.

TRUE   B. These communications are, thankfully, rare, though they should not be
              ignored when varicocele embolization is considered.
              Ch. 106 Gonadal Venography, p 2441.

TRUE   C. This syndrome consists of a cutaneous naevus of one lower limb, varicose
              veins dating from infancy and hypertrophy of the affected limb. These veins
              are *not to be stripped!*
              Ch. 106 Klippel-Trenaunay Syndrome, p 2441.

FALSE   D. Ectopic ACTH syndrome is a subcategory of Cushing's syndrome. The sam-
              pling test differentiates Cushing's *disease* from other causes of increased
              ACTH production.
              Ch. 106 The Pituitary Gland, p 2453.

FALSE   E. *Venogenic* impotence
              Ch. 106 Impotence, p 2455.

A *11.7. Regarding Vascular Disorders*

FALSE   A. Pulmonary sequestration is more common on the left than the right, and
              so is the artery supplying it!
              Ch. 105 Congenital Abnormalities, p 2369.

TRUE   B.
              Ch. 105 Congenital Abnormalities, p 2370.

FALSE   C. A "strawberry naevus" is a true haemangioma that usually proliferates and
              then regresses in childhood. This must be distinguished from an arteriove-
              nous malformation, a lesion that will never spontaneously regress.
              Ch. 105 Vascular Malformations, p 2372.

FALSE   D. Angiodysplasia most commonly affects the caecum.
              Ch. 105 Vascular Malformations, p 2375.

TRUE   E. This sign is thought to be diagnostically useful.
              Ch. 105 Arteriovenous Fistula, p 2375.

Q 11.8. Regarding Vascular Ultrasound

A. Spectral broadening is a feature of flow disturbance

B. A 10% reduction in the diameter area of a vessel will reduce the cross-sectional area by approximately 20%

C. Forward diastolic flow is usually demonstrated in the superficial femoral artery in normal individuals after strenuous exercise

D. When the cross-sectional area of a vessel is reduced by 75% there is an increase in the peak velocity in the proximal vessel, on the spectral trace

E. The resistance index (R.I.) increases with an increase in heart rate

Q 11.9. The Following Are Commonly Accepted Results and Complications for the Procedure of Oesophageal Stent (Uncovered) Placement

A. Central chest pain: less than 1%

B. Technical success rate: 60–70%

C. Stent related mortality: 0–6%

D. Tumour ingrowth between the struts: 5–50%

E. Tumour overgrowth: 5–10%

A 11.8. *Regarding Vascular Ultrasound*

TRUE   A. Severe flow disturbance may produce simultaneous forward and reverse flow in the Doppler signal.
Ch. 107 Turbulent Flow, p 2460.

TRUE   B.
Ch. 107 Doppler USS, Table 107.1.

TRUE   C. This is due to a reduction in the resistance of the vascular bed.
Ch. 107 Doppler USS, p 2462.

FALSE   D. With a 75% reduction in cross-sectional area (i.e., a 50% reduction in diameter) there is a *reduction* in the peak velocity proximal to the vessel.
Ch. 107 Doppler USS, p 2463.

FALSE   E. The opposite. The end-diastolic velocity of blood is higher with decreasing cardiac cycle times; hence the minimum velocity is higher. (See the equation for the R.I.)
Ch. 107 Pulsatility Measurements, p 2464.

A 11.9. *The Following Are Commonly Accepted Results and Complications for the Procedure of Oesophageal Stent (Uncovered) Placement*

FALSE   A. 10–20%
Ch. 108 Dilatation Procedures, p 2490.

FALSE   B. Approaching 100%
Ch. 108 Dilatation Procedures, p 2490.

TRUE   C.
Ch. 108 Dilatation Procedures, p 2490.

TRUE   D.
Ch. 108 Dilatation Procedures, p 2490.

TRUE   E.
Ch. 108 Dilatation Procedures, p 2490.

Q *11.10. Concerning Vascular Embolization*

A. The major vessels arising from the coeliac axis can be embolized with very little risk of organ infarction

B. Embolization is the treatment of choice for femoral arterial pseudoaneurysms

C. Small pulmonary arteriovenous communications are best embolized with large particles which directly occlude the nidus

D. Post-embolization syndrome may be confused with the more serious complications of infection and abscess formation

E. Venous malformations are best demonstrated by selective arteriography

Q *11.11. Regarding Thrombolysis, Thrombosis and Embolism*

A. The procedure of arterial angioplasty is complicated by arterial thrombosis in 15–20% of cases

B. rt-PA activates plasminogen, which in turn lyses thrombin to dissolve clot

C. Cerebral haemorrhage occurs in up to 10–20% of patients undergoing peripheral arterial thrombolysis

D. Patients with an early classical presentation of a proximal embolic arterial occlusion are best treated by surgery

E. Systemic thrombolysis significantly reduces the long term local complications of deep venous thrombosis

A 11.10. Concerning Vascular Embolization

TRUE   A. The operator should be aware, however, that multiple embolizations and/or a background of vascular disease or previous surgery will increase the chances of organ infarction.
Ch. 108 Acute Bleeding, p 2527.

FALSE   B. Direct USS guided local compression is the ideal method.
Ch. 108 Femoral Artery Pseudoaneurysm, p 2531.

FALSE   C. Coils and balloons are the only agents that should be routinely used in the pulmonary circulation. Liquid or particulate agents can pass into the systemic circulation with potentially catastrophic consequences.
Ch. 108 Pulmonary Arteriovenous Communications, p 2531.

TRUE   D. Although this syndrome can last for up to 14 days, the radiologist and the clinician should have a high index of suspicion for infection and abscess formation in the embolized organ/tissue.
Ch. 108 Complications of Embolization, p 2539.

FALSE   E. Many venous malformations are best demonstrated by direct venous puncture and venography.

A 11.11. Regarding Thrombolysis, Thrombosis and Embolism

FALSE   A. The usually quoted figure is between 2 and 3% of patients, although major vascular centres will probably have lower rates.
Ch. 108 Peripheral Arterial Thromboembolism, p 2505.

FALSE   B. rt-PA has a high affinity for fibrin (the polymerized molecule that maintains the integrity of the thrombus). Once the rt-PA is bound, it activates plasminogen to plasmin, which lyses the *fibrin* to dissolve the thrombus. rt-PA enhances the activation of plasminogen by 2–3 orders of magnitude.
Ch. 108 Tissue Plasminogen Activator, p 2504.

FALSE   C. 0–1.3% patients without a history of cerebrovascular disease develop cerebral haemorrhage.
Ch. 108 Haemorrhage, p 2507.

TRUE   D. Thrombolysis may delay reperfusion and may cause distal embolism, which in turn will prolong the duration of treatment and may result in potential complications.
Ch. 108 Acute Thromboembolic Occlusions, p 2505.

TRUE   E. The risks of thrombolysis, however, significantly outweigh this potential benefit.
Ch. 108 Deep Venous Thrombosis, p 2505.

12

The Reticuloendothelial System, Oncology, AIDS

Q *12.1. Regarding Hodgkin's and Non-Hodgkin's Lymphoma*

    A. Haematogenous spread is commoner in non-Hodgkin's lymphoma than in Hodgkin's disease

    B. Lymph node enlargement tends to be greater in non-Hodgkin's lymphoma than in Hodgkin's disease

    C. The upper limit of normal trans-axial diameter for an abdominal or pelvic node is 10 mm

    D. Pulmonary involvement by Hodgkin's disease is almost invariably associated with mediastinal adenopathy

    E. Small bowel lymphoma most frequently affects the duodenum

Q *12.2. Regarding CNS and Head and Neck Lymphoma*

    A. Primary spinal cord lymphoma is commoner than primary cerebral lymphoma

    B. Cerebral lymphoma usually occurs peripherally at the grey/white matter interface

    C. Cerebral lymphoma frequently calcifies

    D. Homogeneous contrast MRI enhancement usually occurs in cerebral lymphoma

    E. The commonest site of head and neck lymphoma is Waldeyer's ring

A 12.1. *Regarding Hodgkin's and non-Hodgkin's Lymphoma*

TRUE

A. Differences between Hodgkin's disease and non-Hodgkin's lymphoma (NHL) are as follows: mediastinal and splenic lesions are commoner in the former; in the latter gastrointestinal, mesenteric, osseous, haematogenous and extranodal involvement are commoner.
Ch. 109A Table 109.3, p 2558.

TRUE

B. Both disease processes may, however, produce huge nodal masses. Conversely, both types of lymphoma may involve nodes without causing them to enlarge.
Ch. 109A, Nodal Disease, p 2559.

FALSE

C. In the retroperitoneum, normal lymph node size increases in a caudal direction: the upper limit of normal in the retrocrural space is 6 mm, in the upper retroperitoneum it is 8 mm, and at the aortic bifurcation is 1 cm. In the pelvis, any node greater than 8 mm in its trans-axial diameter is considered abnormal.
Ch. 109A, Imaging Techniques, p 2559.

TRUE

D. This is in contrast to non-Hodgkin's lymphoma, in which the association between pulmonary involvement and thoracic nodal disease is considerably weaker.
Ch. 109A Pulmonary Involvement, p 2561.

FALSE

E. Small bowel lymphoma most frequently affects the terminal ileum and becomes progressively less common proximally.
Ch. 109A Small Bowel, p 2564.

A 12.2. *Regarding CNS and Head and Neck Lymphoma*

FALSE

A. Primary spinal cord lymphoma is extremely rare—primary CNS lymphoma is confined almost exclusively to the brain.
Ch. 109A Central Nervous System, p 2567.

FALSE

B. The typical position is in the deep white matter of the cerebrum.
Ch. 109A Central Nervous System, p 2568.

FALSE

C. Calcification is not a feature.
Ch. 109A, Central Nervous System, p 2568.

TRUE

D.
Ch. 109A Central Nervous System, p 2568.

TRUE

E. The ring comprises lymphoid tissue in the nasopharynx and oropharynx, the faucial and palatine tonsils and the lingual tonsil on the posterior third of the tongue.
Ch. 109A Waldeyer's Ring, p 2570.

Q *12.3. Regarding the Features of Specific Tumours*

    A. Most ovarian cancers present in FIGO stages I and II

    B. A testicular mass associated with an elevated alpha-feto-protein level (AFP) is likely to be a seminoma

    C. Endorectal ultrasound is more accurate than CT in determining the extent of local spread of early rectal tumours

    D. In lung carcinoma, chest wall involvement precludes surgical resection

    E. In carcinoma of the lung, ipsilateral hilar lymphadenopathy has the same prognostic implications as ipsilateral mediastinal lymphadenopathy

A   *12.3 Regarding the Features of Specific Tumours*

FALSE   A. Ovarian cancer presents late. 55–80% of patients have Stage III or IV disease at presentation. This indicates peritoneal implants outside the pelvis and/or positive retroperitoneal or inguinal nodes (Stage III) or distant metastases, such as cytologically positive pleural effusion or parenchymal liver metastases (Stage IV).
Ch. 110 Early Stage Disease, p 2588.

FALSE   B. AFP is elevated in only 4% of seminomas; the most probable diagnosis in this clinical scenario is teratoma.
Ch. 110 Testicular Germ Cell Tumours, p 2592.

FALSE   C. Unfortunately, early tumours are encountered less frequently than more advanced tumours. The advantage of USS is less clear in the latter, as CT is also accurate in such cases.
Ch. 110 Endorectal Ultrasound, p 2594.

FALSE   D. Chest wall involvement does not preclude resection, but it does alter the prognosis and is associated with significant morbidity and mortality.
Ch. 110 Assessment of Chest Wall Invasion, p 2599.

FALSE   E. Ipsilateral hilar lymphadenopathy constitutes N1 disease using the TNM classification; it does not preclude surgery, but it carries a poorer prognosis. Ipsilateral mediastinal lymphadenopathy indicates N2 disease and, unlike the former, is a contraindication to surgical resection. Contralateral hilar and mediastinal lymphadenopathy are each classed as N3 disease.
Ch. 110 Nodal Involvement, p 2599.

Q *12.4. Regarding the Scintigraphic Imaging of Tumours*

A. ^{111}In DTPA-octreotide has greater sensitivity and specificity for the detection of neuroendocrine tumours than has CT or MRI

B. ^{111}In DTPA-octreotide scanning is better at demonstrating insulinomas than carcinoid tumours

C. Hyperglycaemia decreases the sensitivity of ^{18}F-fluorodeoxy-glucose (FDG) in neuroendocrine tumour detection

D. The rate of glycolysis is faster in tumour cells than in normal tissues

E. FDG scanning differentiates between post-radiotherapy gliosis and recurrent brain tumour

A *12.4. Regarding the Scintigraphic Imaging of Tumours*

TRUE A. The *sensitivity* for the diagnosis and localization of neuroendocrine tumours is about 85% for octreotide scanning. This compares with 68% for CT and MRI. The *specificity* of octreotide scanning is only 50%, but this is far better than that of CT and MRI, which is only 12%.
Ch. 111 Neuroendocrine Tumours, p 2614.

FALSE B. Insulinomas have varying affinities for octreotide. Carcinoid tumours, especially extra-hepatic lesions, can be detected by octreotide scanning in 85–100% of cases.
Ch. 111 Neuroendocrine Tumours, p 2614.

TRUE C. Serum glucose is an important factor in the quantitative assessment of FDG uptake by tumours. FDG imaging of tumours is preferably performed in the fasting state to minimize the competitive inhibition of FDG uptake by serum glucose.
Ch. 111 Neuroendocrine Tumours, p 2614.

TRUE D. This is the basis of FDG scanning. FDG is a glucose analogue labelled with fluorine-18. It is transported into the cell by the same mechanism as glucose but cannot then undergo further metabolism.
Ch. 111 PET: Fluorodeoxyglucose and Cancer Detection, p 2615.

TRUE E. The amount of uptake is greater in viable tumour than in gliosis following radiotherapy.
Ch. 111 Clinical Applications, p 2615.

Q 12.5. *The Following Tumours Can Be Imaged With* ^{111}*InDTPA-Octreotide*

A. Breast cancer

B. Meningioma

C. Paraganglionomas

D. Phaeochromocytoma

E. Small-cell carcinoma of the lung

A 12.5 *The Following Tumours Can Be Imaged with* [111]*InDTPA-Octreotide*

TRUE   A. There is a sensitivity of only 75% in the detection of breast tumours already diagnosed by other means. Octreotide scanning may be more useful in recurrent cancer.
Ch. 111 Non-neuroendocrine Tumours, p 2615.

TRUE   B. These tumours arise outside the blood-brain barrier and contain a high number of somatostatin receptors. They are reported to be detectable with 100% sensitivity irrespective of their location, histology or grade.
Ch. 111 Non-neuroendocrine Tumours, p 2615.

TRUE   C. These can be detected in 94% of cases.
Ch. 111 Neuroendocrine Tumours, p 2614.

TRUE   D. Octreotide can detect phaeochromocytoma with a sensitivity equal to that of MIBG scintigraphy. The same applies to neuroblastomas.
Ch. 111 Neuroendocrine Tumours, p 2615.

TRUE   E. There is a high detection rate for primary and secondary small cell carcinoma of the lung. Adrenal and liver metastases, however, are poorly visualized owing to high abdominal background activity.
Ch. 111 Non-neuroendocrine Tumours, p 2615.

Self Assessment Questions

True False

Test 1.

1. Regarding Periosteal Reaction

A. Periosteal reaction of the newborn may present with several layers of thin new bone along the diaphysis of the humerus

B. Hypervitaminosis A causes painful soft-tissue lumps and periosteal reactions

C. Periosteal elevation caused by pus is usually seen within the first 5 days of symptomatic osteomyelitis

D. Brodie's abscess has some associated periosteal reaction in more than 80% of cases

E. Sclerosing osteitis of Garré is seen most commonly in the mandible

2. Concerning Mammography Technique, Equipment & Quality Control

A. A single film-screen system is used because it allows a lower dose than that obtained by film alone without screen

B. A mediolateral oblique (MLO) view images more of the posterior breast and axillary tail than a 90° lateral view

C. The pectoralis major muscle should be visualized down to the level of the nipple

D. Breast compression reduces geometric unsharpness, motion unsharpness and radiation dose at the expense of reduced tissue contrast

E. At higher kVp settings, the dose is lower because of greater tissue penetration but contrast is reduced

3. Concerning the Radiology of Biliary Disease

A. The commonest enteric site of impaction of a gallstone is the duodenojejunal flexure

509

True	False	
❑	❑	B. The demonstration of a dilated intrahepatic biliary tree is essential to the definitive diagnosis of obstructive jaundice
❑	❑	C. Multiple intra- and extra-hepatic strictures on ERCP are seen exclusively in sclerosing cholangitis
❑	❑	D. Chronic Ascaris Lumbricoides infection is associated with bile duct cancer
❑	❑	E. Atrophy of a lobe of liver occurs as a sequel to portal venous obstruction by tumour

4. Concerning Degenerative Disease of the Spine

True	False	
❑	❑	A. Most acute disc herniations extend through the posterior longitudinal ligament
❑	❑	B. An increased vertebral signal on T_1W and isointensity on T_2W images indicates fatty replacement of red marrow
❑	❑	C. An increased MR signal in an intervertebral disc on T_1W images is a sign of degenerative disease
❑	❑	D. In postoperative MR imaging, recurrent or residual disc material is distinguished reliably from epidural fibrosis by the lack of gadolinium enhancement in the former
❑	❑	E. A mid-sagittal cervical canal diameter of less than 20 mm on the plain film indicates that cord compression is probably present

5. Concerning Paediatric Scintigraphy in Bone Conditions

True	False	
❑	❑	A. It is possible to reliably differentiate septic arthritis from rheumatoid arthritis with multiphase bone imaging
❑	❑	B. Early osteomyelitis appears as a focus of reduced ^{99m}TcMDP uptake
❑	❑	C. MRI is as sensitive as bone scanning in detecting discitis
❑	❑	D. In Perthes' disease, focal photopaenia in an epiphysis means that the loss of the vascular supply to that area must be longstanding
❑	❑	E. Bone scanning is useful for the detection of subtle epiphyseal fractures

6. Multiple Ovarian Cysts are Features of:

True	False	
❑	❑	A. Infantile polycystic kidney disease
❑	❑	B. Oldfield's syndrome
❑	❑	C. Stein-Leventhal syndrome
❑	❑	D. Gardner's syndrome
❑	❑	E. Metropathia haemorrhagia

True	False	

7. Concerning the Neuroradiology of HIV Infection

A. Most asymptomatic HIV positive individuals have some abnormality on cranial MRI

B. CNS tuberculosis indicates probable intravenous drug abuse

C. Multiple high T_2W signal white matter lesions combined with positive JC virus serology is diagnostic of progressive multifocal leukoencephalopathy (PML)

D. Necrotizing ventriculitis is usually caused by cytomegalovirus

E. Kaposi's sarcoma commonly metastasizes to the brain

8. Regarding ENT Radiology

A. Choanal atresia is usually bilateral

B. Choanal atresia is more commonly caused by bony obstruction than membranous obstruction

C. If choanal atresia is present, a thick bony septum is usually identified on plain radiography

D. Uncertainty regarding sinus mucosal thickening is resolved by comparison with the other side

E. A sinus air-fluid level is not a good discriminating feature between infective and allergic sinusitis

9. Regarding Ultrasound of the Infant Brain

A. Transcranial scanning through the temporal bone detects contralateral subdural haematoma

B. The internal carotid bifurcation is regularly seen on coronal section through the anterior fontanelle

C. An isolated hyperreflective focus anterior to the caudothalamic groove at 31 weeks is an indicator of poor prognosis

D. Decreased reflectivity in periventricular white matter is suggestive of early leukomalacia

E. A wedge-shaped area of hyperreflective cortex indicates recent infarction

10. The Following Statements Apply to Ultrasound

A. Diagnostic ultrasound occupies frequencies between 1 and 20 MHz in the electromagnetic spectrum

B. Ultrasound is propagated through tissue as a transverse wave

C. Time gain compensation allows image brightness for superficial and deep structures to be equalized

True	False
☐	☐
☐	☐

D. The prime determinant of the strength of an ultrasound echo is the difference in density between adjacent tissue components

E. A Doppler beam at its highest intensity can cause a significant rise in temperature when directed at a bone surface

11. Concerning Cardiomyopathy

True	False
☐	☐
☐	☐
☐	☐
☐	☐
☐	☐

A. Dilated cardiomyopathy is mimicked by end-stage aortic stenosis

B. Endocardial biopsy should be performed in a young patient with acute-onset heart failure, pyrexia and respiratory symptoms

C. Endocardial fibroelastosis causes mitral stenosis

D. Hypertrophic cardiomyopathy often presents with atypical angina

E. Endomyocardial fibrosis causes subendocardial hyperreflectivity on ultrasound

12. The Following are Normal Features of the Oesophagus on Barium Swallow

True	False
☐	☐
☐	☐
☐	☐
☐	☐
☐	☐

A. The cervical oesophagus starts at the cricopharyngeus impression—usually at C3–C4 level

B. The post-cricoid impression is a small posterior web-like indentation

C. Herring-bone pattern of mucosal folds on double contrast examination

D. The A ring (tubulovestibular junction) varies in calibre during the examination

E. The mucosal gastro-oesophageal junction cannot be identified on double contrast studies

13. Concerning Focal Liver Lesions

True	False
☐	☐
☐	☐
☐	☐
☐	☐
☐	☐

A. Daughter cysts develop within a larger mother cyst in hydatid disease

B. A prominent air-fluid level in an intrahepatic mass implies that it is an abscess

C. "Filling in" of a lesion on delayed contrast-enhanced CT means it is almost certainly a haemangioma

D. A central hyperreflective "punctum" surrounded by echo-poor foci is a feature of fungal abscesses

E. High-attenuation abdominal deposits may occur in angiosarcoma on CT scanning

14. Regarding Ultrasound Imaging of Liver Disease

True	False
☐	☐
☐	☐
☐	☐

A. Regenerating nodules are usually very small and cannot be demonstrated by imaging techniques

B. Acute hepatitis and diffuse tuberculosis are causes of a "bright" liver

C. A fasting portal venous velocity of greater than 12 cm/sec does not occur in portal hypertension

True	False
☐	☐
☐	☐

D. High-velocity spectral traces are seen in relation to most hepatomas

E. Daughter cysts are present in 80-90% of liver hydatid cysts

15. Concerning Obstruction in the Urinary Tract

True	False	
☐	☐	A. Hydronephrosis implies at least a degree of obstruction
☐	☐	B. The degree of dilatation of the collecting system is a useful guide to the severity of the obstruction
☐	☐	C. Primary megaureter occurs in the absence of anatomical or functional obstruction
☐	☐	D. If the 15-minute IVU film fails to show an opacified collecting system, the next film should be taken about one hour later
☐	☐	E. A urinoma, if present in urinary obstruction, opacifies during an IVU in the majority of cases

16. Regarding the Plain Abdominal Radiograph

True	False	
☐	☐	A. The presence of more than two air-fluid levels in dilated small bowel (over 2.5 cm across) is abnormal
☐	☐	B. A caecal fluid level is an abnormal finding
☐	☐	C. It is unusual for the bowel calibre to be less than 5 cm in severe large bowel obstruction
☐	☐	D. Normal fluid levels are usually shorter than 2.5 cm in length
☐	☐	E. A "string of beads" sign caused by bubbles of gas trapped between valvulae conniventes is seen after cleansing enema administration

17. Regarding Large Bowel Obstruction

True	False	
☐	☐	A. In the presence of generalized gaseous bowel distension, a left lateral decubitus radiograph may be helpful in diagnosing large bowel obstruction
☐	☐	B. After carcinoma of the colon, volvulus is the commonest cause of large bowel obstruction in western societies
☐	☐	C. Right-sided large bowel obstruction is almost as common as left-sided obstruction
☐	☐	D. Caecal volvulus occurs only when there is a degree of malrotation
☐	☐	E. Sigmoid volvulus usually has a history of intermittent acute attacks over a period of time

18. Regarding Ultrasound of the Orbit

True	False	
☐	☐	A. The scan is performed through the closed lid
☐	☐	B. A range of 7.5–8 MHz is optimal for examination of the orbit

True   False

C. Ultrasound is the imaging method of choice for demonstrating the degree of retinal detachment

D. "Blow-out" fractures are readily detected

E. Muscles enlarged by Graves' Disease are hyperreflective

19. Regarding the Features of Renal Cystic Masses

A. The collecting system of a multicystic dysplastic kidney does not opacify during intravenous urography

B. Hepatic involvement in multicystic dysplastic kidney is usually confined to a single lobe

C. Multilocular renal cyst (benign cystic nephroma) has a characteristic honeycomb appearance on CT and ultrasound, and requires no further follow-up

D. Hydatid disease commonly affects the kidney

E. Peripelvic cysts are of lymphatic origin and may be confused with hydronephrosis on ultrasound

20. Regarding the Imaging of Prostatic Carcinoma

A. Advanced tumours are often difficult to detect on transrectal ultrasound (TRUS)

B. A serum PSA (prostatic specific antigen) and digital examination are more sensitive than TRUS

C. TRUS should be used to assess the site of the lesion prior to excision biopsy

D. The staging of prostatic cancer is either by the TNM or the Jewitt classification

E. TRUS is as accurate as MRI in staging

21. Regarding the Radiology of Pituitary Tumours

A. Twenty percent of normal people have a 3 mm or greater focal area of low attenuation on CT of the pituitary

B. Eighty to 90% of microadenomas are hypointense on T_1W images

C. MRI is highly accurate at detecting cavernous sinus invasion by pituitary adenoma

D. The pituitary fossa is enlarged on skull radiography in 80% of cases of both acromegaly and Cushing's syndrome

E. In young patients the majority of craniopharyngiomas are cystic and calcified

22. Regarding Phaeochromocytoma

A. The commonest extra-adrenal sites are the renal hilum and the organ of Zuckerkandl

True	False	
❏	❏	B. Calcification is present in about 10%
❏	❏	C. The presence of fat attenuation within an adrenal tumour strongly suggests an alternative diagnosis
❏	❏	D. The use of ^{131}I-MIBG localizes metastatic disease
❏	❏	E. There is an association with angiomyolipoma

23. Regarding the Radiology of Rheumatoid Arthritis

True	False	
❏	❏	A. Acrosclerosis is a feature of rheumatoid arthritis
❏	❏	B. Periosteal reaction occurs in about 15% of cases
❏	❏	C. Rotator cuff atrophy and tearing is a common sequel of shoulder involvement
❏	❏	D. Involvement of the acromioclavicular joint most commonly results in narrowing of the joint space
❏	❏	E. Bony ankylosis of the carpus does not occur

24. Regarding Percutaneous Nephrostomy

True	False	
❏	❏	A. Puncture of an upper-pole calix is preferred as this facilitates wire manipulation into the ureter
❏	❏	B. Passage through the maximum available depth of renal parenchyma is preferred in order to maximise stability of the nephrostomy drain
❏	❏	C. Renal pseudoaneurysms caused by central punctures are best treated by trans-catheter embolisation
❏	❏	D. Percutaneous nephrostomy should be performed in all cases of malignant ureteric obstruction to avoid death from renal failure
❏	❏	E. Percutaneous nephrostomy should not be performed on horseshoe kidneys

25. Regarding Imaging of the Kidney in Renal Failure

True	False	
❏	❏	A. Demonstration of a dilated pelvicalyceal system implies the presence of obstruction
❏	❏	B. Ultrasound is the method of choice for excluding obstruction in polycystic kidney disease
❏	❏	C. High dose urography uses about 60 mg of iodine per kg of patient weight
❏	❏	D. Obstructive renal failure is ruled out when collecting system dilatation is not identified on ultrasound, CT, antegrade or retrograde pyelography
❏	❏	E. High-dose urography should not be used to diagnose obstruction if a definite nephrogram has not been identified on standard dose urography

True	False

26. Concerning MR Imaging of the Spine

A. A band of high signal in the centre of spinal cord on mid-sagittal images is caused by truncation artefact

B. The FLAIR sequence is heavily T2 weighted and CSF appears as a signal void

C. Dura is separated by fat from the bony walls of the spinal canal

D. Dorsal root ganglia enhance strongly with IV gadolinium, unlike normal intradural roots

E. The commonest conjoined roots are L5/S1

27. Regarding MRI of the Female Pelvis

A. The normal uterus has a central low-intensity stripe on T_2W images that represents endometrium

B. On T_1W images the normal uterine body has a homogeneously low signal intensity

C. During staging of cervical carcinoma, on T_2W images the presence of a complete ring of low signal around a tumour mass is an accurate indication of stage 1B

D. Calculated relaxation times allow reliable discrimination between nodes infiltrated by malignancy, non-specific lymphadenopathy and granulomatous disease

E. Brenner tumours of the ovary have a low signal on T_1W and T_2W images

28. Concerning Paediatric Diaphragmatic Disorders

A. Bochdalek hernias are the commonest intrathoracic fetal anomaly

B. Morgagni hernias are most commonly seen anteromedially on the left

C. After repair of a Bochdalek hernia, the mediastinum remains shifted to the contralateral side

D. Diaphragmatic eventration is not associated with pulmonary hypoplasia

E. The scaphoid abdomen usually differentiates diaphragmatic hernia from cystic adenomatoid malformation of the lungs

29. When Monitoring the Response to Therapy in Patients with Bladder Tumours

A. Periodic IVUs are recommended

B. MRI, using contrast medium and a variety of sequences, can reliably distinguish between radiation changes and tumour recurrence

C. CT and MRI are very helpful in differentiating between non-specific granulation tissue and local recurrence

True	False	
❏	❏	D. The typical changes demonstrated on MRI after radiotherapy include abnormal signal intensity of the outer muscle wall on T2-weighted images and mural enhancement (after i/v contrast administration) on T1-weighted images
❏	❏	E. Radiation changes to the bowel are usually demonstrated within one month of treatment

30. Concerning Radionuclide Bone Scanning

True	False	
❏	❏	A. Following injection of ^{99m}Tc labelled MDP, 10% is deposited within bone within one hour
❏	❏	B. The gallium ion shares certain physiological properties with the ferrous ion
❏	❏	C. Gallium localizes to normal bone by binding to phosphate
❏	❏	D. Giant cell tumours of bone demonstrate intense uptake of ^{99m}Tc MDP
❏	❏	E. In patients with bone trauma, a negative bone scan effectively excludes significant bony injury

Test 2.

31. Regarding Imaging of the Small Intestine

True	False	
❏	❏	A. Mesenteric abscesses and mesenteric lymphadenopathy are CT findings of Crohn's disease
❏	❏	B. A "coiled spring" appearance is a sign of coeliac disease on barium follow-through
❏	❏	C. Isolated focal dilation of a small bowel loop is a sign of lymphoma
❏	❏	D. Primary carcinoma is commoner in the ileum than in the jejunum
❏	❏	E. Deep ulceration occurs in 80% of cases of radiation enteritis

32. Regarding the Assessment of Breast Lumps

True	False	
❏	❏	A. The demonstration of fatty density in a circumscribed mass almost certainly excludes the possibility of malignancy
❏	❏	B. Lack of change in a lesion for over 12 months excludes malignancy
❏	❏	C. A rapidly enlarging breast mass occurs in cystosarcoma phylloides
❏	❏	D. Traumatic fat necrosis always has at least some central fat density
❏	❏	E. Ultrasound can detect less than 10% of cancers seen only as areas of microcalcifications on mammography

True	False

33. Regarding Lobar Collapse

A. The more collapsed a lobe is, the more opaque it appears on the chest radiograph

B. Apparent reduction in the size of the hilum occurs in lower-lobe collapse

C. In compensatory hyperinflation, the affected hyperinflated lung fails to deflate normally on expiration

D. Rounded atelectasis is commonest in the lower lobes

E. In left upper-lobe collapse the lower lobe may expand to reach the level of the apex of the hemithorax

34. Regarding the Radiology of Pneumonia

A. A pleural effusion occurs commonly with *Legionella* pneumonia

B. Chest radiograph changes occur in 25% of cases of brucellosis

C. Moderately-sized pleural effusions are a common feature of *Mycoplasma* pneumonia

D. *Leptospira* interrogans infection causes a haemorrhagic pneumonia with small pleural effusions

E. The pattern of consolidation suggests the microbe in most cases

35. Regarding the Findings at ERCP

A. HIV cholangitis resembles sclerosing cholangitis

B. A choledochocele is lined by duodenal mucosa

C. Clonorchis sinensis causes a long linear filling defect in the common bile duct

D. A smooth, tapering stricture of the distal bile duct within the head of the pancreas occurs in chronic pancreatitis

E. Cholangitis is a cause of multiple, contrast-filled intrahepatic cavities

36. Regarding Pancreatic Pathology

A. Fatty replacement of the pancreas occurs in cystic fibrosis

B. There is an association between multiple pancreatic cysts, von Hippel Lindau syndrome and a raised red cell count

C. At least 50% of pancreatic pseudocysts resolve spontaneously without clinical sequelae

D. Acute massive bleeding in a patient with a history of pancreatitis is almost always caused by varices secondary to splenic or mesenteric vein occlusion

E. Most pancreatic cancers are irresectable at the time of diagnosis

True	False

37. Regarding Radiology of the Pericardium

A. A cystic structure arising within the pericardium containing layered calcific deposits is suggestive of a bronchogenic cyst

B. Bilateral hilar overlay occurs in pericardial effusion

C. Chylous pericarditis usually has a negative Hounsfield number on CT

D. Pericardial calcification and thickening are pathognomonic of constrictive pericarditis

E. Malignant mesothelioma is the commonest primary pericardial malignancy

38. Concerning Congenital Anomalies of the Thoracic Aorta

A. An aberrant right subclavian artery causes an anterolateral indentation of the oesophagus on a barium swallow

B. In right-sided aortic arch mirror-image branching is associated with cyanotic congenital heart disease in nearly all cases

C. In right-sided aortic arch, the descending aorta passes to the left of the spine behind the oesophagus

D. In a double aortic arch, the right arch is usually the larger of the two

E. The commonest cause of a tight vascular ring is a right-sided aortic arch with an aberrant left subclavian artery

39. Regarding Imaging of the Large Bowel

A. Umbilication of lymphoid follicles is an abnormal finding in a childhood barium enema

B. On evacuation proctography, the anorectal junction is seen normally above the plane of the ischial tuberosities

C. During evacuation proctography, absence of contraction of the rectum is a cause of incomplete evacuation

D. The major indication for anal endosonography is the assessment of proctalgia

E. Venous intravasation of barium during an enema is a cause of liver abscess

40. Regarding Uncorrected Transposition of the Great Arteries (UTGA)

A. UTGA is the commonest cardiac cause of congenital heart disease central cyanosis at or shortly after birth

B. Isolated UTGA has a better prognosis than one complicated by a VSD

C. The heart size is usually normal at birth

D. Is associated with pulmonary plethora and prominent main pulmonary artery

E. Indomethacin is given at birth to maintain ductal patency

True	False

41. Concerning the Dating of Fractures in Children with Non-Accidental Injury

A. Early periosteal new bone appears between 4 and 21 days

B. Soft callus at 6-8 weeks

C. Loss of fracture-line definition occurs up to 1 week

D. Hard callus may appear at 80 days

E. Remodelling of bone can take up to 2 years

42. Soft-Tissue Tumours Giving a High Signal on T_1W and T_2W Images Include

A. Aggressive fibromatosis (desmoids)

B. Subacute haematoma

C. Giant-cell tumour

D. Melanoma

E. Well-differentiated liposarcoma

43. The Causes of an Enlarged Left Atrium Include

A. Obstruction to left ventricular emptying

B. PDA

C. Tricuspid atresia

D. Aortopulmonary window

E. Non-rheumatic mitral incompetence

44. Concerning Facial Fractures

A. In Le Fort 1 fracture the tooth-bearing part of the maxilla becomes separated from the rest of the maxilla

B. Both zygomatic arches are fractured in Le Fort III fracture

C. When fractured as a result of direct trauma, the zygomatic arch is usually fractured in two places

D. In a "blow-out" fracture the orbital rim remains intact

E. A fracture of the body of mandible which runs inferiorly and anteriorly is more stable than a fracture which runs inferiorly and posteriorly

45. Regarding Imaging of the Salivary Glands

A. The sublingual glands are situated deep to the mylohyoid muscle

B. The facial nerve divides the parotid gland into a larger deep lobe and a much smaller superficial lobe

True	False	
☐	☐	C. Pertechnetate scanning identifies Warthin's tumour as an area of reduced uptake
☐	☐	D. Benign pleomorphic adenoma has a higher attenuation value than normal parotid gland on unenhanced CT scans
☐	☐	E. Sjögren's syndrome is associated with sialectasis

46. Features Consistent with Ectopic Pregnancy on Transvaginal Ultrasound Include

True	False	
☐	☐	A. Uterine decidual thickening
☐	☐	B. Uterine intraluminal fluid
☐	☐	C. An echogenic adnexal ring on the side of the pain
☐	☐	D. A corpus luteal cyst in the ovary contralateral to the side of the pain
☐	☐	E. Absence of fluid in pouch of Douglas

47. The Following Statements Apply to Carcinoma of the Cervix

True	False	
☐	☐	A. Ureteric obstruction is most commonly caused by radiotherapy
☐	☐	B. Vesicovaginal fistula is usually due to direct tumour spread
☐	☐	C. Cavitation in lung metastases suggests the presence of a second, different primary tumour
☐	☐	D. The presence of lymphangitis carcinomatosa suggests a separate pathological process
☐	☐	E. Direct involvement of the rectum is a common finding

48. Concerning Supratentorial Tumours

True	False	
☐	☐	A. Colloid cysts are associated with slit-like third ventricles
☐	☐	B. Colloid cyst has a short T1 and long T2
☐	☐	C. Choroid plexus papillomas are dense on non-contrast-enhanced CT
☐	☐	D. Pineal germinomas are hyperdense on CT but are virtually never calcified
☐	☐	E. Germinomas present as an enhancing suprasellar mass

49. In Non-Accidental Injury of the Infant Brain (NAI)

True	False	
☐	☐	A. Subdural haematomas are most often bilateral
☐	☐	B. Ultrasound is very sensitive at detecting shear injuries
☐	☐	C. CT scanning is mandatory in suspected acute brain injury
☐	☐	D. Hydranencephaly is a potential sequel of NAI
☐	☐	E. Thalamic infarction is characteristic of NAI

True	False	

50. Regarding the Investigation of Urinary Incontinence

A. During cystometrography of a patient with cystitis, no significant rise in intrinsic bladder pressure occurs during filling

B. Reversible bladder instability occurs in bladder outflow obstruction

C. Cystography allows mechanical sphincter problems to be distinguished from bladder instability

D. Stress incontinence in men suggests post-traumatic external sphincter damage

E. The "stop-test" assesses the independent working of the internal and external sphincters

51. Regarding Techniques of Examining the Oesophagus

A. A double-contrast examination is the preferred method of detecting a web

B. A single-contrast study is the best way of demonstrating a sliding hiatus hernia

C. Oesophageal motility is best examined with the patient erect in the LAO position

D. A well-distended, single-contrast study technique is the best way of visualizing oesophageal varices

E. A normal oesophageal scintigram excludes 'nutcracker' oesophagus. (One with abnormally high amplitude contractions.)

52. The Following Statements Apply to Chiari Malformations

A. All the features of a Chiari type 1 malformation may develop after birth

B. Kinking of the medulla oblongata occurs in over 90% of cases of Chiari 1 malformation

C. In Chiari type 2 malformation, a cervical myelomeningocele occurs in over 90–98% of cases

D. Chiari type 2 malformation is associated with basilar invagination

E. Imaging in the sagittal plane is the optimal MRI method of showing the extent of tonsillar descent

53. Dural Ectasia is an Association of

A. Neurofibromatosis

B. Marfan's syndrome

C. Ankylosing spondylitis

D. Gaucher's disease

E. Ehlers-Danlos syndrome

True	False	
		54. Concerning the Extradural Space
☐	☐	A. The commonest extradural tumour of the spine is a metastasis
☐	☐	B. Fifty to 60% of the bone mass of a vertebral body needs to be destroyed before it becomes visible on plain radiography
☐	☐	C. Displacement of the cord substance away from the margin of the thecal sac is the characteristic appearance of an extradural obstruction
☐	☐	D. A densely calcified mass within the spinal canal is likely to be extradural
☐	☐	E. Spinal meningiomas seldom cause conspicuous hyperostosis of adjacent bone
		55. Regarding CT in Urinary Tract Obstruction
☐	☐	A. "Stranding" of peripelvic fat by contrast medium is a recognized sign of obstruction
☐	☐	B. A prolonged cortico-medullary nephrogram occurs in obstruction
☐	☐	C. Modern CT is more sensitive for stone detection than a plain abdominal radiograph
☐	☐	D. Non-contrast enhanced CT rivals the IVU in the assessment of acute obstruction
☐	☐	E. It is the most useful test for the assessment of a transplant kidney
		56. Regarding Graves' Disease
☐	☐	A. The severity of Graves' ophthalmopathy parallels the degree of thyroid dysfunction
☐	☐	B. In Graves' disease glycoprotein deposition in the anterior tendinous parts of the muscles occurs in the majority of cases
☐	☐	C. The MRI signal characteristics allow differentiation of Graves' disease from orbital pseudotumour in over 50% of cases
☐	☐	D. Painful proptosis is commoner with orbital pseudotumour than with Graves' disease
☐	☐	E. Dermoid cyst is the commonest benign tumour of the orbit in adulthood
		57. The Following Statements Apply to Angiomyolipomas
☐	☐	A. Angiomyolipomas contain smooth muscle
☐	☐	B. Adenoma sebaceum is present in 60–70% of patients with this tumour
☐	☐	C. They often present as flank pain, renal mass and haematuria
☐	☐	D. They are usually solitary
☐	☐	E. They may be seen as hyper-reflective masses on ultrasound

True	False

58. Regarding Bone Infection

A. Periosteal reaction is a less prominent feature in the neonate than in the older patient

B. Normal radiographic density in the epiphysis of an involved bone in a young patient is a favourable sign

C. Diaphyseal involvement by tuberculosis is rare

D. Calcific debris around a diseased joint is a reliable indicator of tuberculous, as opposed to pyogenic arthritis

E. The growth plate in childhood provides a potent barrier to the spread of tuberculous infection

59. Regarding Lung Transplantation

A. Acute rejection is the first demonstrable complication following a lung transplant

B. In patients who have undergone transbronchial biopsy, focal nodules in the central portions of lung may be demonstrated

C. The primary reason for lung transplant failure is bronchial dehiscence

D. Bronchial dehiscence is rarely visible on the frontal CXR

E. Chronic lung rejection is defined as obliterative bronchiolitis or accelerated arteriosclerosis or both

60. Regarding the CXR in the Post-Operative Patient

A. About 10% of patients develop visible atelectases after major abdominal surgery

B. Post-operative atelectasis is not usually an infective process

C. Miliary atelectasis can be detected as multiple fine nodules (2–3 mm) throughout the lungs

D. Aspiration pneumonitis tends to clear spontaneously and entirely within 3 days

E. In the presence of a pulmonary capillary wedge pressure below 15 mm/Hg, airspace shadowing is unlikely to be due to cardiac failure

Test 3.

61. In Spinal Injury the Following Features Distinguish Unifacetal Dislocation and Anterior Subluxation from a Hyper-Extension Fracture Dislocation

A. Anterior subluxation is solely a soft-tissue injury

B. Absence of fracture

True	False

C. Subluxation of only the facet joints

D. Anterior displacement of the entire vertebra

E. Neurological symptoms

62. Concerning Tumours of the Bone

A. A vertebral haemangioma has a low signal on T1-weighted images and T2-weighted images owing to the presence of moving blood

B. Angiography of patients with Gorham's disease (vanishing bone disease) demonstrates the arteriovenous malformation

C. An intraosseous lipoma usually arises in the medulla of bone

D. A brown tumour of bone has similar histology to a giant-cell tumour

E. Synovial osteochondromatosis changes to a synovioma in 1–5% of cases

63. Concerning Pulmonary Thromboembolism

A. Of the patients surviving for one hour following acute pulmonary embolism and in whom the correct diagnosis has not been made, 30% will die

B. Haemoptysis occurs in more than 60% of patients with an acute pulmonary embolus

C. Right-sided cardiac failure occurs when more than 50% of the pulmonary vasculature has been occluded by embolus

D. Five to 10% of patients with acute pulmonary embolism may develop chronic pulmonary hypertension

E. The classical ECG findings of pulmonary embolism include sinus tachycardia, right axis deviation, S1Q3T3 and ST changes

64. Concerning External Therapeutic Chest Radiation

A. Symptomatic reactions are uncommon when less than 25% of the lung is irradiated

B. Prednisolone potentiates the pulmonary reaction to chest radiation

C. The changes of radiation pneumonitis tend to be demonstrated on the CXR at 2–3 months

D. Radiation fibrosis is always preceded by radiation pneumonitis on the frontal CXR

E. The fibrotic stage tends to stabilize at 12–24 months

True	False

65. Congenital Lobar Emphysema (CLE)

☐ ☐   A. Is characterized by small cysts in the affected lung

☐ ☐   B. May present with complete opacification of the affected lobe

☐ ☐   C. Affects the lower lobes in more than 25% of cases

☐ ☐   D. Can resemble a tension pneumothorax

☐ ☐   E. Requires surgical treatment in most cases

66. Concerning Chronic Bronchitis and Emphysema

☐ ☐   A. A normal CXR is found in 40–60% of patients

☐ ☐   B. Over-inflation and pulmonary plethora are radiological features present in the affected areas of the lung

☐ ☐   C. The "dirty chest" is a typical finding

☐ ☐   D. Upper-zone blood diversion is found in some cases of emphysema

☐ ☐   E. Well-defined cysts on HRCT are a feature

67. In Avulsion Fractures the Following Muscles and Bony Sites are Associated.

☐ ☐   A. Sartorius and anterior inferior iliac spine

☐ ☐   B. The reflected head of rectus femoris and the anterior inferior iliac spine

☐ ☐   C. The hamstrings and the ischial spine

☐ ☐   D. Adductor avulsion and the inferior pubic ramus

☐ ☐   E. Iliopsoas and the lesser femoral trochanter

68. Concerning the Hip

☐ ☐   A. A frog lateral view requires the femora to be abducted and externally rotated

☐ ☐   B. The Garden classification is used for trochanteric fractures

☐ ☐   C. A subcapital fracture is more likely to produce AVN (avascular necrosis) of the femoral head than a basal fracture

☐ ☐   D. There is a significant risk of AVN with intertrochanteric fractures

☐ ☐   E. An isolated fracture of the lesser trochanter should be regarded as an uncommon injury in the elderly and warrants further investigation

69. Concerning the Radiology of Bronchogenic Carcinoma

☐ ☐   A. Tumours that have more than 90 degrees of circumferential contact with the aorta should be regarded as irresectable

True	False	
❏	❏	B. Mediastinal fat plane obliteration suggests irresectability of the tumour
❏	❏	C. MRI has proved to be of little help in distinguishing T3 from T4 tumours
❏	❏	D. Contact with the visceral pleura is often associated with pain
❏	❏	E. All Pancoast's tumours should be imaged with MRI if there is no obvious bone destruction

70. Concerning the Diagnosis and Staging of Lung Cancer

True	False	
❏	❏	A. A negative CXR with positive cytology suggests a better prognosis than a positive CXR with positive cytology
❏	❏	B. Approximately 30–40% of potentially visible primary peripheral pulmonary cancers had been missed on at least one previous CXR in the NCI (National Cancer Institute) screening programme
❏	❏	C. The TNM classification does not apply to small-cell cancer of the lung
❏	❏	D. The sensitivity and specificity of nodal enlargement, as demonstrated by CT, tend to be better in Europe and Japan than in the USA
❏	❏	E. Pre-operative nodal sampling (biopsy) should be undertaken in nodes <10 mm in transaxial diameter if they receive lymph from the region of the tumour

71. Concerning the Pulmonary Eosinophilias

True	False	
❏	❏	A. A peripheral eosinophil count of less than 500 mm³ does not exclude the diagnosis
❏	❏	B. The pulmonary infiltrates with eosinophilia (PIE) syndrome is associated with *Schistosoma japonicum*
❏	❏	C. There is an association with bronchoceles
❏	❏	D. Chlorpromazine is associated with pulmonary eosinophilia
❏	❏	E. Chronic pulmonary eosinophilia associated with allergic bronchopulmonary aspergillosis produces upper-zone fibrosis

72. Concerning Pulmonary Parenchymal Disease Caused by Organic Material (Extrinsic Allergic Alveolitis) EAA

True	False	
❏	❏	A. It is commonly associated with eosinophilia
❏	❏	B. It produces lower-zone changes in the acute phase
❏	❏	C. It can produce a honeycomb lung
❏	❏	D. It produces a distribution of fibrosis similar to that seen with interstitial pneumonitis (fibrosing alveolitis)
❏	❏	E. It is invariably associated with finger clubbing

True	False	

73. The Following Are Features of Collagen Vascular Disease in the Chest

A. Basal pulmonary fibrosis occurs in more than 30% of patients with systemic lupus erythematosus

B. Pleural effusion is the commonest radiographic manifestation of rheumatoid disease

C. Caplan's nodules occur in patients who have been exposed to silicone

D. The fibrosis demonstrated in patients with systemic sclerosis can be readily differentiated from other causes of basal fibrosis

E. The apparent reduction in lung volume in patients with dermatomyositis and polymyositis is commonly due to basal fibrosis

74. Regarding Sarcoidosis

A. The commonest presentation in the UK is one of bilateral hilar adenopathy

B. A stage III presentation is when the CXR demonstrates a pulmonary opacity in the absence of any hilar adenopathy

C. Asymmetrical mediastinal adenopathy occurs in less than 10% of patients

D. Nodal enlargement disappears within 6–12 months in over 80% of cases

E. Ten to 20% of patients develop intra-pulmonary opacities on CXR prior to nodal enlargement

75. Industrial/Occupational Lung Disease

A. Is a group of disorders that results solely from inorganic dust exposure

B. When due to coal worker's pneumoconiosis (CWP), is characterized by discrete nodules (1–4 mm) often most profuse in the upper zones

C. May be associated with large spiculated intra-pulmonary masses (1–10 cm) in the late phase of the disease

D. Induces extensive fibrosis when produced by silica (SiO_2)

E. Is treated with antibiotics in some instances

76. Regarding Asbestos-Related Thoracic Disease

A. The short fibres of crocidolite are more likely to induce chest disease than the longer fibres of chrysotile

B. Classical signs of asbestosis are the "holly leaf" pleural plaque and the diaphragmatic calcification

C. Malignancy should be suspected in all patients who develop a pleural effusion

D. Malignant mesotheliomas usually arise independently from pleural plaques

E. Severe pulmonary asbestosis tends to affect the whole lung

True	False

77. The Following Are Common Features of Large Airway Obstruction

A. Hyperinflation

B. Hypoinflation

C. A normal inspiratory chest radiograph

D. Bronchogenic cyst formation

E. A bronchocele

78. Concerning Neurogenic Tumours of the Thorax

A. Neuroblastoma does not occur in the anterior mediastinum

B. A thoracic neuroblastoma is likely to be of higher stage (i.e., INSS 3 or 4) than an abdominal tumour

C. Nerve-sheath tumours are generally spherical

D. Calcification in a tumour suggests that it is more likely to be benign than malignant

E. Lateral thoracic meningoceles almost always communicate with the subarachnoid space

79. Regarding CNS Mass Lesions

A. In children, raised intracranial pressure is associated with thickening of the skull vault

B. Most brain tumours in children are primary CNS tumours

C. Most astrocytomas are cortically based

D. T_2W images allow tumour to be differentiated from oedema

E. Oligodendrogliomas enhance with GdDTPA in under 10% of cases

80. A Morgagni Hernia

A. Commonly presents in childhood after streptococcal infections

B. Occurs through a defect in the posterior pleuroperitoneal fold

C. Contains large bowel in over 90% of cases

D. May extend into the pericardium

E. Is optimally diagnosed with an oral water-soluble contrast medium study

81. Regarding Scintigraphy in Children

A. A dilated, unobstructed pelvicaliceal system with preserved renal function will show half of its activity washed out within 10 minutes of administering a diuretic agent

True	False	

B. In the presence of reduced renal function, an unobstructed kidney will yield quantitative data which simulates an obstructed system

C. Lack of ^{99m}Tc sulphur colloid uptake by the spleen in an adult is a feature of sickle cell disease

D. Absence of ^{99m}Tc HIDA in the gastrointestinal tract on the images obtained at 24 hours implies the presence of biliary atresia

E. In Barrett's oesophagus there is an accumulation of ^{99m}Tc pertechnetate

82. Concerning Pulmonary Consolidation

A. The consolidation associated with pulmonary sarcoidosis is due to granulomata within the alveoli

B. A segmental distribution is characteristic

C. Desquamative insterstitial pneumonitis (DIP) is a predominantly interstitial process producing alveolar compression

D. There is usually associated loss of volume

E. Early changes include acinar nodules/shadows 1–4 mm in diameter

83. Concerning the Principles of Magnetic Resonance Imaging

A. The frequency of precession of a nucleus is inversely proportional to the applied magnetic field

B. Spin Echo sequences utilize an initial 180° pulse followed at a specific time by a 90° pulse

C. A decrease in mobile proton density is seen in acute demyelination

D. Extracellular methaemoglobin exhibits a high signal on both T_1W and T_2W images

E. In the STIR sequence, the TI is reduced to 100–150 ms in order to null the signal from fat

84. Regarding Localized Loss of Bone Density

A. Patients with reflex sympathetic dystrophy and disuse osteoporosis cannot be differentiated clinically

B. Reflex sympathetic dystrophy is associated with thinning of the soft tissues

C. Gorham's disease demonstrates progressive involvement of contiguous bones

D. Transient regional osteoporosis is characterized by high levels of alkaline phosphatase

E. Bilateral transient osteoporosis of the hips tends to occur in the first trimester of pregnancy

True   **False**

85. Concerning Patients with Osteogenesis Imperfecta

☐ ☐   A. There is an abnormality of type II collagen

☐ ☐   B. Patients with type I osteogenesis imperfecta are stillborn

☐ ☐   C. The sclerae of patients with type IV osteogenesis imperfecta are normal in colour

☐ ☐   D. Patients with type III osteogenesis imperfecta have normal dentition

☐ ☐   E. Type IV is the commonest of these disorders

86. Regarding Langerhans Cell Histiocytosis

☐ ☐   A. Bone lesions predominate in Letterer-Siwe syndrome

☐ ☐   B. The triad of calvarial lesions, exomphalos and diabetes insipidus suggests the diagnosis of Hand-Schüller-Christian disease

☐ ☐   C. The typical bony sites for eosinophilic granuloma include the skull and proximal femur

☐ ☐   D. Vertebra plana is often associated with a soft-tissue mass

☐ ☐   E. Eosinophilic granuloma is a self-limiting disorder

87. Typical Features of Multiple Myeloma Include

☐ ☐   A. A 5 year survival rate in excess of 50%

☐ ☐   B. Ten to 20% of cases demonstrate Bence-Jones proteinuria

☐ ☐   C. Amyloidosis is reported in about 20% of patients

☐ ☐   D. Complete absence of lesions on scintigraphic imaging

☐ ☐   E. A periosteal reaction

88. The Following are Typical Bone Changes Demonstrated in Children with Leukaemia

☐ ☐   A. Epiphyseal lucencies

☐ ☐   B. Osteolytic lesions

☐ ☐   C. Osteoblastic lesions

☐ ☐   D. Soft-tissue mass with periosteal reaction

☐ ☐   E. Diffuse bony destruction

89. Concerning Sickle Cell Disease

☐ ☐   A. The presence of the haematobium parasite within red blood cells causes them to sickle

True	False	
☐	☐	B. Cardiomegaly is only present in 20–30% of homozygotic sickle-cell subjects
☐	☐	C. Most homozygotic subjects die before the age of 40 years
☐	☐	D. Bone infarction tends to occur in the epiphyses and metaphyses of bones in adolescents and adults
☐	☐	E. Stepped-end plate depression of the vertebrae is unique to sickle cell disease

90. The Following are Features of the Prune Belly Syndrome (PBS)

True	False	
☐	☐	A. Undescended testes
☐	☐	B. Renal dysplasia
☐	☐	C. The disorder is unique to males
☐	☐	D. The upper ureters are disproportionately dilated in comparison with the lower ureters
☐	☐	E. A posterior urethral valve on MCUG is pathognomonic of this condition

Test 4.

91. Concerning Non-Hodgkin's Lymphoma of the Bone

True	False	
☐	☐	A. Bone lesions are commoner than lesions in other organ systems in HIV related lymphoma
☐	☐	B. Bone involvement is commoner in children than in adults
☐	☐	C. The commonest sites affected by Burkitt's lymphoma are the bones of the jaw and the abdominal viscera
☐	☐	D. The treatment of Burkitt's lymphoma is primarily surgical
☐	☐	E. Floating teeth are pathognomonic of Burkitt's lymphoma

92. Regarding the Diagnosis of Metastatic Disease of Bone

True	False	
☐	☐	A. Bony metastases are rarely demonstrated by conventional radiography when less than 2 cm in diameter
☐	☐	B. A blastic metastasis is produced as a result of tumour laying down bone
☐	☐	C. MRI is more sensitive than scintigraphy and more specific than radiography
☐	☐	D. MRI high-signal return can be expected on STIR images
☐	☐	E. Uterine carcinoma produces bony metastases more commonly than does thyroid carcinoma

True   False

93. Regarding the Frequency of Urothelial Tumours

A. Bladder tumours are about five times commoner than renal pelvic tumours.

B. Simultaneous bilateral ureteric tumours occur in approximately 1/1000 patients with urothelial malignancy

C. Five percent of patients will have multiple lesions

D. Ten percent of patients with renal pelvic urothelial tumours will develop bladder tumours in less than 15 months

E. About 20% of affected patients have carcinoma in situ

94. The Following are More Commonly Associated with Upper Renal Tract Urothelial Tumours Than Bladder Tumours

A. Finnish nephrosis

B. Phenacetin abuse

C. Cyclophosphamide

D. Balkan nephropathy

E. Medullary sponge kidney

95. Concerning the Investigation of Metastatic Bone Disease

A. A skeletal survey is recommended to establish the diagnosis of metastases in all patients with a known primary carcinoma

B. The site of the primary tumour is not found in 1–5% of patients

C. The Gd-DTPA-enhanced MRI, in most instances, distinguishes between benign and malignant bone lesions

D. The metastases from Ewing's sarcoma tend to resemble those of leukaemia on plain radiography in children

E. Medulloblastoma only metastasizes after surgery

96. Concerning Osteosarcoma

A. It is the commonest malignant lesion of bone

B. It can only arise in bone

C. It is uncommon under the age of 10 years

D. When the jaw is affected, it carries a poor prognosis

E. Systemic symptoms are uncommon

True	False

97. The Following Criteria Have to be Satisfied to Diagnose a Sarcoma in an Irradiated Bone as Having Arisen as a Result of the Radiation

A. A previous radiograph without any evidence of disease

B. Evidence of radiation osteitis must be present

C. A latent period of at least 10 years

D. Histological evidence of a sarcoma

E. A recorded minimum dose of 30 Gy

98. Regarding Ewing's Sarcoma

A. There is an associated chromosomal abnormality

B. Most tumours occur between the ages of 5 and 15 years

C. Asiatic races are more commonly affected than other racial groups

D. The tumour readily metastasizes to bone

E. The tumour is usually medullary in origin

99. Concerning the Diagnosis of Pregnancy and Assessment of Gestational Age

A. Using transvaginal sonography, a gestational sac can be seen only when the Beta Human Chorionic Gonadotrophin (βHCG) level is greater than 1500 mlu/ml

B. Transabdominal scanning can detect a gestational sac within the choriodecidual mass at 4–5 weeks amenorrhoea

C. Between 8 and 10 weeks transvaginal assessment of crown rump length is the preferred method of determining gestational age

D. Abdominal circumference is a reliable measurement of the assessment of gestational age after 12 weeks

E. A crescentic hyporeflective area beneath the choriodecidua is an abnormal finding

100. Concerning the Radiological Assessment of Bladder Tumours

A. The IVU and cystogram are still useful in the staging of bladder carcinoma

B. Transurethal and transrectal USS have staging accuracies of 75–95%

C. The major role of CT is to stage the bladder tumour

D. Angiography plays an important role in preoperative assessment

E. Loss of the fat plane between the seminal vesicles and the bladder invariably suggests tumour invasion

True	False

101. The Following Imaging Criteria are Used in the Staging of Bladder Tumours

A. CT cannot differentiate tumours between stages T1 and T3b

B. T1 to T3a tumours are best demonstrated using an SE T1-weighted MRI sequence

C. A T3b tumour is easily demonstrable on a T1-weighted image sequence

D. Pelvic lymph node(s) of 12 mm in their trans-axial diameter would not be regarded as significant using MRI criteria

E. Tis (carcinoma in situ; TMN staging) is demonstrated on T2-weighted images as an area of reduced signal intensity after gadolinium contrast enhancement

102. Concerning Abdominal Masses in the Neonate

A. The commonest abdominal mass in an apparently healthy neonate is a Wilms' tumour

B. Mesoblastic nephroma is the commonest solid renal mass in the neonate

C. Urgent surgery is required for most cases of multicystic dysplastic kidneys

D. A mesoblastic nephroma is benign

E. Myelolipomas are demonstrated in patients with tuberose sclerosis

103. Concerning Urinary Calculi

A. Calcium oxalate and phosphate stones are commoner in males than females

B. Peanuts and spinach increase the urinary excretion of oxalate

C. Triple phosphate stones are seen in over 50% of patients with hyperphosphatasia

D. Struvite stones are commoner in women than men

E. Cystinosis is associated with the excessive excretion of dibasic amino acids

104. Regarding Renal Tract Calculi

A. About 10% of renal tract stones occur as a result of primary hyperparathyroidism

B. Urinary calculi are usually an admixture of organic and inorganic complexes

C. The nidus of the stone may have a different chemical composition to the main bulk of the stone

D. About 50% of stone formers may expect a recurrence in their lifetime

E. The ingestion of large amounts of protein and purine account for the high incidence of stone disease in the USA

105. Regarding MRI of the Cardiovascular System

A. Blood moving at 5 cm/sec yields no signal on spin echo sequences

True	False	
☐	☐	B. Nonturbulent blood flow on gradient echo sequences has a uniformly high signal
☐	☐	C. Pericardium is readily distinguished from pericardial effusion
☐	☐	D. Spin echo is the method of choice for imaging an aortic dissection flap
☐	☐	E. Implantable pacemakers are generally not a contraindication to MRI

106. The Following Produce Cortical Nephrocalcinosis

True	False	
☐	☐	A. Nephrotic syndrome due to glomerulonephritis
☐	☐	B. Obstetric shock
☐	☐	C. Nail patella syndrome
☐	☐	D. Paget's disease
☐	☐	E. Oxalosis

107. There is an Association Between the Following Disorders

True	False	
☐	☐	A. Bladder agenesis: absence of the urethra
☐	☐	B. Dwarf bladder: achondroplasia
☐	☐	C. Hutch diverticulum: bladder outflow obstruction
☐	☐	D. Bladder exstrophy: cleidocranial dysostosis
☐	☐	E. Double bladder: penis didelphys

108. The Following Features are Associated with Changes in the Urinary Tract Related to Pregnancy

True	False	
☐	☐	A. The ureters dilate throughout their length
☐	☐	B. Dilatation is greater on the left than the right
☐	☐	C. Dilatation of the ureters may persist long after the pregnancy
☐	☐	D. Prolonged dilatation is not associated with an increased incidence of re-infection
☐	☐	E. Ovarian vein syndrome is pain in the right iliolumbar nerve ascribed to pressure from an aberrant right ovarian vein

109. Regarding Imaging Techniques of the Skull and Brain

True	False	
☐	☐	A. The anteroposterior projection is generally preferable to the postero anterior in frontal skull radiography
☐	☐	B. Contrast-enhanced MRI is more sensitive than contrast-enhanced CT for detecting breakdown in the blood-brain barrier

True   False

☐ ☐ C. Cochlear implants are an absolute contraindication to MRI

☐ ☐ D. A 15 ml bolus of intravenous GdDTPA is adequate for MR angiography

☐ ☐ E. In the investigation of clinically typical Bell's palsy, MRI of the petrous temporal bone has replaced CT

110. Bronchogenic Carcinoma

☐ ☐ A. May present with multiple primary tumours in 10–15% of patients

☐ ☐ B. Is very rare under the age of 25 years

☐ ☐ C. Typically presents clinically with pneumonia or, radiologically, as a solitary pulmonary nodule

☐ ☐ D. Is typically asymptomatic in about 40–60% of patients

☐ ☐ E. In the superior sulcus may present with brachial plexus neuropathy

111. Concerning Pulmonary Haemorrhage

☐ ☐ A. Haemoptysis is a common presentation

☐ ☐ B. Air-space shadowing tends to clear within 5–10 days

☐ ☐ C. There is an increase in the KCO_2

☐ ☐ D. Systemic lupus erythematosus nephritis with pulmonary haemorrhage is associated with antiglomerular basement membrane antibodies

☐ ☐ E. Cardiac enlargement is an important sign when deciding the aetiology of pulmonary haemorrhage

112. Regarding the Thymus

☐ ☐ A. Prior to puberty the thymus occupies most of the mediastinum in front of the great vessels as seen on the CXR

☐ ☐ B. The CT density (HU) of the thymus tends to decrease with age

☐ ☐ C. Thymomas tend to occur in patients less than 20 years of age

☐ ☐ D. ACTH is the commonest ectopic hormone to be produced by thymic carcinoid tumours

☐ ☐ E. Eighty to 90% of patients with thymomas have myasthenia gravis

113. The Following are Causes of an Air Bronchogram on the CXR

☐ ☐ A. Non-obstructive collapse

☐ ☐ B. Passive atelectasis

☐ ☐ C. Lymphoma

True	False	
☐	☐	D. Progressive massive fibrosis
☐	☐	E. Alveolar cell carcinoma

114. The Following are Regarded as Routine Indications for a Micturating Cystogram

True	False	
☐	☐	A. A urinary tract infection in a child under the age of 1 year
☐	☐	B. The follow-up of vesico-ureteric reflux
☐	☐	C. The screening of girls with UTI
☐	☐	D. The demonstration of a thick-walled bladder on USS
☐	☐	E. The investigation of children with renal failure of unknown cause

115. Concerning Polycystic Renal Disease

True	False	
☐	☐	A. There is a significant number of children in whom the differentiation between the dominant and recessive forms is impossible
☐	☐	B. Hepatic fibrosis is always associated with autosomal recessive polycystic disease (ARPD)
☐	☐	C. ARPD is generally associated with a family history
☐	☐	D. Potassium loss is a common complication in children with ARPD
☐	☐	E. Autosomal dominant polycystic disease (ADPD) presents in infancy in 30–40% of cases

116. Concerning Ectopic or Hamartomatous Development of the Lung

True	False	
☐	☐	A. Cystic adenomatoid malformation of the lung (CAM) is a lesion containing all the components of normal lung
☐	☐	B. The mass of CAM is always predominantly cystic
☐	☐	C. Occasionally CAM may present with a large single cyst
☐	☐	D. The cysts of CAM may communicate with the bronchial tree
☐	☐	E. Pulmonary hypoplasia is an associated finding in some patients

117. Concerning Congenital Pulmonary Anomalies

True	False	
☐	☐	A. Swyer-James syndrome is the commonest congenital pulmonary anomaly
☐	☐	B. Tracheal agenesis is incompatible with life
☐	☐	C. Bronchial stenosis may be produced by an aberrant left main pulmonary artery
☐	☐	D. Bronchial atresia tends to present in the older child or the adult
☐	☐	E. The normal trachea expands 50% in diameter during expiration whereas in children with tracheomalacia there is an expansion of 70% or greater

True	False

118. Regarding Injuries to the Foot

☐ ☐ A. The Lisfranc fracture dislocation is associated with a fracture at the base of the second metatarsal

☐ ☐ B. A march fracture most commonly occurs in the first metatarsal

☐ ☐ C. Freiberg's infarction occurs in the first metatarsal head

☐ ☐ D. The Jones' fracture is situated transversely across the base of the fifth metatarsal

☐ ☐ E. Fractures of the phalanges require prolonged immobilization

119. Concerning Fractures of the Spine

☐ ☐ A. Compression fractures usually involve the superior vertebral endplate and do not disrupt the inferior endplate

☐ ☐ B. The commonest sites for fracture dislocation are the lower cervical spine and the thoracolumbar junction

☐ ☐ C. Fractures of the posterior elements commonly occur without accompanying fractures of the vertebral bodies

☐ ☐ D. A gap in the neural arch of C1 may be a normal variant

☐ ☐ E. The cervicodorsal junction must be demonstrated at all costs in cases of suspected traumatic damage

120. Regarding Urinary Schistosomiasis

☐ ☐ A. It is very common on the west coast of Africa

☐ ☐ B. It is caused by the ova descending from the kidney in the ureter and embedding in the bladder

☐ ☐ C. The intermediate host is the snail

☐ ☐ D. The worms incite a severe local inflammatory reaction

☐ ☐ E. The calcified bladder is small and rigid and its function is impaired

Answers to Self Assessment Questions

Test 1.

1. A. False
    B. True
    C. False
    D. False
    E. True
    (see question 7.91)

2. A. True
    B. True
    C. True
    D. False
    E. True
    (see question 8.17)

3. A. False
    B. False
    C. False
    D. False
    E. True
    (see question 5.11)

4. A. False
    B. True
    C. True
    D. True
    E. False
    (see question 9.21)

5. A. False
    B. True
    C. True
    D. False
    E. False
    (see question 1.3)

6. A. True
    B. False
    C. True
    D. False
    E. True
    (see question 8.14)

7. A. False
    B. True
    C. False
    D. True
    E. False
    (see question 9.11)

8. A. True
    B. True
    C. False
    D. False
    E. False
    (see question 10.7)

9. A. True
    B. True
    C. False
    D. False
    E. True
    (see question 9.27)

10. A. False
    B. False
    C. True
    D. False
    E. True
    (see question 1.2)

11. A. True
    B. True
    C. False
    D. True
    E. True
    (see question 3.19)

12. A. False
    B. False
    C. True
    D. True
    E. False
    (see question 4.11)

13. A. True
    B. False
    C. False
    D. True
    E. True
    (see question 5.2)

14. A. True
    B. True
    C. False
    D. True
    E. False
    (see question 5.3)

15. A. False
    B. False
    C. True
    D. False
    E. False
    (see question 6.39)

16. A. True
    B. False
    C. True
    D. True
    E. False
    (see question 4.1)

17. A. True
    B. False
    C. False
    D. True
    E. True
    (see question 4.6)

18. A. True
    B. True
    C. True
    D. False
    E. True
    (see question 10.2)

19. A. True
    B. False
    C. False
    D. False
    E. True
    (see question 6.24)

20. A. True
    B. True
    C. False
    D. True
    E. True
    (see question 6.47)

21. A. True
    B. True
    C. False
    D. False
    E. True
    (see question 5.14)

22. A. True
    B. True
    C. True
    D. True
    E. True
    (see question 5.21)

23. A. True
    B. False
    C. True
    D. False
    E. False
    (see question 7.74)

24. A. False
    B. False
    C. True
    D. False
    E. False
    (see question 6.90)

25. A. False
    B. False
    C. False
    D. False
    E. True
    (see question 6.65)

26. A. True
    B. True
    C. True
    D. True
    E. True
    (see question 9.14)

27. A. False
    B. True
    C. True
    D. False
    E. True
    (see question 8.15)

28. A. True
    B. False
    C. True
    D. False
    E. True
    (see question 2.68)

29. A. True
    B. False
    C. False
    D. True
    E. False
    (see question 6.54)

30. A. False
    B. False
    C. True
    D. True
    E. True
    (see question 7.100)

Test 2.

31. A. True
    B. True
    C. True
    D. False
    E. False
    (see question 4.14)

32. A. True
    B. False
    C. True
    D. False
    E. True
    (see question 8.19)

33. A. False
    B. True
    C. False
    D. True
    E. True
    (see question 2.21)

34. A. True
    B. False
    C. False
    D. True
    E. False
    (see question 2.14)

35. A. True
    B. True
    C. False
    D. True
    E. True
    (see question 4.20)

36. A. True
    B. True
    C. True
    D. False
    E. True
    (see question 5.12)

37. A. True
    B. True
    C. False
    D. False
    E. True
    (see question 3.22)

38. A. False
    B. True
    C. True
    D. True
    E. False
    (see question 3.23)

39. A. False
    B. True
    C. False
    D. False
    E. True
    (see question 4.15)

40. A. True
    B. False
    C. True
    D. False
    E. False
    (see question 3.1)

41. A. True
    B. False
    C. False
    D. True
    E. True
    (see question 7.90)

42. A. False
    B. True
    C. False
    D. True
    E. True
    (see question 7.86)

43. A. True
    B. True
    C. True
    D. True
    E. True
    (see question 3.15)

44. A. True
    B. True
    C. False
    D. True
    E. True
    (see question 10.15)

45. A. False
    B. False
    C. False
    D. True
    E. True
    (see question 10.17)

46. A. True
    B. True
    C. True
    D. True
    E. True
    (see question 8.2)

47. A. False
    B. False
    C. False
    D. False
    E. False
    (see question 8.12)

48. A. True
    B. True
    C. True
    D. True
    E. True
    (see question 9.4)

49. A. True
    B. True
    C. True
    D. False
    E. False
    (see question 9.28)

50. A. True
    B. True
    C. False
    D. True
    E. True
    (see question 6.6)

51. A. False
    B. True
    C. False
    D. False
    E. True
    (see question 4.12)

52. A. True
    B. False
    C. False
    D. False
    E. False
    (see question 9.18)

53. A. True
    B. True
    C. True
    D. False
    E. True
    (see question 9.19)

54. A. True
    B. True
    C. False
    D. True
    E. True
    (see question 9.22)

55. A. True
    B. True
    C. True
    D. True
    E. False
    (see question 6.40)

56. A. False
    B. False
    C. False
    D. True
    E. False
    (see question 10.5)

57. A. True
    B. False
    C. True
    D. True
    E. True
    (see question 6.26)

58. A. False
    B. False
    C. True
    D. True
    E. False
    (see question 7.95)

59. A. False
    B. False
    C. True
    D. True
    E. True
    (see question 2.55)

60. A. False
    B. True
    C. False
    D. False
    E. True
    (see question 2.51)

Test 3.

61. A. True
    B. True
    C. True
    D. True
    E. False
    (see question 7.16)

62. A. False
    B. False
    C. True
    D. True
    E. False
    (see question 7.18)

63. A. True
    B. False
    C. True
    D. True
    E. True
    (see question 2.48)

64. A. True
    B. False
    C. True
    D. True
    E. True
    (see question 2.53)

65. A. False
    B. True
    C. False
    D. True
    E. False
    (see question 2.64)

66. A. True
    B. False
    C. True
    D. True
    E. False
    (see question 2.22)

67. A. False
    B. False
    C. False
    D. False
    E. True
    (see question 7.3)

68. A. True
    B. False
    C. True
    D. False
    E. True
    (see question 7.10)

69. A. False
    B. True
    C. False
    D. False
    E. True
    (see question 2.26)

70. A. True
    B. False
    C. True
    D. True
    E. False
    (see question 2.27)

71. A. True
    B. False
    C. True
    D. False
    E. True
    (see question 2.35)

72. A. False
    B. True
    C. True
    D. False
    E. False
    (see question 2.39)

73. A. False
    B. True
    C. False
    D. False
    E. False
    (see question 2.41)

74. A. False
    B. True
    C. True
    D. True
    E. False
    (see question 2.40)

75. A. False
    B. True
    C. True
    D. True
    E. True
    (see question 2.44)

76. A. True
    B. False
    C. True
    D. True
    E. False
    (see question 2.45)

77. A. True
    B. True
    C. True
    D. False
    E. True
    (see question 2.19)

78. A. False
    B. False
    C. True
    D. False
    E. True
    (see question 2.12)

79. A. True
    B. True
    C. False
    D. False
    E. False
    (see question 9.3)

80. A. False
    B. False
    C. False
    D. True
    E. False
    (see question 2.8)

81. A. True
    B. True
    C. True
    D. False
    E. True
    (see question 1.4)

82. A. False
    B. False
    C. False
    D. False
    E. False
    (see question 2.5)

83. A. False
    B. False
    C. False
    D. True
    E. True
    (see question 1.1)

84. A. False
    B. False
    C. True
    D. False
    E. False
    (see question 7.65)

85. A. False
    B. False
    C. True
    D. True
    E. False
    (see question 7.72)

86. A. False
    B. False
    C. True
    D. True
    E. True
    (see question 7.44)

87. A. False
    B. False
    C. True
    D. False
    E. False
    (see question 7.46)

88. A. False
    B. True
    C. True
    D. False
    E. True
    (see question 7.50)

89. A. False
    B. False
    C. True
    D. True
    E. False
    (see question 7.52)

90. A. True
    B. True
    C. False
    D. False
    E. False
    (see question 6.76)

Test 4.

91. A. False
    B. True
    C. True
    D. False
    E. False
    (see question 7.55)

92. A. True
    B. False
    C. False
    D. True
    E. True
    (see question 7.25)

93. A. False
    B. False
    C. False
    D. False
    E. False
    (see question 6.28)

94. A. False
    B. True
    C. False
    D. True
    E. False
    (see question 6.29)

95. A. False
    B. False
    C. True
    D. True
    E. False
    (see question 7.29)

96. A. False
    B. False
    C. True
    D. False
    E. False
    (see question 7.33)

97. A. True
    B. False
    C. False
    D. True
    E. False
    (see question 7.37)

98. A. True
    B. True
    C. False
    D. True
    E. True
    (see question 7.39)

99. A. False
    B. False
    C. False
    D. False
    E. True
    (see question 8.1)

100. A. False
     B. True
     C. True
     D. False
     E. False
     (see question 6.56)

101. A. False
     B. False
     C. True
     D. False
     E. False
     (see question 6.57)

102. A. False
     B. True
     C. False
     D. False
     E. False
     (see question 6.75)

103. A. True
     B. True
     C. False
     D. True
     E. False
     (see question 6.31)

104. A. True
     B. True
     C. True
     D. True
     E. True
     (see question 6.34)

105. A. True
     B. True
     C. False
     D. False
     E. False
     (see question 3.11)

106. A. True
     B. True
     C. False
     D. False
     E. True
     (see question 6.37)

107. A. True
     B. False
     C. False
     D. False
     E. True
     (see question 6.44)

108. A. False
     B. False
     C. True
     D. True
     E. False
     (see question 6.7)

109. A. False
     B. True
     C. True
     D. False
     E. False
     (see question 9.1)

110. A. False
     B. True
     C. True
     D. False
     E. True
     (see question 2.28)

111. A. False
     B. True
     C. False
     D. False
     E. False
     (see question 2.32)

112. A. True
     B. True
     C. False
     D. True
     E. False
     (see question 2.2)

113. A. True
     B. True
     C. True
     D. True
     E. True
     (see question 2.6)

114. A. True
     B. False
     C. False
     D. True
     E. True
     (see question 6.80)

115. A. True
     B. False
     C. False
     D. False
     E. False
     (see question 6.87)

116. A. False
     B. False
     C. True
     D. True
     E. True
     (see question 2.56)

117. A. False
     B. True
     C. True
     D. True
     E. False
     (see question 2.60)

118. A. True
     B. False
     C. False
     D. True
     E. False
     (see question 7.13)

119. A. True
     B. True
     C. False
     D. True
     E. True
     (see question 7.14)

120. A. False
     B. False
     C. True
     D. False
     E. False
     (see question 6.19)